THE AN VACCINE

Is It Safe? Does It Work?

Lois M. Joellenbeck, Lee L. Zwanziger,
Jane S. Durch, and Brian L. Strom, *Editors*

Committee to Assess the Safety and Efficacy of the Anthrax Vaccine

Medical Follow-up Agency

INSTITUTE OF MEDICINE

NATIONAL ACADEMY PRESS
Washington, D.C.

NATIONAL ACADEMY PRESS • 2101 Constitution Avenue, N.W. • Washington, DC 20418

NOTICE: The project that is the subject of this report was approved by the Governing Board of the National Research Council, whose members are drawn from the councils of the National Academy of Sciences, the National Academy of Engineering, and the Institute of Medicine. The members of the committee responsible for the report were chosen for their special competences and with regard for appropriate balance.

Support for this project was provided by the Department of Defense (Contract No. DASW01-00-6-3045). The views presented in this report are those of the Institute of Medicine Committee to Assess the Safety and Efficacy of the Anthrax Vaccine and are not necessarily those of the funding agency.

International Standard Book Number 0-309-08309-5
Library of Congress Control Number 2002104241

Additional copies of this report are available for sale from the National Academy Press, 2101 Constitution Avenue, N.W., Box 285, Washington, DC 20055. Call (800) 624-6242 or (202) 334-3313 (in the Washington metropolitan area), or visit the NAP's home page at www.nap.edu. The full text of this report is available at www.nap.edu.

For more information about the Institute of Medicine, visit the IOM home page at www.iom.edu.

Copyright 2002 by the National Academy of Sciences. All rights reserved.

Printed in the United States of America.

The serpent has been a symbol of long life, healing, and knowledge among almost all cultures and religions since the beginning of recorded history. The serpent adopted as a logotype by the Institute of Medicine is a relief carving from ancient Greece, now held by the Staatliche Museen in Berlin.

*"Knowing is not enough; we must apply.
Willing is not enough; we must do."*
—Goethe

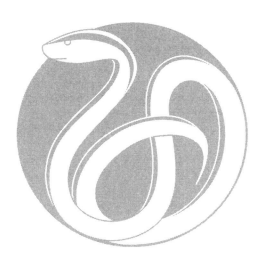

INSTITUTE OF MEDICINE

Shaping the Future for Health

THE NATIONAL ACADEMIES

National Academy of Sciences
National Academy of Engineering
Institute of Medicine
National Research Council

The **National Academy of Sciences** is a private, nonprofit, self-perpetuating society of distinguished scholars engaged in scientific and engineering research, dedicated to the furtherance of science and technology and to their use for the general welfare. Upon the authority of the charter granted to it by the Congress in 1863, the Academy has a mandate that requires it to advise the federal government on scientific and technical matters. Dr. Bruce M. Alberts is president of the National Academy of Sciences.

The **National Academy of Engineering** was established in 1964, under the charter of the National Academy of Sciences, as a parallel organization of outstanding engineers. It is autonomous in its administration and in the selection of its members, sharing with the National Academy of Sciences the responsibility for advising the federal government. The National Academy of Engineering also sponsors engineering programs aimed at meeting national needs, encourages education and research, and recognizes the superior achievements of engineers. Dr. Wm. A. Wulf is president of the National Academy of Engineering.

The **Institute of Medicine** was established in 1970 by the National Academy of Sciences to secure the services of eminent members of appropriate professions in the examination of policy matters pertaining to the health of the public. The Institute acts under the responsibility given to the National Academy of Sciences by its congressional charter to be an adviser to the federal government and, upon its own initiative, to identify issues of medical care, research, and education. Dr. Kenneth I. Shine is president of the Institute of Medicine.

The **National Research Council** was organized by the National Academy of Sciences in 1916 to associate the broad community of science and technology with the Academy's purposes of furthering knowledge and advising the federal government. Functioning in accordance with general policies determined by the Academy, the Council has become the principal operating agency of both the National Academy of Sciences and the National Academy of Engineering in providing services to the government, the public, and the scientific and engineering communities. The Council is administered jointly by both Academies and the Institute of Medicine. Dr. Bruce M. Alberts and Dr. Wm. A. Wulf are chairman and vice chairman, respectively, of the National Research Council.

COMMITTEE TO ASSESS THE SAFETY AND EFFICACY OF THE ANTHRAX VACCINE

BRIAN L. STROM (*Chair*), Professor and Chair, Biostatistics & Epidemiology, University of Pennsylvania School of Medicine
WILLIAM E. BARLOW, Senior Scientific Investigator, Center for Health Studies, Group Health Cooperative, and Research Professor, Biostatistics Department, University of Washington
DAN G. BLAZER II, J. P. Gibbons Professor of Psychiatry, Duke University Medical Center
LINDA D. COWAN, Professor of Biostatistics and Epidemiology, University of Oklahoma College of Public Health
KATHRYN M. EDWARDS, Professor of Pediatrics, Division of Infectious Diseases, Vanderbilt University School of Medicine
DENISE L. FAUSTMAN, Associate Professor of Medicine, Harvard Medical School, and Director, Immunobiology Laboratory, Massachusetts General Hospital
EMIL C. GOTSCHLICH, Vice President for Medical Sciences and R. Gwin Follis-Chevron Professor, The Rockefeller University
DENNIS L. KASPER, Executive Dean for Academic Programs, William Ellery Channing Professor of Medicine, and Professor of Microbiology and Molecular Genetics, Harvard Medical School
DON P. METZGAR, Scientific Consultant
HUGH H. TILSON, Clinical Professor of Epidemiology and Health Policy and Senior Adviser to the Dean, University of North Carolina School of Public Health

Consultants

STANLEY A. PLOTKIN, Medical and Scientific Consultant, Aventis Pasteur, and Emeritus Professor of Pediatrics, University of Pennsylvania
GEORGE A. ROBERTSON, Senior Manager of Biological Quality Control, Wyeth-Ayerst Pharmaceuticals

Staff

LOIS JOELLENBECK, Senior Program Officer (Study Director)
LEE ZWANZIGER, Senior Program Officer (until January 2002)
JANE DURCH, Freelance Writer and Editor
KAREN KAZMERZAK, Research Assistant
PHILLIP BAILEY, Project Assistant
RICHARD MILLER, Director, Medical Follow-up Agency

Preface

The Institute of Medicine convened the Committee to Assess the Safety and Efficacy of the Anthrax Vaccine in October 2000 to prepare a congressionally mandated report for the Department of Defense. The committee was charged with reviewing data regarding the efficacy and safety of the currently licensed anthrax vaccine—Anthrax Vaccine Adsorbed (AVA)—and assessing the efforts to resolve manufacturing issues and resume production and distribution of the vaccine. This report is a summary of the committee's deliberations.

As the committee completed its work, the nation experienced the traumas of not only the attacks of September 11, 2001, but also the distribution of potent anthrax spores through the U.S. mail, which resulted in 5 deaths, at least 13 nonfatal confirmed cases, and the exposure of more than 30,000 other people. The nation and public health and health care professionals found themselves with much new but hard-won knowledge about anthrax, as well as many new questions about the disease and its prevention and treatment, including the merits of vaccination following exposure.

These events lent urgency to the committee's work. However, the study charge already reflected concerns that arose in the context of discussions of the risk of exposure to anthrax spores and the merits of vaccination for military personnel, given the perceived threat of battlefield exposure to anthrax. The Department of Defense had begun to implement a plan to vaccinate all military personnel, but some service members were sufficiently concerned about the efficacy or safety of AVA that they chose to resign or even undergo court-martial to avoid vaccination. Some have also questioned whether the vaccine might be related to the health problems experienced by some Gulf War veterans. In addition, the manufacturing plant producing the vaccine failed to pass Food and Drug Administration inspection until very recently. As a result of the limited supply of the vaccine, the Department of Defense's Anthrax Vaccine Immunization Program was proceeding at a very reduced rate. These manufacturing issues further accentuated the questions about the vaccine.

Vaccines are critically important tools for the prevention of serious infectious diseases. As with any pharmaceutical product or medical procedure, however, the use of vaccines carries a risk of adverse health effects, which must be weighed against the expected health benefit. Safety expectations for vaccines are especially high because they are usually given to healthy people to protect them against a disease that they may not be exposed to in the future.

In approaching its task, the committee recognized that it was dealing with difficult issues, both scientifically and politically. Scientifically, it was dealing with a series of questions on which the published data were limited. Politically, it was operating in a charged arena, where strong positions had been taken and strong emotions expressed, even in the absence of convincing data. In response, the committee chose to embark on a process that would be as open as possible while maintaining maximum scientific rigor. It elected to hear from all who had anything to contribute, whether the contributions were concerns, complaints, or data. All available data were sought and reviewed and were then weighed in the committee's scientific assessment. Through its questions and initiatives the committee even triggered the development of significant new data on these questions.

Of course, upon starting its work, the committee never foresaw how timely its efforts would be. In the wake of the attacks of September 11 and especially the subsequent use of anthrax as a bioterrorist weapon, the committee debated how and when to accelerate the release of its findings and recommendations, whether through an abbreviated interim report or through normal channels. In the end, it chose to complete its full report but to accelerate the timetable. We are grateful to the Institute of Medicine for providing us the extra staff support necessary to achieve this.

Recent events, including the deployment of U.S. troops to Afghanistan and surrounding areas and contamination of the U.S. mail with items containing anthrax spores, all strongly suggest not only the possibility of resumption of anthrax vaccination for military personnel but also the possibility of expanding vaccination to newly recognized high-risk persons in the civilian population. To the degree that our efforts will assist in these future decisions, we are grateful for having had the opportunity to help.

Brian L. Strom
Chair

Acknowledgments

The committee has been honored and privileged to be able to contribute to this important effort and wishes to acknowledge the valuable contributions and assistance from many individuals who shared their experiences and their expertise. We are especially grateful for the perspectives provided by individuals who took their own time to provide information to the committee through presentations or testimony. Personal and written testimony from members of the military, former members of the military, and family members of those who had been vaccinated with Anthrax Vaccine Adsorbed (AVA) provided important information to the committee. The committee also appreciates the extra work and efforts of many scientific investigators, both military and civilian, who shared their work with the committee both through scientific presentations and through their manuscripts. (Agendas for the committee's information-gathering sessions are found in Appendix C, which also includes the names of the many individuals who generously provided testimony and presentations.) The Department of Defense (particularly the Anthrax Vaccine Immunization Program Agency, the Army Medical Surveillance Activity, and the U.S. Army Medical Research Institute of Infectious Diseases) and the Department of Health and Human Services (particularly the Food and Drug Administration and the Centers for Disease Control and Prevention) provided valuable information throughout the study, as well as technical review of some background portions of the report. As our study contact with the Department of Defense, LTC John Grabenstein was very helpful and responsive in his efforts to provide information to the committee. BioPort Corporation also provided a tremendous amount of information to the committee in the form of reports and correspondence relevant to its product, AVA; technical review of some background information for the report; and last-minute information about the newly approved license supplement.

The committee also appreciates the valuable contributions of two unpaid consultants. Stanley Plotkin shared some of his wisdom and experience in vaccinology with the group, and George Robertson provided useful expertise in the area of biologics manufacture. We are also grateful to John Treanor who furthered our study with a very helpful commissioned paper on adverse events associated with adult vaccines.

We also would like to thank our tireless staff, who made this possible. Lois Joellenbeck was terrific to work with as our project director, providing guidance and assistance as we gathered data and then enormous assistance as we crafted our final language. We were particularly delighted, as well, when our committee's family was increased in size with the arrival of her first child. Lee Zwanziger was generous as she stepped in while Lois was on maternity leave, taking on our work along with that of our sister committee, the Committee to Review the CDC Anthrax Vaccine Safety and Efficacy Research Program. We also appreciated her continued assistance, along with the skilled assistance of Jane Durch, as we moved to accelerate our timetable. Karen Kazmerzak was extremely helpful in gathering and keeping track of the array of references, handouts, and other materials used during the study. Phillip Bailey was always a great help, assisting with the myriad logistical arrangements needed for the committee's meetings. In addition, IOM staff Andrea Cohen, Bronwyn Schrecker, Paige Baldwin, Jennifer Otten, Hallie Wilfert, and Clyde Behney provided important assistance in the report review, preproduction, and dissemination processes. Finally, we would like to thank our peer reviewers and our review coordinator and monitor for their useful and constructive suggestions.

Reviewers

This report has been reviewed in draft form by individuals chosen for their diverse perspectives and technical expertise, in accordance with procedures approved by the National Research Council's Report Review Committee. The purpose of this independent review is to provide candid and critical comments that will assist the institution in making its published report as sound as possible and to ensure that the report meets institutional standards for objectivity, evidence, and responsiveness to the study charge. The review comments and draft manuscript remain confidential to protect the integrity of the deliberative process. We wish to thank the following individuals for their review of this report:

KEN ALIBEK, President, Advanced Biosystems, Inc.
R. JOHN COLLIER, Presley Professor of Microbiology and Molecular Genetics, Department of Microbiology and Molecular Genetics, Harvard Medical School
DOUGLAS T. GOLENBOCK, Chief, Division of Infectious Diseases and Immunology, University of Massachusetts Medical School
HARRY A. GUESS, Vice President, Epidemiology, Merck Research Laboratories
FLORENCE P. HASELTINE, Director, Center for Population Research, National Institute of Child Health and Human Development, National Institutes of Health
SAMUEL L. KATZ, Wilburt C. Davison Professor Emeritus, Department of Pediatrics, Duke University Medical Center

MYRON M. LEVINE, Professor and Director, Center for Vaccine Development, School of Medicine, University of Maryland at Baltimore
PAUL PARKMAN, Parkman Associates
RICHARD PLATT, Professor of Ambulatory Care and Prevention, Harvard Medical School and Harvard Pilgrim Health Care
ART REINGOLD, Epidemiology Department, University of California, Berkeley
RONALD J. SALDARINI, President, Wyeth Lederle Vaccines and Pediatrics (Retired)
FRANKLIN H. TOP, JR., Executive Vice President and Medical Director, MedImmune, Inc.

Although the reviewers listed above have provided many constructive comments and suggestions, they were not asked to endorse the conclusions or recommendations, nor did they see the final draft of the report before its release. The review of this report was overseen by Leslie Z. Benet, professor, Department of Biopharmaceutical Sciences, School of Pharmacy, University of California, San Francisco, and Enriqueta C. Bond, Burroughs Wellcome Fund. Appointed by the National Research Council and Institute of Medicine, they were responsible for making certain that an independent examination of this report was carried out in accordance with institutional procedures and that all review comments were carefully considered. Responsibility for the final content of this report rests entirely with the authoring committee and the institution.

Contents

EXECUTIVE SUMMARY   1
Abstract, 1
Study Process and Information Sources, 3
Anthrax and Anthrax Vaccine, 5
Anthrax Vaccine Efficacy, 5
Anthrax Vaccine Safety, 10
Anthrax Vaccine Manufacture, 14
Future Needs, 15
References, 28

1 INTRODUCTION   33
Study Process and Information Sources, 34
Related Reports, 35
General Principles Regarding Use of Vaccines, 37
Organization of the Report, 38
References, 39

2 BACKGROUND   40
The Disease, 41
Anthrax Vaccine Development, 48
Use of Anthrax Vaccine, 49
Concerns About Use of AVA, 50
Available Data on AVA, 51
References, 53

3 ANTHRAX VACCINE EFFICACY 56
Evaluating Efficacy of AVA for Inhalational Anthrax, 57
Efficacy of AVA Against All Known *B. anthracis* Strains, 69
Correlation of Protection: Animal Models and Human Immunity, 72
Postexposure Use of Anthrax Vaccine, 75
Conclusions Regarding Efficacy, 76
References, 78

4 SAFETY: INTRODUCTION 83
Safety Concerns About the Anthrax Vaccine, 84
Identifying Vaccine-Related Adverse Events, 85
Gaining Perspective on Adverse Events Following Vaccination, 88
Sources of Information Regarding the Safety of AVA, 93
Testing for Vaccine Contamination, 95
References, 97

5 SAFETY: CASE REPORTS 102
Vaccine Adverse Event Reporting System, 102
DoD and VAERS, 107
Reports to VAERS Related to AVA, 112
References, 115

6 SAFETY: EPIDEMIOLOGIC STUDIES 118
Ad Hoc Studies, 119
Record-Linkage Studies, 155
Preliminary Information on Analysis of Data on Birth Defects, 171
Conclusions Regarding AVA Vaccination and Adverse Events, 172
Findings and Recommendations, 175
References, 176

7 ANTHRAX VACCINE MANUFACTURE 180
Committee's Interpretation of the Charge, 180
Regulatory Oversight of Vaccine Manufacture, 181
Anthrax Vaccine Development, 183
Regulatory Actions Concerning AVA Manufacture, 190
Findings and Recommendations, 194
References, 195

8 FUTURE NEEDS 198
Future Use of AVA, 199
Surveillance for Adverse Events, 201
New Anthrax Vaccine Development, 207
References, 210

APPENDIXES
A Statement of Task, 213
B Biographical Sketches, 214
C Information-Gathering Meeting Agendas, 218
D Anthrax Vaccine Adsorbed Package Inserts, 227
E Vaccine Adverse Event Reporting System (VAERS) Form, 239
F Anthrax Vaccine Expert Committee (AVEC) Case Assessment Form, 243
G DMSS Analyses Requested by the IOM Committee to Assess the Safety and Efficacy of the Anthrax Vaccine, 245
H *An Assessment of the Safety of the Anthrax Vaccine: A Letter Report,* 251

Figures, Tables, and Boxes

FIGURES

ES-1 Model of anthrax toxin action, 8

2-1 Cutaneous anthrax lesion, 43
2-2 Chest radiograph characteristic of inhalational anthrax, 45
2-3 Hemorrhagic meningitis caused by anthrax, 45
2-4 Model of anthrax toxin action, 47

5-1 VAERS information flowchart. AVEC is unique to the anthrax vaccine, 104

7-1 Changes to parameters of the Anthrax Vaccine Adsorbed manufacturing process, 191

TABLES

4-1 Local and Systemic Event Rates Reported in Selected Prospective Vaccine Trials, 90

5-1 AVEC Classification of Hospitalizations Reported to VAERS (as of October 2, 2001) Following Anthrax Vaccination and Not Classified as "Very Likely/Certainly" or "Probably" Caused by Anthrax Vaccine Adsorbed, 113

5-2   Adverse Events Reported to VAERS (as of October 2, 2001) Involving Loss of Time from Duty of 24 Hours or More and Considered by AVEC as Certainly or Probably Caused by Anthrax Vaccine Adsorbed, 114

6-1   Ad Hoc Studies of Immediate-Onset Adverse Events Following Anthrax Vaccination: Local Events, 120
6-2   Ad Hoc Studies of Immediate-Onset Adverse Events Following Anthrax Vaccination: Systemic Events, 128
6-3   Ad Hoc Studies of Later-Onset Adverse Events Following Anthrax Vaccination, 134
6-4   Record-Linkage Studies of Adverse Events Following Anthrax Vaccination, 136

7-1   Events in AVA Development and Manufacture, 184
7-2   Comparison of AVA and Merck Vaccine, 185
7-3   Timeline for Production of AVA, 189

8-1   Functions of AVEC and Post-AVEC Panels, 203

BOXES

ES-1   Chapter 3 Findings and Recommendations, 22
ES-2   Chapter 5 Findings and Recommendations, 23
ES-3   Chapter 6 Findings and Recommendations, 24
ES-4   Chapter 7 Findings, 25
ES-5   Chapter 8 Findings, 26
ES-6   Chapter 8 Recommendations, 27

8-1   Goals of Anthrax Vaccine Development, 209

Abbreviations and Acronyms

ACCA	Advisory Committee on Causality Assessment
ACIP	Advisory Committee on Immunization Practices
AMSA	Army Medical Surveillance Activity
ATR	anthrax toxin receptor
AVA	Anthrax Vaccine Adsorbed
AVEC	Anthrax Vaccine Expert Committee
AVIP	Anthrax Vaccine Immunization Program
BLA	Biologics License Application
CBER	Center for Biologics Evaluation and Research
CDC	Centers for Disease Control and Prevention
C.F.R.	Code of Federal Regulations
CI	confidence interval
cm	centimeter
DBS	Division of Biologics Standards, National Institutes of Health
DEERS	Defense Enrollment Eligibility Reporting System
DHHS	Department of Health and Human Services
DMSS	Defense Medical Surveillance System
DNA	deoxyribonucleic acid
DoD	Department of Defense
DTaP	diphtheria and tetanus toxoid and acellular pertussis

EF	edema factor
E/I	erythema and/or induration
EIR	Establishment Inspection Report
ELISA	enzyme-linked immunosorbent assay
FDA	Food and Drug Administration
GAO	General Accounting Office
GMPs	good manufacturing practices
ICD-9-CM	*International Classification of Diseases, Ninth Revision, Clinical Modification*
IgG	immunoglobulin G
IND	Investigational New Drug
IOM	Institute of Medicine
kDa	kilodalton
LF	lethal factor
MBPI	Michigan Biologic Products Institute
MDPH	Michigan Department of Public Health
ml	milliliter
NCDC	National Communicable Disease Center
NIH	National Institutes of Health
NOIR	Notice of Intent to Revoke
OR	odds ratio
PA	protective antigen
PBT	pentavalent botulinum toxoid
PCR	polymerase chain reaction
ROTC	Reserve Officer Training Corps
SDS-PAGE	sodium dodecyl sulfate-polyacrylamide gel electrophoresis
SWA	Southwest Asia
Td	tetanus and diphtheria toxoid
TNA	toxin neutralizing antibody
µg	microgram

μm	micrometer
USAMRIID	U.S. Army Medical Research Institute of Infectious Diseases
VA	Department of Veterans Affairs
VAERS	Vaccine Adverse Event Reporting System
VNTR	variable-nucleotide tandem repeat

Executive Summary

ABSTRACT

Anthrax Vaccine Adsorbed (AVA) was licensed in 1970 to provide protection against infection with Bacillus anthracis. *AVA was initially administered on a limited basis, primarily to protect veterinarians and workers processing animal products such as hair or hides that could be contaminated with anthrax spores. In the 1990s, with growing concerns about the possible use of anthrax as a biological weapon, use of the vaccine was substantially expanded. The Department of Defense (DoD) vaccinated some of the military personnel deployed for the Gulf War in 1991 and in 1998 initiated the Anthrax Vaccine Immunization Program, calling for mandatory vaccination of all U.S. service members. By late 2001, roughly 2.1 million doses of AVA had been administered. Production of AVA was suspended in 1998 when the facility manufacturing the vaccine was closed for renovations, which were undertaken to meet regulatory requirements of the Food and Drug Administration (FDA).*

Concerns about the efficacy and safety of AVA, and about vaccine production, led Congress to direct the DoD to support an independent examination of AVA by the Institute of Medicine. In October 2000, the Institute of Medicine convened the Committee to Assess the Safety and Efficacy of the Anthrax Vaccine. The committee reviewed all available data, both published and unpub-

lished, and heard from representatives of DoD, FDA, and other federal agencies; from the vaccine manufacturer BioPort; from researchers studying the efficacy and safety of the vaccine; and from service members and others with concerns about the safety or efficacy of the vaccine. After the bioterrorism of fall 2001, the committee accelerated its original timetable for its review.

As indicated by evidence from studies in both humans and animals, the committee concluded that AVA, as licensed, is an effective vaccine to protect humans against anthrax, including inhalational anthrax. Moreover, because the vaccine exerts its protection via an antigen crucial to the action of the bacterium's toxins, AVA should be effective against anthrax toxicity from all known strains of B. anthracis, *as well as from any potential bio-engineered strains.*

After examining data from numerous case reports and especially epidemiologic studies, the committee also concluded that AVA is reasonably safe. Within hours or days following vaccination, it is fairly common for recipients to experience some local events (e.g., redness, itching, swelling, or tenderness at the injection site), while a smaller number of vaccine recipients experience some systemic events (e.g., fever and malaise). But these immediate reactions, and the rates at which they occur, are comparable to those observed with other vaccines regularly administered to adults. The committee found no evidence that vaccine recipients face an increased risk of experiencing life-threatening or permanently disabling adverse events immediately after receiving AVA, when compared with the general population. Nor did it find any convincing evidence that vaccine recipients face elevated risk of developing adverse health effects over the longer term, although data are limited in this regard (as they are for all vaccines).

Regarding manufacture of AVA, the committee reviewed and evaluated the steps taken by BioPort to win FDA approval of its production process. With the newly validated manufacturing process being used in a renovated facility, AVA will be produced under strict controls according to current FDA requirements. The newly produced vaccine is expected to have greater assurance of consistency than the vaccine produced at the time of its original licensure.

It remains important to continue and improve monitoring efforts to detect any adverse health effects caused by AVA and other vaccines. Also needed are studies to establish a quantitative correlation of protective levels of antibodies in animals with antibody levels in humans after full immunization. Direct tests of the efficacy of AVA are neither feasible nor ethical in humans. However, corre-

lates of protection in animal models can be used to test the efficacy of AVA, as well as new vaccines against anthrax. The production, testing, and licensure of a new vaccine requiring fewer doses and producing fewer local reactions are needed.

Anthrax Vaccine Adsorbed[1] (AVA) was licensed in 1970. More than 2 million doses have been administered, and most of those doses have been given since 1998 to U.S. military personnel to protect them against possible exposure to anthrax spores used as biological weapons. The terrorist attacks of September 11, 2001, and the subsequent distribution through the U.S. mail of potent doses of anthrax spores drew new attention to the risks of anthrax exposure and to questions about the anthrax vaccine.

Until the 1990s, AVA had primarily been used by a small population with a risk of occupational exposure to anthrax (e.g., textile mill workers and veterinarians). In 1990, concerns that Iraq had biological weapons containing anthrax spores motivated the U.S. military to administer AVA to an estimated 150,000 service members deployed for the Gulf War. The existence of an Iraqi biological weapons program was confirmed in the mid-1990s (Henderson, 1999; Zilinskas, 1997), and in 1997 the Department of Defense (DoD) announced a plan to vaccinate all U.S. service members with the licensed anthrax vaccine. DoD's Anthrax Vaccine Immunization Program (AVIP) began in March 1998 with personnel scheduled for deployment to higher-risk areas (e.g., Korea and Southwest Asia). In 2000 a limited vaccine supply, the result of delays in federal approval for release of newly manufactured vaccine lots, began slowing plans to vaccinate all military personnel. As more service members were vaccinated under the mandatory AVIP, some raised concerns about the safety or the efficacy of AVA, and more than 400 personnel refused vaccination (Weiss, 2001). Some had also suggested a link between vaccination with AVA and illnesses in Gulf War veterans.

STUDY PROCESS AND INFORMATION SOURCES

Responding to the concerns about the anthrax vaccine and AVIP, the U.S. Congress directed DoD to enter into a contract with the National Research Council for a study of the vaccine's efficacy and safety.[2] In October 2000 the Institute of Medicine (IOM) convened the Committee to

---

[1]As of January 31, 2002, AVA will be manufactured under the name Biothrax.
[2]The study was called for in the conference report accompanying the 2000 DoD appropriations act P. L. No. 106-79 (1999).

Assess the Safety and Efficacy of the Anthrax Vaccine to carry out that study. Committee members were selected for their expertise in microbiology; vaccine research, development, manufacture, and evaluation; postmarketing surveillance of adverse events; regulatory and licensing procedures; epidemiology; biostatistics; immunology; and health surveillance.

The charge to the committee included consideration of the types and severity of adverse reactions, sex differences in adverse reactions, long-term health implications, the efficacy of AVA against inhalational exposure to all known anthrax strains, and the correlation of the safety and efficacy of the vaccine in animal models to its safety and efficacy in humans. The study was also to address the issue of validation of the manufacturing process, with consideration of discrepancies identified by the Food and Drug Administration (FDA) in February 1998, the definition of vaccine components, and identification of gaps in existing research. (See Appendix A for the Statement of Task.) The charge did not include evaluation of the DoD policy to vaccinate all service members, so the committee did not include an evaluation of the threat from biological warfare agents in its purview. Similarly, the committee was not asked to address the challenges in bioweapons vaccine development and procurement generally, which have recently been discussed in a statement from the Council of the Institute of Medicine (http://www.iom.edu/IOM/IOMHome.nsf/Pages/Vaccine+ Development) and in reports by the Gilmore Commission (http://www.rand.org/nsrd/terrpanel/) and DoD (http://www.defenselink.mil/pubs/Reporton BiologicalWarfareDefenseVaccineRDPrgras-July2001.pdf).

Since the terrorist attacks of September 11, 2001, and subsequent mail distribution of anthrax spores, interest in AVA has greatly increased. Consideration of the full range of topics concerning civilian use of the anthrax vaccine was beyond the purview of this report. However, some of the issues that the committee did address should also be of interest for civilians.

The committee held eight deliberative meetings plus four public workshops. At those workshops, the committee heard from representatives of DoD, FDA, and other federal agencies; from the manufacturer of AVA, BioPort; from researchers studying the efficacy and safety of the vaccine; and from service members and others with concerns about the safety or efficacy of the vaccine. The committee also commissioned a review of the available literature on adverse events associated with other vaccines routinely administered to adults.

The committee examined both published and unpublished data from studies of the safety and efficacy of AVA. The investigators involved in many of those studies presented their data and discussed their findings at committee workshops. In addition, several analyses of existing data were carried out at the committee's request.

ANTHRAX AND ANTHRAX VACCINE

Anthrax is caused by infection with *Bacillus anthracis*, a gram-positive, nonmotile, spore-forming organism (Brachman and Friedlander, 1999; Dixon et al., 1999). It is primarily a disease of wild and domestic animals. Historically, humans have contracted the disease through contact with infected animals or animal products, such as hair or hides, contaminated with anthrax spores. Depending on the site of infection, anthrax can occur in a cutaneous, gastrointestinal, or inhalational form. The disease had become extremely uncommon in any form in the United States until the bioterrorist incidents of the autumn of 2001 caused an outbreak of both cutaneous and inhalational cases of the disease. As of November 28, 2001, there had been 11 cases of inhalational anthrax, 5 of which were fatal, and 7 confirmed and 5 suspected cutaneous anthrax infections (CDC, 2001b). More than 30,000 people may have been exposed to anthrax spores (CDC, 2001a,b).

The virulence of *B. anthracis* derives from the production of a capsule and three toxin proteins: protective antigen (PA), edema factor (EF), and lethal factor (LF). To produce active toxins, PA must bind to cellular receptors and then to either EF or LF. AVA, the vaccine currently licensed for human use in the United States, is a cell-free filtrate containing PA as the principal immunogen. It is administered in six subcutaneous injections of 0.5 milliliters each. The first three doses are given 2 weeks apart, and the following doses are given 6, 12, and 18 months after administration of the first dose. Annual booster doses are required.

ANTHRAX VACCINE EFFICACY

The committee's observations and findings addressed the efficacy of immunization with the licensed vaccine, AVA, against inhalational anthrax and all known anthrax strains (see Chapter 3). Of particular concern is exposure to anthrax spores processed for use in biological weapons. The committee also examined what is known and what must still be established regarding the correlation of protection in animal models with immunity in humans.

It is important to note that efficacy is relative, not absolute. The degree of protection provided by a vaccine is determined by a variety of factors, which can include the size of the inoculum of exposure, the strain of the pathogen, and the host response. Even a vaccine considered highly effective may fail to protect some individuals under some circumstances.

Evaluating Efficacy of AVA

The efficacy of a PA-containing anthrax vaccine similar to AVA against anthrax infection was established by a randomized controlled field study of textile mill workers (Brachman et al., 1962). Subsequent data from the Centers for Disease Control and Prevention (CDC) support the results of that study (FDA, 1985). The small number of inhalational cases in those studies provides insufficient information to establish the vaccine's efficacy against inhalational infection, but the data suggest that the vaccine has a protective effect.

Animal studies are essential for further investigation of the efficacy of AVA and other anthrax vaccines against inhalational disease because studies with humans are neither feasible nor ethical. Cases of inhalational anthrax are very rare, even where anthrax occurs naturally in the environment or as an occupational hazard. Moreover, human research subjects cannot be deliberately exposed to potentially lethal agents, such as anthrax spores, for no therapeutic reason and without the availability of a proven treatment.

> **Finding:** Because additional clinical trials to test the efficacy of AVA in humans are not feasible and challenge trials with volunteers are unethical, by necessity animal models represent the only sources of the supplementary data needed to evaluate AVA's efficacy.

Animal models with pathological and immunological characteristics similar to those of humans could be considered the most appropriate ones for the evaluation of vaccine efficacy. The pathophysiology of anthrax in nonhuman primates, such as the macaque, most closely resembles the pathophysiology of anthrax in humans. Among the smaller and more available laboratory animals, rabbits most closely resemble nonhuman primates in terms of the pathology of anthrax and their response to the anthrax vaccine.

> **Finding:** The macaque and the rabbit are adequate animal models for evaluation of the efficacy of AVA for the prevention of inhalational anthrax.

Efficacy of AVA Against All Known *B. anthracis* Strains

Several different *B. anthracis* strains are found in nature worldwide (Fellows et al., 2001; Keim et al., 2000), and analysis of tissue samples from victims of the release of anthrax spores from the Soviet biological weapons facility at Sverdlovsk in 1979 indicated the presence of several *B. anthracis* strains (Grinberg et al., 2001; Jackson et al., 1998). It is important to establish whether AVA can afford protection against the full range of naturally occurring or engineered *B. anthracis* strains.

Studies have shown that the protection that AVA affords guinea pigs differs by bacterial strain (Auerbach and Wright, 1955; Fellows et al., 2001; Ivins et al., 1994; Little and Knudson, 1986; Turnbull et al., 1986), but AVA and a predecessor vaccine protected rabbits and monkeys against the numerous strains tested (Auerbach and Wright, 1955), including those that defeated the vaccine in guinea pigs (Fellows et al., 2001). No AVA-resistant strains have been demonstrated in nonhuman primates. Observational data from studies with humans also support the efficacy of AVA against a variety of strains, though exposure strains were not evaluated in the studies (Brachman et al., 1962; CDC, 1967–1971).

PA is the principal immunogen in AVA, and the efficacy of AVA against a broad spectrum of *B. anthracis* strains is consistent with the critical role of PA in the pathogenesis of anthrax (Bhatnagar and Batra, 2001; Cataldi et al., 1990; Smith and Keppie, 1954). As shown in Figure ES-1, PA must be competent to carry out multiple complicated tasks: it must bind to its receptor, form a heptamer, and bring EF and LF into the cell.

There is concern that natural mutations or bioengineered alterations of the PA component of anthrax could result in vaccine-resistant strains. Studies (Sellman et al., 2001; see also Mogridge et al., 2001) have shown, however, that a PA heptamer is deactivated by the presence of even a few mutant subunits. A deactivated heptamer is unlikely to be able to deliver EF and LF to the cytosol. The committee considers it improbable that a mutant PA that retains its function yet escapes the vaccine-elicited protective antibodies directed to the wild-type PA could be constructed at this time.

The likely difficulty of successfully altering PA is supported by evidence that the *B. anthracis* genome is highly conserved among strains isolated across a wide geographical area (Jackson, 2001; Keim et al., 1997) and that PA is also highly conserved (Jackson, 2001; Price et al., 1999). Because PA is critical to virulence and because its structure is so highly conserved, it appears likely that changing its structure would alter and thus eliminate its toxic action.

Finding: It is unlikely that either naturally occurring or anthrax strains with bioengineered protective antigen could both evade AVA and cause the toxicity associated with anthrax.

Establishing Animal Model Correlates of Anthrax Vaccine Efficacy

Several recent studies have used passive protection to demonstrate a relationship between levels of circulating anti-PA antibody and protection from challenge with anthrax spores (Barnard and Friedlander, 1999; Beedham et al., 2001; Little et al., 1997; McBride et al., 1998; Pitt et al., 2001; Reuveny et al., 2001).

Finding: The available data indicate that immunity to anthrax is associated with the presence of antibody to protective antigen.

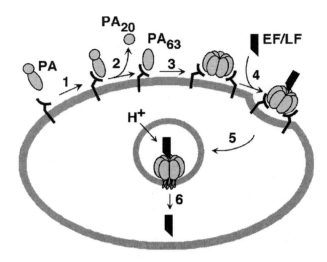

FIGURE ES-1 Model of anthrax toxin action. (1) PA binds to cellular receptor. (2–3) The protein is cleaved and activated to form a heptameric prepore. (4) LF, EF, or both bind to the heptamer, and the resulting complex is taken into an acidic compartment in the cell through endocytosis. (5–6) The acidic pH initiates the heptamer to pierce the membrane of the cell and translocate LF, EF, or both into the cytosol, where the toxins lead to damage. [Reprinted, with permission, from *Biochemistry* 38:10432–10441 (1999). Copyright 1999 by American Chemical Society.]

The information reviewed by the committee demonstrates that both humans and certain laboratory animals manifest the same disease after infection with the same anthrax organism and that both are protected by immunization with AVA, which elicits the production of antibodies to PA. This information establishes a *qualitative* correlation between protection in animal models and protection in humans. To move forward with research on the current anthrax vaccine or any new vaccines, however, a *quantitative* correlation of the protective levels of antibodies in animals with the antibody titers obtained after full immunization in humans is needed. Those correlates in animal models can then be used to test new vaccines for efficacy with confidence that the data from studies with animals will be predictive of the clinical results for immunized humans. The data from animal studies already developed suggest that serological correlates of human immunity can be developed in appropriate animal models. The committee commends this work and encourages its further development.

Recommendation: Additional passive protection studies with rabbits

and monkeys including the transfer of animal and human sera are urgently needed to quantify the protective levels of antibody in vivo against different challenge doses of anthrax spores.

Recommendation: Additional active protection studies should be conducted or supported to develop data that describe the relationship between immunity and both specific and functional quantitative antibody levels, including studies of

- the relationship between the vaccine dose and the resulting level of antibody in the blood of test animals that protects the animals from challenge;
- the relationship between the level of antibody that protects animals from challenge and the level of antibody present in humans vaccinated by the regimen currently recommended for the licensed product; and
- the vaccine dose that results in a level of antibody in the blood of human volunteers similar to that in the blood of protected animals.

Postexposure Use of Anthrax Vaccine

As a result of the inhalational exposure to anthrax spores from letters mailed in the autumn of 2001, questions about the postexposure efficacy of AVA have arisen. No data from studies with humans are available, but two papers provide information from studies with rhesus monkeys.

These limited data suggest that use of the vaccine in combination with an appropriate antibiotic for 30 days could provide excellent postexposure protection against inhalational anthrax. Although the additional benefit from receiving the vaccine after a prolonged period of antibiotic use is not proven, reliance on the vaccine alone after exposure is clearly insufficient, as some protection is needed during the time required for an immune response to develop. Additional studies on the postexposure use of AVA with antibiotics are needed.

Recommendation: DoD should pursue or support additional research with laboratory animals on the efficacy of AVA in combination with antibiotics administered following inhalational exposure to anthrax spores. Studies should focus on establishment of an appropriate duration for antibiotic prophylaxis after vaccine administration.

Conclusions Regarding Efficacy

A vaccine similar to AVA was shown to be effective against cutaneous anthrax in humans in the field trial supporting the original application for licensure of AVA (Brachman et al., 1962). Although that study had too few cases to evaluate the vaccine's efficacy for the prevention of inhalational disease, the five inhalational cases observed during the trial occurred only among nonvaccinated or placebo recipients. Data from CDC on cases reported between 1962 and 1974 also indicated that the vaccine offered protection against the cutaneous form of the disease (FDA, 1985). Furthermore, laboratory experiments indicate that AVA provides effective protection against inhalational challenge in rabbits and macaques, the animal models in which the disease is most reflective of the disease in humans (Fellows et al., 2001; Ivins et al., 1996, 1998; Pitt et al., 2001). Because PA is critical to the virulence of *B. anthracis* and because PA's structure is so highly conserved, it appears likely that changing its structure would alter and thus eliminate its toxic action. Data from studies with animals suggest that AVA will offer protection against strains with PA-based toxicity. Finally, the available data indicate that immunity to anthrax is associated with the presence of antibodies to PA, such as those stimulated by the anthrax vaccine.

> Finding: The committee finds that the available evidence from studies with humans and animals, coupled with reasonable assumptions of analogy, shows that AVA as licensed is an effective vaccine for the protection of humans against anthrax, including inhalational anthrax, caused by any known or plausible engineered strains of *B. anthracis*.

ANTHRAX VACCINE SAFETY

As with any pharmaceutical product or medical procedure, the use of vaccines carries a risk of adverse health effects that must be weighed against the expected health benefit. Expectations for the safety[3] of vaccines are especially high because, in contrast to therapeutic agents, which are given when a disease is known to be present (or at least suspected), vaccines are usually given to people who are healthy to protect them against a disease that they may not be exposed to in the future.

The committee evaluated case reports and epidemiologic studies providing information about the safety of the anthrax vaccine. Case reports can help to generate hypotheses about possible associations but are rarely sufficient by themselves to confirm such associations. Formal epidemiologic studies are usually needed to determine whether those adverse events iden-

---

[3] For this report, safety reflects expectations of relative freedom from harmful effects when a product is used prudently, considering the condition of the recipient and the health risk the product is directed against.

tified in case reports occur in exposed populations at a rate that exceeds the background rate in unexposed populations.

The case reports relating to AVA come primarily from the Vaccine Adverse Event Reporting System (VAERS), a passive surveillance system that collects reports on adverse events following the use of any vaccine licensed in the United States (see Chapter 5). A subset of the committee reviewed each of 120 VAERS reports on serious adverse events associated with AVA. The committee also heard testimony regarding adverse events following vaccination with AVA. These statements, some of which concerned cases reported to VAERS, added valuable insight into the conditions that some military personnel are experiencing.

In evaluating the epidemiologic studies of adverse events following receipt of AVA (see Chapter 6), the committee gave additional weight to those that (1) used active surveillance rather than self-reports of postimmunization events; (2) included sufficiently large numbers of subjects; (3) had clearly specified, objective criteria for the definition of adverse events; and (4) had sufficiently long postimmunization follow-up intervals to allow identification of later-onset events. Those studies that included a suitable unimmunized comparison group or in which evaluators were blinded to vaccination status were especially useful to the committee.

Conclusions Regarding AVA Vaccination and Adverse Events

Substantial data are now available from VAERS, epidemiologic studies with data from the Defense Medical Surveillance System (DMSS), and other epidemiologic studies for assessments of the health outcomes following vaccination with AVA. Immediate-onset health events are observable within hours or days following vaccination; later-onset events would be observable only months or years following vaccination.

Epidemiologic studies that have used either active surveillance (Brachman et al., 1962; Pittman, 2001b,c; Pittman et al., 1997, 2002, in press) or passive surveillance (Hoffman et al., submitted for publication; Pittman, 2001a; Pittman et al., 2001a,b; Wasserman, 2001) have consistently found local injection-site reactions, including redness, induration, edema, itching, or tenderness (see Table 6-1 for details). Systemic events, such as fever, malaise, and myalgia, are also associated with vaccination with AVA but are generally less common than injection-site reactions. The types of local and systemic reactions associated with AVA and the rates at which they were observed are comparable to those observed with other vaccines regularly administered to adults, such as diphtheria and tetanus toxoids and influenza vaccines (Treanor, 2001). Although these immediate-onset health effects can result in brief limitation of activities or the loss of time from work (Hoffman et al., submitted for publication; Wasserman,

2001), they are self-limited and result in no serious, permanent health impairments (AMSA, 2001a,b,c; Grabenstein, 2000; Lange et al., 2001a,b; Rehme, 2001; Rehme et al., 2002; Mason et al., 2001, submitted for publication; Sato, 2001a,b; Sato et al., 2001).

> Finding: The data available from VAERS, DMSS, and epidemiologic studies indicate the following regarding immediate-onset health events following receipt of AVA:
>
> - Local events, especially redness, swelling, or nodules at the injection site, are associated with receipt of AVA, are similar to the events observed following receipt of other vaccines currently in use by adults, and are fairly common.
> - Systemic events, such as fever, malaise, and myalgia, are associated with receipt of AVA, are similar to the events observed following receipt of other vaccines currently in use by adults but are much less common than local events.
> - Immediate-onset health effects can be severe enough in some individuals to result in brief functional impairment, but these effects are self-limited and result in no permanent health impairments.
> - There is no evidence that life-threatening or permanently disabling immediate-onset adverse events occur at higher rates in individuals who have received AVA than in the general population.

Sex differences are seen in local injection-site reactions. Women are more likely than men to experience and report erythema, local tenderness, subcutaneous nodules, itching, and edema (Hoffman et al., submitted for publication; Pittman, 2001a,b; Pittman et al., 2001a,b, 2002; Wasserman, 2001). In addition, some systemic effects, including fever, headache, malaise, and chills, were sometimes more often reported by women than by men (Hoffman et al., submitted for publication; Pittman, 2001a; Pittman et al., 2001a,b), but rates of clinically observed systemic reactions generally did not differ substantially between men and women (Pittman, 2001b; Pittman et al., 2002). For female service members, reactions following vaccination against anthrax may be more likely to have an adverse effect on their ability to perform their duties (Hoffman et al., submitted for publication; Wasserman, 2001). Studies of other vaccines have also generally found higher rates of local reactions among women but similar rates of systemic reactions between men and women (Treanor, 2001). The factors that account for these sex differences are not known, but they could be a function of differences in muscle mass, differences in the doses per unit of body mass, physiologic factors, or differences in care-seeking behavior. Future studies of vaccination against anthrax should continue to analyze data for men and women separately.

Finding: The available data from both active and passive surveillance indicate that there are sex differences in local reactions following vaccination with AVA, as there are following administration of other vaccines. For female service members, reactions following vaccination with AVA can have a transient adverse impact on their ability to perform their duties. The factors that account for these sex differences are not known.

Recommendation: Future monitoring and study of health events following vaccination(s) with AVA (and other vaccines) should continue to include separate analyses of data for men and women.

Some of the data reviewed by the committee showed lot-to-lot differences in the reactogenicities of AVA doses (CDC, 1967–1971; Pittman, 2001a; Pittman et al., 2001a,b).

Unlike most vaccines, AVA is licensed for subcutaneous rather than intramuscular administration. The limited evidence from a small study that tested changes in the AVA dosing schedule and route of administration (Pittman, 2001b; Pittman et al., 2002) suggests that subcutaneous administration contributes to the local reactions but not systemic reactions associated with AVA. With other vaccines, subcutaneous administration is also associated with higher rates of local erythema or induration (Treanor, 2001), reactions commonly reported following the administration of AVA.

Finding: The currently licensed subcutaneous route of administration of AVA and the six-dose vaccination schedule appear to be associated with a higher incidence of immediate-onset, local effects than is intramuscular administration or a vaccination schedule with fewer doses of AVA. The frequencies of immediate-onset, systemic events were low and were not affected by the route of administration.

Recommendation: DoD should continue to support the efforts of CDC to study the reactogenicity and immunogenicity of an alternative route of AVA administration and of a reduced number of vaccine doses.

Some have expressed concerns about potential later-onset and chronic health effects resulting from AVA use. The available information regarding later-onset health effects is limited, as for all vaccines, but provides no convincing evidence of elevated risks of later-onset health events (AMSA, 2001a,b,c; Grabenstein, 2000; Lange et al., 2001a,b; Mason et al., 2001, submitted for publication; Peeler et al., 1958, 1965; Rehme, 2001; Rehme et al., 2002; Sato, 2001a,b; Sato et al., 2001; White et al., 1974). DMSS, which provides the best source of data for studying later-onset health effects, provides data on service personnel who have documented histories of vaccination with AVA and who have been observed for up to 3 years.

Although AVA has been administered to military personnel for more than 3 years, unreliable documentation of vaccinations before 1998 limits analysis of DMSS data for observation of potential vaccine-related health effects over longer periods.

> **Finding:** The available data are limited but show no convincing evidence at this time that personnel who have received AVA have elevated risks of later-onset health events.

> **Recommendation:** DoD should develop systems to enhance the capacity to monitor the occurrence of later-onset health conditions that might be associated with the receipt of any vaccine; the data reviewed by the committee do not suggest the need for special efforts of this sort for AVA.

The studies reviewed did not examine the use of AVA in children, the elderly, or individuals with chronic illnesses. In addition, information regarding the outcomes of pregnancy following use of the vaccine is limited. These limitations should be taken into account if AVA is considered for use in the general population.

ANTHRAX VACCINE MANUFACTURE

The committee was charged with addressing "validation of the manufacturing process focusing on, but not limited to, discrepancies identified by the Food and Drug Administration in February 1998." The committee could not directly validate the manufacturing process and did not wish to second-guess FDA's inspection and determination of validity. It was possible, however, to review and evaluate the steps by which BioPort worked to validate the AVA manufacturing process (see Chapter 7).

Documents that BioPort provided to the committee gave detailed information about findings from FDA inspections conducted since 1998, the company's responses to those findings, and FDA's evaluation of BioPort's progress. The committee paid special attention to materials on product characterization and process validation. It also considered the recent and increasing investments by BioPort and DoD in facility renovations and improvements in documentation of the manufacturing process, as well as the transfer, with approval from FDA's Center for Biologics Research (CBER), of filling operations to a contractor meeting Good Manufacturing Practices standards. The committee noted BioPort's access to technical support and assistance from CBER and DoD research and development resources. The results of these efforts were reflected in BioPort's reports of progress in correcting deficiencies previously noted by FDA, as reported at the committee's July 2001 meeting. This progress was confirmed by FDA.

On January 31, 2002, FDA approved BioPort's supplements to its Biologics License Application covering facility renovations, changes to the package label, and the contracted filling operations.

In evaluating BioPort's efforts to meet the manufacturing requirements for AVA, the committee noted FDA's changes and modernizations and improvements in the regulation of biologics, as well as the continuing effort at constructive criticism and response between the agency and the manufacturer. The committee also considered the history of the AVA manufacturer—in particular, the switch from a state-owned to a privately owned and operated interstate commercial venture—and the coincident changes in FDA oversight and validation requirements. Finally, the committee was mindful of the scientific and technical advances in vaccine manufacture and characterization that have occurred since the original licensure of the AVA product.

> **Finding:** FDA's process of plant inspection and FDA's validation of the vaccine manufacturing process have changed and have become more stringent with time.

> **Finding:** With high-priority efforts by the manufacturer and FDA, the manufacturing process for AVA has been validated so that vaccine manufactured postrenovation has been approved for release and distribution.

BioPort has responded to numerous specific citations from FDA regarding the manufacturing process and equipment and has now received FDA approval of its license supplements. In the committee's judgment, the cumulative effects of the changes in materials, equipment, and processes in response to FDA citations, as well as the changes in the regulatory climate and in scientific knowledge, are likely to result in greater assurance of consistency in the final AVA product.

> **Finding:** AVA will now be produced by a newly validated manufacturing process under strict controls, according to current FDA requirements. As a result, the postrenovation product has greater assurance of consistency than that produced at the time of original licensure.

FUTURE NEEDS

Despite recent FDA approval of the license supplement for AVA manufacturing renovations, package insert, and contract filler, the committee is convinced that relying on AVA and the current specifications for its use is far from satisfactory. There is a need for research toward the development of a different and better anthrax vaccine, as well as a need for improvements in monitoring the safety of the current vaccine.

Future Use of AVA

Finding: Current events in both the military and civilian arenas highlight and confirm the importance of ensuring both the availability and the quality of the nation's anthrax vaccine.

With the deployment of U.S. troops to Afghanistan and surrounding areas and domestic bioterrorism incidents involving exposure to *B. anthracis* spores, vaccination against anthrax is likely to resume and possibly expand. This means that AVA is likely to be given to a much larger population than was anticipated at the time that the vaccine was licensed.

Meanwhile, the current supply of AVA is limited because of manufacturing difficulties, which have now been overcome. On the basis of information provided by BioPort and FDA, the committee notes that the AVA manufacturing process has been modified to incorporate more modern technology and procedures. These changes are expected to increase assurance of the consistency of the final product, which remains a relatively crude vaccine by current standards.

Although greater assurance of product consistency will occur, the levels of immunogenicity, safety, and stability of the postrenovation AVA product must be characterized. The committee emphasizes that the surveillance methods recommended below are the same as those that would be expected for any widely used vaccine and are not unique to AVA.

Finding: The AVA product produced in a renovated facility by a newly validated manufacturing process could differ from the prerenovation product in terms of its reactogenicity, immunogenicity, and stability. The information available to the committee suggests that AVA lots manufactured postrenovation may show less variation in reactogenicity because of greater consistency in the production process, and there is no a priori basis to believe that the postrenovation product will be more reactogenic or less immunogenic than the older vaccine.

Recommendation: As with all vaccines, AVA lots produced postrenovation should be monitored for immunogenicity and stability, and individuals receiving these lots should be monitored for possible acute or chronic adverse events of immediate or later onset.

Surveillance for Adverse Events

DoD has supported an independent civilian advisory panel called the Anthrax Vaccine Expert Committee (AVEC) to review each VAERS report associated with AVA.

The Future and AVEC

The committee found AVEC's expert scrutiny of VAERS reports for signals that might require further action to be an important component of surveillance for the safety of AVA. However, the value of such a review process may not be limited to AVA. Furthermore, the IOM committee is generally skeptical about attribution of causality, such as those that AVEC makes, from reports to a surveillance system like VAERS, especially given the potential for misclassification of reported events when considering them as possibly related or unrelated to vaccination. The committee emphasizes that a review of case reports to VAERS is appropriate only for the generation of hypotheses. More emphasis should therefore be placed on the use of AVEC-derived hypotheses to trigger additional analyses, such as those that can be performed with data from DMSS. Toward that end, AVEC and the Army Medical Surveillance Activity (the office responsible for DMSS) should maintain regular and frequent communication, with signals from the former leading to analyses by the latter. "Signals" are the earliest indication of a possible causal relationship between an exposure and a health event. Such signals can come from the anecdotal experiences of patients with an adverse event after the exposure or from preliminary analyses of data. A signal does not mean that a causal relationship exists, as there may be other explanations for the apparent association. Instead, a signal is merely an indication that further investigation is needed.

Although AVA appears to be associated with certain undesirable but self-limited or easily treated adverse events, the committee saw no indication from the currently available data of a need to continue special monitoring programs for AVA. Nevertheless, monitoring of vaccine safety in general and the safety of vaccines for use by members of the military in particular must be a priority. The committee observed several areas in which surveillance for the safety of vaccines in general and AVA in particular might be improved.

> **Finding: Given the concerns raised by some service members about the safety of the anthrax vaccine, the creation of AVEC was an appropriate complement to other resources in FDA, CDC, and DoD for the monitoring of vaccine safety concerns. The results of the extra monitoring did not indicate the existence of any sentinel events that were not detected in the existing FDA and CDC reviews. The committee finds no scientific reason for the continued operation of AVEC in its present form.**

The IOM committee's observations about AVEC reflect no fault with the members of AVEC or its performance as that committee is constituted; rather, the IOM committee observes that AVEC was designed to pay extra attention to safety concerns regarding the safety of AVA and that the data do not warrant the continuation of such exceptional attention. The resources supporting AVEC activities related to AVA alone could be more wisely invested in improved monitoring of the safety of vaccines in general.

> **Recommendation:** DoD should disband AVEC in its current form and instead assist FDA and CDC in establishing an independent advisory committee charged with overseeing the entire process of evaluating vaccine safety. The proposed advisory committee can also assist on an ad hoc basis in the interpretation of potential signals detected in VAERS or other sources regarding the safety of any vaccine. The newly established FDA drug safety committee might be an appropriate model.

Should DoD choose to continue AVEC, the committee urges DoD to recommend a shift in AVEC's focus from making attributions of causality in individual cases to seeking any patterns or rate thresholds that have been crossed in terms of the serious adverse events reported to VAERS. AVEC could then develop criteria for signals from VAERS data for any vaccine that warrants additional follow-up and could in general further systematize its processes by developing standard operating procedures and a regular schedule for examination of aggregate VAERS data. Background rates of illnesses as well as the biological plausibility of hypothesized effects must be taken into consideration as part of the method used to identify signals of possible safety concerns.

> **Recommendation:** If DoD chooses to continue AVEC, DoD should consider redefining the panel's role so that it serves as an independent advisory committee that responds on an ad hoc basis to specific requests to assist in the interpretation of potential signals detected by others (e.g., CDC and FDA) and reported to VAERS or other sources regarding the safety of all vaccines administered to service personnel rather than continuing the panel's current role of rereviewing each VAERS report related to AVA.

Additional Sources of Data on Adverse Events

Ensuring the best use and interpretation of VAERS reports requires complementary information from other sources that can be used to help analyze the signals that may be suggested by VAERS reports. One such resource is DMSS. DMSS can be used both to generate and test hypotheses. If VAERS raises a hypothesis, it can be further evaluated in DMSS. DMSS data can also be used to generate hypotheses (as in its quarterly screening reports); these then need to be evaluated in more detail within DMSS, including more detailed data analyses and efforts that might involve review

EXECUTIVE SUMMARY

of medical records, for example. Formal testing of these hypotheses would require additional studies, however, in separate data sets.

Finding: DMSS is a unique and promising population-based resource for monitoring the emergence of both immediate-onset and later-onset (perhaps up to 5 years) health concerns among military personnel and for testing hypothesized associations between such health concerns and exposures resulting from military service, including vaccines.

Because DMSS is designed to record all medical encounters without depending on the decision of a patient or a physician to report a particular encounter, DMSS data may be cross-checked with the more open-ended but much less complete case reports collected through VAERS.

Recommendation: DoD should develop a capability for the effective use of DMSS to regularly test hypotheses that emerge from VAERS and other sources regarding vaccine-related adverse events.

Finding: DoD personnel have used DMSS to conduct valuable analyses in response to concerns about health effects that might be associated with vaccination with AVA. Yet DoD personnel working with DMSS data are necessarily limited in time and focus. DMSS data could therefore yield valuable insights in the hands of civilian researchers.

Recommendation: DoD should actively support and advance the development of DMSS data resources and the staffing of units that will allow the continuing rapid and careful analysis of these data, including but not limited to the proposed collaboration between CDC and the Army Medical Surveillance Activity.

Recommendation: DoD should investigate mechanisms that can be used to make DMSS data available to civilian researchers, as is done by civilian agencies, with appropriate controls and protections for privacy.

As discussed in Chapter 6, data on the later-onset adverse effects of vaccines are available for few, if any, vaccines. Although the committee found no data indicating that vaccination with AVA is associated with any later-onset adverse events or with any severe or lasting adverse events, some service members have had serious concerns about possible links between AVA and such adverse events. To make it possible to conduct studies of later-onset health concerns, DoD could take steps to improve access to data on the chronic or later-onset effects, if any, of vaccines in general.

Recommendation: DoD should carefully evaluate options for longer-term follow-up of the possible health effects of vaccination against anthrax (and other service-related exposures). The committee recommends consideration of the following specific steps:

- Encourage participation in the Millennium Cohort Study[4] as part of a program to ensure adequate monitoring for any possible later-onset health effects that might be associated with vaccination with AVA or other service-related exposures.
- Collaborate with the Department of Veterans Affairs (VA) to monitor service members who receive medical care through VA facilities after separation from military service. Linking of data from DMSS to data from VA is a possible tool. Even though those who receive their medical care through VA may be an unrepresentative minority of all former military personnel, valid comparisons may be possible between those within that population who received a vaccine or other exposure and those who did not.
- Collaborate with VA to obtain fact-of-death information from the Beneficiary and Records Locator System and with the Social Security Administration to obtain death files. Data on the cause of death should be obtained from the National Death Index as needed.
- Ensure the long-term maintenance of DMSS and other relevant paper and electronic records so that retrospective studies will be feasible if health concerns are identified in the future.

New Anthrax Vaccine Development

Although AVA appears to be sufficiently safe and effective for use, it is far from optimal.

Finding: The current anthrax vaccine is difficult to standardize, is incompletely characterized, and is relatively reactogenic (probably even more so because it is administered subcutaneously), and the dose schedule is long and challenging. An anthrax vaccine free of these drawbacks is needed, and such improvements are feasible.

Initially, the committee urges that improvements to the currently licensed vaccine, AVA, be made as quickly as possible. The committee welcomes anticipated improvements in the assurance of lot-to-lot consis-

---

[4]The Millennium Cohort Study is a survey recommended by the U.S. Congress and sponsored by DoD. The study will monitor a total of 140,000 U.S. military personnel during and after their military service for up to 21 years to evaluate the health risks of military deployment, military occupations, and general military service (see http://www.millenniumcohort.org/about.html).

tency in the postrenovation vaccine. The committee also believes that it is likely that the rates of adverse events and the general acceptability of AVA will improve with a change in the route of administration (from the subcutaneous to the intramuscular route) and with a reduction in the total number of injections required and that such improvements would be desirable. Research to assess the effects of those changes in vaccine administration was under way as this report was being written.

The committee concluded, however, that a new vaccine, developed according to more modern principles of vaccinology, is urgently needed. The committee did not comment on any particular new vaccine development program, and a review of research related to the development of a new vaccine was beyond its charge. The committee recognizes that research on new vaccines against anthrax is under way at DoD, the National Institutes of Health, and various university laboratories and strongly encourages continued and further support of work on promising new vaccines. Further research with AVA on topics such as correlates of immunity in animals, the components necessary to stimulate protective immunity, and the best way to administer the vaccine should aid in the development of new and improved vaccine products for protection against anthrax.

> Recommendation: DoD should continue and further expedite its research efforts pertaining to anthrax disease, the *B. anthracis* organism, and vaccines against anthrax. Research related to anthrax should include, in particular, efforts such as the following:
>
> • DoD should pursue and encourage research to develop an anthrax vaccine product that can be produced more consistently and that is less reactogenic than AVA;
> • DoD should pursue and encourage research regarding the *B. anthracis* capsule;
> • DoD should pursue and encourage research on the mechanisms of action of the anthrax toxins; such research could lead to the development of small-molecule inhibitors;
> • DoD should pursue and encourage research to map the epitopes of the protective antigen that correlate with specific functional activities;
> • DoD should pursue and encourage research to test the therapeutic potential of antitoxin proteins or antibodies; and
> • DoD should pursue and encourage research into additional potential virulence factors in *B. anthracis,* and into other possible vaccine candidates.

BOX ES-1
Chapter 3 Findings and Recommendations

Findings

- The randomized field study carried out by Brachman and colleagues (1962) provides solid evidence indicating the efficacy of a vaccine similar to AVA against *B. anthracis* infection. The subsequent CDC data are supportive. However, the small number of inhalational cases in those studies provides insufficient information to allow a conclusion about the vaccine's efficacy against inhalational infection to be made.
- Because additional clinical trials to test the efficacy of AVA in humans are not feasible and challenge trials with volunteers are unethical, by necessity animal models represent the only sources of the supplementary data needed to evaluate AVA's efficacy.
- The macaque and the rabbit are adequate animal models for evaluation of the efficacy of AVA for the prevention of inhalational anthrax.
- It is unlikely that either naturally occurring or anthrax strains with bioengineered protective antigen could both evade AVA and cause the toxicity associated with anthrax.
- The available data indicate that immunity to anthrax is associated with the presence of antibody to protective antigen.
- The committee finds that the available evidence from studies with humans and animals, coupled with reasonable assumptions of analogy, shows that AVA as licensed is an effective vaccine for the protection of humans against anthrax, including inhalational anthrax, caused by any known or plausible engineered strains of *B. anthracis* .

Recommendations

- Additional passive protection studies with rabbits and monkeys, including the transfer of animal and human sera, are urgently needed to quantify the protective levels of antibody in vivo against different challenge doses of anthrax spores.
- Additional active protection studies should be conducted or supported to develop data that describe the relationship between immunity and both specific and functional quantitative antibody levels, including studies of
    - the relationship between the vaccine dose and the resulting level of antibody in the blood of test animals that protects the animals from challenge;
    - the relationship between the level of antibody that protects animals from challenge and the level of antibody present in humans vaccinated by the regimen currently recommended for the licensed product; and
    - the vaccine dose that results in a level of antibody in the blood of human volunteers similar to that in the blood of protected animals.
- The Department of Defense should support efforts to standardize an assay for quantitation of antibody levels that can be used across laboratories carrying out research on anthrax vaccines.
- The Department of Defense should pursue or support additional research with laboratory animals on the efficacy of AVA in combination with antibiotics administered following inhalational exposure to anthrax spores. Studies should focus on establishment of an appropriate duration for antibiotic prophylaxis after vaccine administration.

> **BOX ES-2**
> **Chapter 5 Findings and Recommendations**
>
> **Findings**
>
> - The presence or absence of VAERS reports (or other case reports) cannot be considered in and of itself to provide adequate evidence of causal associations or its absence. Reports may suggest hypotheses for further investigation, but it must be borne in mind that many different factors beyond the presence of health symptoms can influence whether a report is filed.
> - Concerns of service members that reporting to VAERS is sometimes discouraged within the military setting have been responded to appropriately with reminders to physicians that DoD policy requires submission of a VAERS report for postvaccination health events that result in hospitalization or the loss of time from duty of more than 24 hours. Additional steps, however, are possible to facilitate reporting to VAERS, including improvements in the coding of health care visits that are potentially vaccine related.
> - The committee has reviewed the case materials and the methods applied by VAERS and AVEC to evaluate those materials and concurs with their conclusions that those materials present no signals of previously undescribed serious adverse reactions associated with exposure to AVA.
>
> **Recommendations**
>
> - DoD should develop and implement a system to automate the generation of VAERS reports within the military health care system, using codes to identify from automated records those health care visits that are potentially vaccine related. Use of these codes should generate an automatic filing of a VAERS report that includes the specific diagnoses for the clinical event(s) that prompted the health care visit. However, the submission of reports to VAERS should not be restricted to visits assigned codes that identify them as potentially vaccine related.

> **BOX ES-3**
> **Chapter 6 Findings and Recommendations**
>
> **Findings**
>
> - DMSS data are screened quarterly to identify statistically significant elevations in hospitalization and outpatient visit rate ratios associated with receipt of AVA. In this way, DMSS promises to be very useful as a tool for hypothesis generation.
> - The elevated rates of specific diagnoses in the various analyses of DMSS data are not unexpected per se; that is, they appear to be explicable by chance alone. The bias of selection of healthy individuals for receipt of AVA is also a likely explanation for some observed associations. Thus these elevated rate ratios should not be automatically viewed as an indication of a causal association with the receipt of AVA. However, additional follow-up is needed.
> - Examination of data from the DMSS database to investigate potential signals suggested by VAERS reports related to vaccination with AVA has not detected elevated risks for any of these signals for the vaccinated population, although continued monitoring is warranted.
> - The data available from VAERS, DMSS, and epidemiologic studies indicate the following regarding immediate-onset health events following receipt of AVA:
>   - Local events, especially redness, swelling, or nodules at the injection site, are associated with receipt of AVA, are similar to the events observed following receipt of other vaccines currently in use by adults, and are fairly common.
>   - Systemic events, such as fever, malaise, and myalgia, are associated with receipt of AVA, are similar to the events observed following receipt of other vaccines currently in use by adults, but are much less common than local events.
>   - Immediate-onset health effects can be severe enough in some individuals to result in brief functional impairment, but these effects are self-limited and result in no permanent health impairments.
>   - There is no evidence that life-threatening or permanently disabling immediate-onset adverse events occur at higher rates in individuals who have received AVA than in the general population.
>   - The available data from both active and passive surveillance indicate that there are sex differences in local reactions following vaccination with AVA, as there are following the administration of other vaccines. For female service members, reactions following vaccination with AVA can have a transient adverse impact on their ability to perform their duties. The factors that account for these sex differences are not known.
>   - The currently licensed subcutaneous route of administration of AVA and the six-dose vaccination schedule appear to be associated with a higher incidence of immediate-onset, local effects than is intramuscular administration or a vaccination schedule with fewer doses of AVA. The frequencies of immediate-onset, systemic events were low and were not affected by the route of administration.
> - The available data are limited but show no convincing evidence at this time that personnel who have received AVA have elevated risks of later-onset health events.

Recommendations

- AMSA staff should follow up the currently unexplained elevations in hospitalization rate ratios for certain diagnostic categories among the cohorts of AVA recipients. Studies might include additional analyses with the database or examination of medical records to validate and better understand the exposures and outcomes in question. A protocol should be developed to ensure that such follow-up regularly and reliably occurs after a potential signal is generated.
- Future monitoring and study of health events following vaccination(s) with AVA (and other vaccines) should continue to include separate analyses of data for men and women.
- DoD should continue to support the efforts of CDC to study the reactogenicity and immunogenicity of an alternative route of AVA administration and of a reduced number of vaccine doses.
- DoD should develop systems to enhance the capacity to monitor the occurrence of later-onset health conditions that might be associated with the receipt of any vaccine; the data reviewed by the committee do not suggest the need for special efforts of this sort for AVA.

BOX ES-4
Chapter 7 Findings

- FDA's process of plant inspection and FDA's validation of the vaccine manufacturing process have changed and have become more stringent with time.
- With high-priority efforts by the manufacturer and FDA, the manufacturing process for AVA has been validated so that vaccine manufactured postrenovation has been approved for release and distribution.
- AVA will now be produced by a newly validated manufacturing process under strict controls, according to current FDA requirements. As a result the postrenovation product has greater assurance of consistency than that produced at the time of original licensure.

BOX ES-5
Chapter 8 Findings

- Current events in both the military and the civilian arenas highlight and confirm the importance of ensuring both the availability and the quality of the nation's anthrax vaccine.
- The AVA product produced in a renovated facility by a newly validated manufacturing process could differ from the prerenovation product in terms of its reactogenicity, immunogenicity, and stability. The information available to the committee suggests that AVA lots manufactured postrenovation may show less variation in reactogenicity because of greater consistency in the production process, and there is no a priori basis to believe that the postrenovation product will be more reactogenic or less immunogenic than the older vaccine.
- Given the concerns raised by some service members about the safety of the anthrax vaccine, the creation of AVEC was an appropriate complement to other resources in FDA, the Centers for Disease Control and Prevention (CDC), and DoD for the monitoring of vaccine safety concerns. The results of the extra monitoring did not indicate the existence of any sentinel events that were not detected in the existing FDA and CDC reviews. The committee finds no scientific reason for the continued operation of AVEC in its present form.
- The possibility of detecting a signal in VAERS will be even more limited for AVA than for many other vaccines, given the relatively small population (primarily military personnel) exposed to the vaccine and the low rates at which the hypothesized health effects of greatest concern might be expected to occur in that population.
- VAERS is a critically important source of signals, that is, hypotheses about potential associations between a vaccine and a health event, but these hypotheses must be tested through other means. DMSS gives DoD a unique resource with which to conduct such testing.
- DMSS is a unique and promising population-based resource for monitoring the emergence of both immediate-onset and later-onset (perhaps up to 5 years) health concerns among military personnel and for testing hypothesized associations between such health concerns and exposures resulting from military service, including vaccines.
- DoD personnel have used DMSS to conduct valuable analyses in response to concerns about health effects that might be associated with vaccination with AVA. Yet DoD personnel working with DMSS data are necessarily limited in time and focus. DMSS data could therefore yield valuable insights in the hands of civilian researchers.
- DMSS cannot be used to study mild adverse events, even if they are common.
- Because DMSS captures health care data only for military personnel on active duty, it cannot be used to study the later-onset effects of vaccines over periods of time beyond the normal length of active military service.
- The current anthrax vaccine is difficult to standardize, is incompletely characterized, and is relatively reactogenic (probably even more so because it is administered subcutaneously), and the dose schedule is long and challenging. An anthrax vaccine free of these drawbacks is needed, and such improvements are feasible.

> **BOX ES-6**
> **Chapter 8 Recommendations**
>
> - As with all vaccines, AVA lots produced postrenovation should continue to be monitored for immunogenicity and stability, and individuals receiving these lots should be monitored for possible acute or chronic events of immediate or later onset.
> - DoD should disband AVEC in its current form and instead assist FDA and CDC in establishing an independent advisory committee charged with overseeing the entire process of evaluating vaccine safety. The proposed advisory committee can also assist on an ad hoc basis in the interpretation of potential signals detected in VAERS or other sources regarding the safety of any vaccine. The newly established FDA drug safety committee might be an appropriate model.
> - If DoD chooses to continue AVEC, DoD should consider redefining the panel's role so that it serves as an independent advisory committee that responds on an ad hoc basis to specific requests to assist in the interpretation of potential signals detected by others (e.g., CDC and FDA) and reported to VAERS or other sources regarding the safety of all vaccines administered to service personnel rather than continuing the panel's current role of rereviewing each VAERS report related to AVA.
> - DoD should develop a capability for the effective use of DMSS to regularly test hypotheses that emerge from VAERS and other sources regarding vaccine-related adverse events.
> - DoD should actively support and advance the development of DMSS data resources and the staffing of units that will allow the continuing rapid and careful analysis of these data, including but not limited to the proposed collaboration between CDC and the Army Medical Surveillance Activity.
> - DoD should investigate mechanisms that can be used to make DMSS data available to civilian researchers, as is done by civilian agencies, with appropriate controls and protections for privacy.
> - DoD should develop ad hoc prospective cohort studies in one or more military settings to test hypotheses that emerge from VAERS, DMSS, or other sources. However, the committee does not recommend that such studies targeted at AVA be conducted at present since no convincing evidence of new adverse events in AVA recipients sufficient to merit a prospective investigation has been presented. Rather, further studies of the effects of AVA should be performed in the context of studies of the effects of all vaccines administered to members of the military.
> - DoD should carefully evaluate options for longer-term follow-up of the possible health effects of vaccination against anthrax (and other service-related exposures). The committee recommends consideration of the following specific steps:
>   - Encourage participation in the Millennium Cohort Study as part of a program to ensure adequate monitoring for any possible later-onset health effects that might be associated with vaccination with AVA or other service-related exposures.
>   - Collaborate with the Department of Veterans Affairs (VA) to monitor service members who receive medical care through VA facilities after separation from military service. Linking of data from DMSS to data from VA is a possible tool. Even though those who receive their medical care through VA may be an unrepresentative minority of all former military personnel, valid comparisons may be pos-

> **BOX ES-6 Continued**
>
> sible between those within that population who received a vaccine or other exposure and those who did not.
> - Collaborate with VA to obtain fact-of-death information from the Beneficiary Identification and Records Locator System and with the Social Security Administration to obtain death files. Data on the cause of death should be obtained from the National Death Index as needed.
> - Ensure the long-term maintenance of DMSS and other relevant paper and electronic records so that retrospective studies will be feasible if health concerns are identified in the future.
> - DoD should continue and further expedite its research efforts pertaining to anthrax disease, the *B. anthracis* organism, and vaccines against anthrax. Research related to anthrax should include, in particular, efforts such as the following:
> - DoD should pursue and encourage research to develop an anthrax vaccine product that can be produced more consistently and that is less reactogenic than AVA;
> - DoD should pursue and encourage research regarding the *B. anthracis* capsule;
> - DoD should pursue and encourage research on the mechanisms of action of the anthrax toxins; such research could lead to the development of small-molecule inhibitors;
> - DoD should pursue and encourage research to map the epitopes of the protective antigen that correlate with specific functional activities;
> - DoD should pursue and encourage research to test the therapeutic potential of antitoxin proteins or antibodies; and
> - DoD should pursue and encourage research into additional potential virulence factors in *B. anthracis* and into other possible vaccine candidates.

REFERENCES

AMSA (Army Medical Surveillance Activity). 2001a. *Quarterly Report—January 2001. Surveillance of Adverse Effects of Anthrax Vaccine Adsorbed.* Washington, D.C.: Army Medical Surveillance Activity, U.S. Army Center for Health Promotion and Preventive Medicine.

AMSA. 2001b. *Quarterly Report—April 2001. Surveillance of Adverse Effects of Anthrax Vaccine Adsorbed.* Washington, D.C.: Army Medical Surveillance Activity, U.S. Army Center for Health Promotion and Preventive Medicine.

AMSA. 2001c. *Surveillance of Adverse Effects of Anthrax Vaccine Adsorbed: Results of Analyses Requested by the Institute of Medicine Committee to Assess the Safety and Efficacy of the Anthrax Vaccine.* Washington, D.C.: Army Medical Surveillance Activity, U.S. Army Center for Health Promotion and Preventive Medicine.

Auerbach BA, Wright GG. 1955. Studies on immunity in anthrax. VI. Immunizing activity of protective antigen against various strains of *Bacillus anthracis*. *Journal of Immunology* 75:129–133.

Barnard JP, Friedlander AM. 1999. Vaccination against anthrax with attenuated recombinant strains of *Bacillus anthracis* that produce protective antigen. *Infection and Immunity* 67(2):562–567.

Beedham RJ, Turnbull PC, Williamson ED. 2001. Passive transfer of protection against *Bacillus anthracis* infection in a murine model. *Vaccine* 19(31):4409–4416.

Bhatnagar R, Batra S. 2001. Anthrax toxin. *Critical Reviews in Microbiology* 27(3):167–200.

Brachman PS, Friedlander AM. 1999. Anthrax. In: Plotkin SA, Orenstein WA, eds. *Vaccines*, 3rd ed. Philadelphia, Pa.: W. B. Saunders Co. Pp. 629–637.

Brachman PS, Gold H, Plotkin S, Fekety FR, Werrin M, Ingraham NR. 1962. Field evaluation of a human anthrax vaccine. *American Journal of Public Health* 52:632–645.

Cataldi A, Labruyere E, Mock M. 1990. Construction and characterization of a protective antigen-deficient *Bacillus anthracis* strain. *Molecular Microbiology* 4(7):1111–1117.

CDC (Centers for Disease Control and Prevention). 1967–1971. *Application and Report on Manufacture of Anthrax Protective Antigen, Aluminum Hydroxide Adsorbed (DBS-IND 180). Observational Study*. Atlanta, Ga.: Centers for Disease Control and Prevention.

CDC. 2001a. Update: investigation of bioterrorism-related anthrax and adverse events from antimicrobial prophylaxis. *MMWR (Morbidity and Mortality Weekly Report)* 50(44): 973–976.

CDC. 2001b. Update: investigation of bioterrorism-related inhalational anthrax—Connecticut, 2001. *MMWR (Morbidity and Mortality Weekly Report)* 50(47):1049–1051.

Dixon TC, Meselson M, Guillemin J, Hanna PC. 1999. Anthrax. *New England Journal of Medicine* 341(11):815–826.

FDA (Food and Drug Administration). 1985. Biological products: bacterial vaccines and toxoids: implementation of efficacy review. Proposed rule. *Federal Register* 50(240): 51002–51117.

Fellows PF, Linscott MK, Ivins BE, Pitt ML, Rossi CA, Gibbs PH, Friedlander AM. 2001. Efficacy of a human anthrax vaccine in guinea pigs, rabbits, and rhesus macaques against challenge by *Bacillus anthracis* isolates of diverse geographical origin. *Vaccine* 19(23–24):3241–3247.

Grabenstein JD. 2000. The AVIP: status and future. Presentation to the Institute of Medicine Committee to Assess the Safety and Efficacy of the Anthrax Vaccine, Meeting I, Washington, D.C.

Grinberg LM, Abramova FA, Yampolskaya OV, Walker DH, Smith JH. 2001. Quantitative pathology of inhalational anthrax. I. Quantitative microscopic findings. *Modern Pathology* 14(5):482–495.

Henderson DA. 1999. The looming threat of bioterrorism. *Science* 283(5406):1279–1282.

Hoffman K, Costello C, Engler RJM, Grabenstein J. Submitted for publication. Using a patient-centered structured medical note for aggregate analysis: determining the side-effect profile of anthrax vaccine at a mass immunization site.

Ivins BE, Fellows PF, Nelson GO. 1994. Efficacy of a standard human anthrax vaccine against *Bacillus anthracis* spore challenge in guinea pigs. *Vaccine* 12(10):872–874.

Ivins BE, Fellows PF, Pitt MLM, Estep JE, Welkos SL, Worsham PL, Friedlander AM. 1996. Efficacy of a standard human anthrax vaccine against *Bacillus anthracis* aerosol spore challenge in rhesus monkeys. *Salisbury Medical Bulletin* 87(suppl):125–126.

Ivins BE, Pitt ML, Fellows PF, Farchaus JW, Benner GE, Waag DM, Little SF, Anderson GW Jr, Gibbs PH, Friedlander AM. 1998. Comparative efficacy of experimental anthrax vaccine candidates against inhalation anthrax in rhesus macaques. *Vaccine* 16(11–12): 1141–1148.

Jackson PJ. 2001. Genetic diversity in *B. anthracis*. Presentation to the Institute of Medicine Committee to Assess the Safety and Efficacy of the Anthrax Vaccine, Meeting III, Washington, D.C.

Jackson PJ, Hugh-Jones ME, Adair DM, Green G, Hill KK, Kuske CR, Grinberg LM, Abramova FA, Keim P. 1998. PCR analysis of tissue samples from the 1979 Sverdlovsk anthrax victims: the presence of multiple *Bacillus anthracis* strains in different victims. *Proceedings of the National Academy of Sciences USA* 95(3):1224–1229.

Keim P, Kalif A, Schupp J, Hill K, Travis SE, Richmond K, Adair DM, Hugh-Jones M, Kuske CR, Jackson P. 1997. Molecular evolution and diversity in *Bacillus anthracis* as detected by amplified fragment length polymorphism markers. *Journal of Bacteriology* 179(3): 818–824.

Keim P, Price LB, Klevytska AM, Smith KL, Schupp JM, Okinaka R, Jackson PJ, Hugh-Jones ME. 2000. Multiple-locus variable-number tandem repeat analysis reveals genetic relationships within *Bacillus anthracis*. *Journal of Bacteriology* 182(10):2928–2936.

Lange JL, Lesikar SE, Brundage JF, Rubertone MV. 2001a. Screening for adverse events following anthrax immunization using the Defense Medical Surveillance System. Presentation to the Institute of Medicine Committee to Assess the Safety and Efficacy of the Anthrax Vaccine, Meeting II, Washington, D.C.

Lange JL, Lesikar SE, Brundage JF, Rubertone MV. 2001b. Update: surveillance of adverse events of Anthrax Vaccine Adsorbed. Presentation to the Institute of Medicine Committee to Assess the Safety and Efficacy of the Anthrax Vaccine, Meeting IV, Washington, D.C.

Little SF, Knudson GB. 1986. Comparative efficacy of *Bacillus anthracis* live spore vaccine and protective antigen vaccine against anthrax in the guinea pig. *Infection and Immunity* 52(2):509–512.

Little SF, Ivins BE, Fellows PF, Friedlander AM. 1997. Passive protection by polyclonal antibodies against *Bacillus anthracis* infection in guinea pigs. *Infection and Immunity* 65(12):5171–5175.

Mason KT, Grabenstein JD, McCracken LR. 2001. Hearing loss after anthrax vaccination among US Army aircrew members. Unpublished manuscript.

Mason KT, Grabenstein JD, McCracken LR. Submitted for publication. US Army Aviation Epidemiology Data Register: physical findings after anthrax vaccination among US Army aircrew members, a prospective matched-pair, case-control study.

McBride BW, Mogg A, Telfer JL, Lever MS, Miller J, Turnbull PC, Baillie L. 1998. Protective efficacy of a recombinant protective antigen against *Bacillus anthracis* challenge and assessment of immunological markers. *Vaccine* 16(8):810–817.

Mogridge J, Mourez M, Lacy B, Collier RJ. 2001. Role of protective antigen oligomerization in anthrax toxin action. In: *Program and Abstracts of the Fourth Annual Conference on Anthrax*. Washington, D.C.: American Society for Microbiology.

Peeler RN, Cluff LE, Trever RW. 1958. Hyper-immunization of man. *Bulletin of the Johns Hopkins Hospital* 103:183–198.

Peeler RN, Kadull PJ, Cluff LE. 1965. Intensive immunization of man: evaluation of possible adverse consequences. *Annals of Internal Medicine* 63(1):44–57.

Pitt ML, Little SF, Ivins BE, Fellows P, Barth J, Hewetson J, Gibbs P, Dertzbaugh M, Friedlander AM. 2001. In vitro correlate of immunity in a rabbit model of inhalational anthrax. *Vaccine* 19(32):4768–4773.

Pittman PR. 2001a. Anthrax vaccine: an analysis of short-term adverse events in an occupational setting—the Special Immunization Program experience over 30 years. Presentation to the Institute of Medicine Committee to Assess the Safety and Efficacy of the Anthrax Vaccine, Meeting II, Washington, D.C.

Pittman PR. 2001b. Anthrax vaccine: dose reduction/route change pilot study. Presentation to the Institute of Medicine Committee to Assess the Safety and Efficacy of the Anthrax Vaccine, Meeting II, Washington, D.C.

Pittman PR. 2001c. Anthrax vaccine: the Fort Bragg Booster Study. Presentation to the Institute of Medicine Committee to Assess the Safety and Efficacy of the Anthrax Vaccine, Meeting II, Washington, D.C.

Pittman PR, Sjogren MH, Hack D, Franz D, Makuch RS, Arthur JS. 1997. *Serologic Response to Anthrax and Botulinum Vaccines.* Protocol No. FY92-5, M109, Log No. A-5747. Final report to the Food and Drug Administration. Fort Detrick, Md.: U.S. Army Medical Research Institute of Infectious Diseases.

Pittman PR, Gibbs PH, Cannon TL, Friedlander AM. 2001a. Anthrax vaccine: short-term safety experience in humans. Manuscript.

Pittman PR, Gibbs PH, Cannon TL, Friedlander AM. 2001b. Anthrax vaccine: short-term safety experience in humans. *Vaccine* 20(5–6):972–978.

Pittman PR, Kim-Ahn G, Pifat DY, Coon K, Gibbs P, Little S, Pace-Templeton J, Myers R, Parker GW, Friedlander AM. 2002. Anthrax vaccine: safety and immunogenicity of a dose-reduction, route comparison study in humans. *Vaccine* 20(9–10):1412–1420.

Pittman PR, Hack D, Mangiafico J, Gibbs P, McKee KT Jr., Friedlander AM, Sjogren MH. In press. Antibody response to a delayed booster dose of anthrax vaccine and botulinum toxoid. *Vaccine.*

Price LB, Hugh-Jones M, Jackson PJ, Keim P. 1999. Genetic diversity in the protective antigen gene of *Bacillus anthracis. Journal of Bacteriology* 181(8):2358–2362.

Rehme P. 2001. Ambulatory medical visits among anthrax-vaccinated and unvaccinated personnel after return from Southwest Asia. Presentation to the Institute of Medicine Committee to Assess the Safety and Efficacy of the Anthrax Vaccine, Meeting IV, Washington, D.C.

Rehme PA, Williams R, Grabenstein JD. 2002. Ambulatory medical visits among anthrax-vaccinated and unvaccinated personnel after return from Southwest Asia. *Military Medicine* 167(3):205–210.

Reuveny S, White MD, Adar YY, Kafri Y, Altboum Z, Gozes Y, Kobiler D, Shafferman A, Velan B. 2001. Search for correlates of protective immunity conferred by anthrax vaccine. *Infection and Immunity* 69(5):2888–2893.

Sato PA. 2001a. DoD-wide surveillance of hospitalizations for long-term adverse events potentially associated with anthrax immunization. Presentation to the Institute of Medicine Committee to Assess the Safety and Efficacy of the Anthrax Vaccine, Meeting IV, Washington, D.C.

Sato PA. 2001b. Questions on updated data. E-mail to Joellenbeck L, Institute of Medicine, Washington, D.C., November 21.

Sato PA, Reed RJ, Smith TC, Wang LZ. 2001. *DoD-wide medical surveillance for potential long-term adverse events associated with anthrax immunization: hospitalizations. Provisional report for IOM of data from January 1998 to March 2000.* San Diego, Calif.: U.S. Department of Defense Center for Deployment Health Research at the Naval Health Research Center.

Sellman BR, Mourez M, Collier RJ. 2001. Dominant-negative mutants of a toxin subunit: an approach to therapy of anthrax. *Science* 292(5517):695–697.

Smith H, Keppie J. 1954. Observations on experimental anthrax: demonstration of a specific lethal factor produced in vivo by *Bacillus anthracis. Nature* 173:869–870.

Treanor JJ. 2001. Adverse reactions following vaccination of adults. Commissioned paper. Committee to Assess the Safety and Efficacy of the Anthrax Vaccine, Institute of Medicine, Washington, D.C.

Turnbull PC, Broster MG, Carman JA, Manchee RJ, Melling J. 1986. Development of antibodies to protective antigen and lethal factor components of anthrax toxin in humans and guinea pigs and their relevance to protective immunity. *Infection and Immunity* 52(2):356–363.

Wasserman GM. 2001. Analysis of adverse events after anthrax vaccination in U.S. Army medical personnel. Presentation to the Institute of Medicine Committee to Assess the Safety and Efficacy of the Anthrax Vaccine, Meeting IV, Washington, D.C.

Weiss R. 2001, September 29. Demand growing for anthrax vaccine: fear of bioterrorism attack spurs requests for controversial shot. *Washington Post.* p. A16.

White CS, Adler WH, McGann VG. 1974. Repeated immunization: possible adverse effects. *Annals of Internal Medicine* 81(5):594–600.

Zilinskas RA. 1997. Iraq's biological weapons: the past as future? *JAMA* 278(5):418–424.

1

Introduction

In the autumn of 2001, following the terrorist attacks of September 11, anthrax and the anthrax vaccine became prominent national concerns. The deliberate distribution of anthrax spores through the U.S. mail resulted in 5 deaths from inhalational anthrax, 6 additional cases of inhalational anthrax that were successfully treated, 12 cutaneous anthrax infections (confirmed and suspected; CDC, 2001), and the treatment of thousands of others with known or suspected exposure to anthrax spores. Previously, concerns about anthrax had focused on its possible use as a biological weapon in a military context.

During the 1991 Gulf War, concerns that Iraq had prepared anthrax spores for use as a biological weapon motivated the U.S. military to administer the licensed anthrax vaccine to an estimated 150,000 service members. After the war, admission by Iraq that it had indeed produced weapons containing anthrax spores confirmed fears of the potential use of anthrax as a biological weapon (Henderson, 1999; Zilinskas, 1997). As a response to this threat, in December 1997 Secretary of Defense William Cohen announced a plan to vaccinate all U.S. service members for anthrax using the licensed anthrax vaccine. The universal vaccination plan was to be phased in gradually, starting with service members judged most likely to encounter the threat. Service members scheduled for deployment to areas considered to be "high risk" began to receive vaccinations through the Department of Defense's (DoD's) Anthrax Vaccine Immunization Program starting in March 1998. As more service members received the mandatory vaccines, however, some raised concerns about the safety and the efficacy of the vaccine being administered.

Responding to those concerns, the U.S. Congress included language in the conference report accompanying the 2000 DoD appropriations legislation directing DoD to enter into a contract with the National Research Council to study the effectiveness and safety of the anthrax vaccine.[1] Congress called for the study to examine the safety and efficacy of the licensed vaccine, including consideration of the types and severities of adverse reactions, differences in reactions by sex, long-term health implications, its efficacy against inhalational exposure to all known anthrax strains, and correlation of the safety and efficacy of the vaccine in animal models to its safety and efficacy in humans. The study was also to address the issue of the validation of the manufacturing process, with consideration of discrepancies identified by the Food and Drug Administration in February 1998, definition of vaccine components, and identification of gaps in existing research. (See Appendix A for the Statement of Task.)

In June 2000 a contract between DoD and the Institute of Medicine (IOM) was finalized to carry out the study requested by Congress. IOM convened the Committee to Assess the Safety and Efficacy of the Anthrax Vaccine, and this report reflects the work of that committee.

STUDY PROCESS AND INFORMATION SOURCES

Reflecting the components of the statement of task, the members of the Committee to Assess the Safety and Efficacy of the Anthrax Vaccine brought expertise in microbiology; vaccine research, development, manufacture, and evaluation; postmarketing surveillance of adverse events; regulatory and licensing procedures; epidemiology; biostatistics; immunology; and health surveillance (see Appendix B for biographical sketches of the committee members). The committee's charge did not include evaluation of the DoD policy to vaccinate all service members, so the committee did not include an evaluation of the threat from biological warfare agents in its purview. Similarly, the committee was not asked to address the challenges in bioweapons vaccine development and procurement generally, which have recently been discussed in a statement from the Council of the Institute of Medicine (http://www.iom.edu/IOM/IOMHome.nsf/Pages/Vaccine+ Development) and in reports by the Gilmore Commission (http://www.rand.org/nsrd/terrpanel/) and DoD (http://www.defenselink.mil/pubs/Reporton BiologicalWarfareDefenseVaccineRDPrgras-July2001.pdf).

---

[1]Making Appropriations for the Department of Defense for the Fiscal Year Ending September 30, 2000, and for Other Purposes, P. L. No. 106-79 (1999).

INTRODUCTION 35

Since the terrorist attacks of September 11, 2001, and subsequent mail distribution of anthrax spores, interest in AVA has greatly increased. Consideration of the full range of topics concerning civilian use of the anthrax vaccine was beyond the purview of this report. However, some of the issues that the committee did address should also be of interest for civilians.

The committee gathered information for the study through several means. The committee held a total of four public workshops to collect relevant information; the dates and locations of these meetings are provided in Appendix C. At these meetings, researchers presented the committee with data gathered in studies of the safety of the vaccine. In addition, the committee heard from service members and others with concerns about the safety and efficacy of the vaccine, as well as additional information about the manufacture of the vaccine and the disease itself. The committee also commissioned a paper to review the available literature regarding the rates of adverse events associated with several vaccines routinely administered to adults. Information on the anthrax vaccine was obtained from DoD, the Food and Drug Administration, and BioPort, the current manufacturer. In addition to its four public workshops, the committee met in two additional meetings and two conference calls.

The committee sought access to all possible data, not just published data. Only a few studies on the safety of the anthrax vaccine had been published by the time the committee preparing this report began its work in October 2000. However, several studies had been conducted by DoD investigators, who were urged by IOM and DoD to publish their work. Over the course of this study, investigators made available to the committee several manuscripts submitted or planned for submission for publication. The investigators involved in many of the studies, published or unpublished, also attended open committee meetings to present their data and discuss their findings with the committee. In addition, several analyses of existing data were carried out at the committee's request, and these provided some of the most compelling information supporting the committee's findings on safety.

RELATED REPORTS

IOM Letter Report on Anthrax Vaccine

The conference report mandating the current study required that a preliminary report be submitted to Congress by April 1, 2000. At the time of the legislation, the IOM Committee on Health Effects Associated with Exposures During the Gulf War was active in its work to evaluate the published scientific literature concerning the agents to which Gulf War veterans may have been exposed. Since the anthrax vaccine was among these exposures, the committee had already reviewed the available database regarding the safety, but not the efficacy, of the vaccine. To be responsive to Congress and DoD, that committee issued a letter report on March 30, 2000 (see Appendix H).

The letter report summarized the IOM committee's review of the literature on the safety of the anthrax vaccine. After a review of only primary peer-reviewed literature, the committee concluded that there was inadequate or insufficient evidence to determine whether an association does or does not exist between vaccination against anthrax and long-term adverse health outcomes. The committee noted the large body of results that had not yet been published and strongly urged investigators conducting relevant studies to submit their results to peer-reviewed scientific journals for publication.

The same committee released the first volume of its full report in September 2000 (IOM, 2000). In its chapter on vaccines, the Committee on Health Effects Associated with Exposures During the Gulf War provided a review of the published studies available. In addition to the conclusion about long-term health outcomes noted above, the committee concluded that "there is sufficient evidence of an association between anthrax vaccination and transient acute local and systemic effects (e.g., redness, swelling, fever) typically associated with vaccination" (IOM, 2000, p. 16). Again, that committee urged publication of additional studies in peer-reviewed scientific journals.

IOM Committee to Review the CDC Anthrax Vaccine Safety and Efficacy Research Program

In the 2000 Department of Health and Human Services appropriations legislation, Congress provided funding to the Centers for Disease Control and Prevention (CDC) for an effort to study the safety and efficacy of vaccines used against biological agents. The mandate was to (1) address risk factors for adverse events, (2) determine immunological correlates of protection and document vaccine efficacy, and (3) determine the optimal vaccination schedule and routes of administration.[2] CDC contracted with IOM to establish an expert panel to review the completeness and appropriateness of the CDC plan for responding to the congressional mandate. The IOM Committee to Review the CDC Anthrax Vaccine Safety and Efficacy Research Program began its work in October 2000. The committee's interim report, which provided preliminary findings and recommendations about the CDC research plans, was released to the public on July 2, 2001

---

[2]An Act Making Consolidated Appropriations for the Fiscal Year Ending September 30, 2000, and for Other Purposes, P. L. No. 106-113 (1999).

(IOM, 2001). Four members of the committee also serve on the IOM Committee to Evaluate the Safety and Efficacy of the Anthrax Vaccine, which carried out the study described in this report.

ACIP Recommendations

In December 2000 a report regarding recommendations for use of the anthrax vaccine was released by the Advisory Committee on Immunization Practices (ACIP) (CDC, 2000). This committee consists of 15 experts selected to provide advice to the Secretary of Health and Human Services and CDC regarding the routine use of vaccines (http://www.cdc.gov/nip/ACIP/). In *Use of Anthrax Vaccine in the United States*, ACIP reviewed safety and efficacy data and recommended routine vaccination with Anthrax Vaccine Adsorbed (AVA) for those working with large quantities or concentrations of *Bacillus anthracis* and those conducting activities with a high potential for *B. anthracis* aerosol production (CDC, 2000). ACIP did not recommend preexposure vaccination for emergency first responders, federal responders, medical practitioners, or private citizens for bioterrorism preparedness because "the target population for bioterrorist release of *B. anthracis* cannot be predetermined, and the risk of exposure cannot be calculated. . . . For the military and other select populations or for groups for which a calculable risk can be assessed, pre-exposure vaccination may be indicated" (CDC, 2000, p. 12).

Since the release of that report, the intentional mailing of anthrax spores in letters in October 2001 and the subsequent illnesses and deaths from anthrax have heightened interest in the use of AVA for a wider population. At the time of this writing, however, ACIP had not altered its recommendations regarding the populations for whom vaccination would be indicated.

GENERAL PRINCIPLES REGARDING USE OF VACCINES

Like all medical interventions, vaccines should be used only when the potential benefits from the intervention warrant the risks of adverse effects. Vaccines, however, differ from drugs used for treatment, and in the case of a vaccine against anthrax, some additional special considerations affect the trade-off.

First, vaccines share with other preventive interventions the burden of being used prophylactically for otherwise healthy individuals. Their use is intended for prevention rather than treatment. As such, they are given to healthy individuals, so it is less tolerable if they cause adverse effects in the course of promoting overall health. The burden of proof for the safety of vaccines is therefore even higher than the burden of proof for the safety of other medical interventions. This makes it even more important that their risk-benefit balance be as favorable as possible.

Second, one must consider very carefully the appropriate target group that should receive the vaccine. For some vaccines, the target group is the entire population. Often, that is because of the phenomenon of "herd immunity"; that is, for diseases that can be transmitted from person to person (e.g., poliomyelitis), it benefits the entire population to have others protected from the disease, as it reduces the risk to the population as well as to the individual. For other vaccines (e.g., tetanus toxoid), the illness cannot be passed from person to person, but the vaccine is nevertheless recommended for use by everyone since everyone is at sufficiently high risk of the disease. For still other vaccines, there are clearly identifiable target groups at higher risk; for example, typhoid vaccine is recommended for use by travelers to developing countries.

In the case of a vaccine against anthrax, the situation is even more complex. The illness cannot be transmitted from person to person. Therefore, there is no possibility of herd immunity, nor is there a reason to vaccinate the entire population. Thus, the vaccine should be targeted to those at higher risk of disease. In light of recent events, however, that target population has become very fluid, whereas formerly it was definable. Historically, the licensed vaccine was recommended only for those at risk for occupational exposure to anthrax bacteria or spores. However, in recent years the risk of biological warfare led to a judgment that military personnel were at occupational risk of exposure and should receive the anthrax vaccine. Recent bioterrorist use of anthrax spores in the U.S. mail system has indicated that some civilian populations might even be considered at sufficient risk to warrant their use of an anthrax vaccine, if one were available, sufficiently safe, and sufficiently effective.

As noted earlier, this report does not address the military policy to vaccinate all service members, nor does it consider which other populations should be considered for vaccination. These questions were not part of the charge to the committee, nor is biological warfare or bioterrorist risk assessment part of its expertise. Rather, the report focuses on the efficacy and safety of the current licensed vaccine and provides information for those who must establish vaccination policy.

ORGANIZATION OF THE REPORT

The varied components of the committee's statement of task (see Appendix A) fall into broad categories of efficacy, safety, manufacturing, and future needs. This report is organized into these categories as well. Chapter 2 provides background material about the disease known as anthrax, the licensed anthrax vaccine, and the data available for evaluation of its safety and efficacy. Information relevant to assessing the efficacy of the vaccine is presented in Chapter 3. The establishment of efficacy is crucial before one can consider the use of any such intervention, and no safety risk is tolerable in the absence of efficacy. Chapter 4 introduces the types of information available concerning the assessment of vaccine safety, whereas Chapters 5 and 6 review the safety data available on this vaccine from case reports and from epidemiologic studies, respectively. Issues related to manufacturing are reviewed in Chapter 7, and in Chapter 8 the committee discusses needs for future efforts, including gaps in research.

REFERENCES

CDC (Centers for Disease Control and Prevention). 2000. Use of anthrax vaccine in the United States: recommendations of the Advisory Committee on Immunization Practices (ACIP). *MMWR (Morbidity and Mortality Weekly Report)* 49(RR-15):1–20.

CDC. 2001. Update: investigation of bioterrorism-related inhalational anthrax—Connecticut, 2001. *MMWR (Morbidity and Mortality Weekly Report)* 50(47):1049–1051.

Henderson DA. 1999. The looming threat of bioterrorism. *Science* 283(5406):1279–1282.

IOM (Institute of Medicine). 2000. *Gulf War and Health.* Washington, D.C.: National Academy Press.

IOM. 2001. *CDC Anthrax Vaccine Safety & Efficacy Research Program. Interim Report.* Washington, D.C.: National Academy Press.

Zilinskas RA. 1997. Iraq's biological weapons: the past as future? *JAMA* 278(5):418–424.

2

Background

Anthrax is primarily a disease of animals, and historically, humans have generally contracted the disease through contact with infected animals or contaminated animal products. The disease had become extremely uncommon in any form in the United States until the intentional mailings of anthrax spores caused an outbreak in the autumn of 2001 that resulted in five deaths from the inhalational form of the disease.

Anthrax vaccines for use in animals were first developed in the late 19th century. Work on vaccines suitable for human use gained urgency in the 1940s, with fears that anthrax would be used as a biological warfare agent. The current vaccine, Anthrax Vaccine Adsorbed (AVA), was licensed in 1970 and was recommended for use by a small population of textile mill workers, veterinarians, laboratory scientists, and other workers with occupational risk of exposure to anthrax. In the 1990s, increased concern about the use of biological weapons led the Department of Defense (DoD) to begin vaccination of U.S. military personnel. Some troops were given anthrax vaccine in the 1991 Gulf War, and a large program to vaccinate all service members was begun in 1998. By 2001 a limited vaccine supply, the result of delays in federal approval for release of newly manufactured vaccine lots, had significantly slowed plans to vaccinate all military personnel. After the deliberate distribution of anthrax spores in bioterrorist incidents in the autumn of 2001, the vaccine was offered as part of the treatment for as many as 10,000 of the civilians who had been exposed.

This chapter summarizes the basic pathophysiology of anthrax, reviews the history of anthrax vaccine development, and outlines the concerns that have emerged on the part of some people about the adverse health outcomes that might be associated with use of the vaccine.

THE DISEASE

Anthrax is caused by infection with *Bacillus anthracis*, a gram-positive, nonmotile, spore-forming organism (Brachman and Friedlander, 1999; Dixon et al., 1999). Exposure to the spores of this one organism can cause three different forms of disease—cutaneous, gastrointestinal, or inhalational anthrax—depending on the site of infection. Cutaneous anthrax is the most common and the most treatable form; inhalational anthrax is rare but poses a much greater risk of death.

Epidemiology

Anthrax is found worldwide and is transmitted primarily through spores that are highly resistant to heat, drought, and many disinfectants (Dixon et al., 1999). It is primarily a disease of wild and domestic animals, especially herbivores such as cattle, sheep, and goats. Animals can be infected through exposure to spores in contaminated grazing areas, contaminated feed, or infected carcasses (Friedlander, 2000). Humans in agricultural settings can be infected through contact with infected animals or contaminated animal products. Human infections also occur in industrial settings where contaminated animal products such as wool, hair, hides, or meat are processed. Most human cases in either agricultural or industrial settings are cutaneous. Inhalational anthrax is generally seen only in industrial settings because conditions where a sufficiently large number of spores are aerosolized in an enclosed area do not generally occur naturally (Brachman and Friedlander, 1999). Person-to-person transmission is not known to occur with inhalational anthrax and has rarely been reported with other forms of the disease (Friedlander, 2000).

The worldwide incidence of anthrax in humans is difficult to determine, but the annual number of cases in the 1980s and 1990s is estimated to have been about 2,000, down from an estimated 20,000 to 100,000 cases in 1958 (Brachman and Friedlander, 1999). During the 19th century, "wool-sorters' disease," or inhalational anthrax, was fairly common among workers handling animal hides, hairs, or wools. Approximately 200 cases were reported in the United States before 1900 (Plotkin et al., 1960). Only 18 cases of inhalational anthrax were reported in the United States in the 20th century, despite evidence of extensive exposure of workers in goat hair-processing mills to aerosolized spores (Inglesby et al., 1999). In 1957, five cases of inhalational anthrax, four of them fatal, occurred at a goat hair-processing mill in New Hampshire. Vaccination did not become mandatory for these workers until the 1960s and so cannot account for the low rate of inhalational disease (Inglesby et al., 1999).

Other forms of anthrax are also rare in the United States. Until the bioterrorist events in the autumn of 2001, a total of 238 anthrax cases had been reported since 1955; of those, 95 percent were cutaneous infections (Brachman and Friedlander, 1999; CDC, 2001a). In 2000, one reported case of cutaneous anthrax occurred (CDC, 2001a) and possible cases of gastrointestinal infection were associated with the consumption of contaminated meat (CDC, 2000b).

In the autumn of 2001 the United States experienced an outbreak of anthrax due to bioterrorism. Exposure to letters containing B. *anthracis* spores sent through the U.S. mail resulted in seven confirmed and five suspected cutaneous cases and 11 confirmed inhalational cases (CDC, 2001e). The victims included postal workers (Gallagher and Strober, 2001), employees of print and broadcast media organizations, and at least one infant (Roche et al., 2001).

Anthrax has also been part of biological warfare programs in some countries. In 1979 in Sverdlovsk, Russia, an apparently accidental release of aerosolized spores from a military facility resulted in 68 deaths among 79 individuals with reported cases of inhalational anthrax (Meselson et al., 1994).

Clinical Features

The outbreak of inhalational and cutaneous anthrax in the United States during the autumn of 2001 produced far more clinical and public health experience with the disease than had occurred in many decades. Both the outbreak and the outcomes of individual cases showed considerable differences from previous classic descriptions. The anthrax spores appeared to have been processed intentionally to enhance their most dangerous properties. They were finely milled and rendered nonpolar to maintain the very small particle size necessary for inhalation and to promote prolonged aerosolization. Naturally occurring spores tend to adhere quickly to each other and to surfaces.

Improvements in both the speed of diagnosis and clinical management resulted in the survival of at least some of those who contracted inhalational anthrax, which would not have been expected on the basis of earlier experience (Brown, 2001). Analysis of this new information on the clinical course of disease was continuing as the committee completed this report. In particular, both the inoculum associated with infection in different individuals and the duration of antibiotic treatment necessary for survival after infection remain uncertain. Although every effort was made to include

Cutaneous Anthrax

Cutaneous anthrax results from the introduction of spores through the skin, generally at the site of a minor injury. After an incubation period, typically 2 to 5 days, a small pruritic (itchy) papule appears (Brachman and Friedlander, 1999). In 1 to 2 days, the site develops one or more vesicles filled with clear or serous fluid containing numerous anthrax bacilli. Within a week, the vesicle erodes, leaving a necrotic ulcer with a characteristic black eschar at the center (see Figure 2-1). The lesion then heals in another 2 to 3 weeks. Edema may develop around a lesion and can become extensive in some cases. Other symptoms including malaise, low-grade fever, and swelling of adjacent lymph glands may occur, but anthrax lesions are generally painless unless a secondary infection is present. Without antibiotic treatment, up to 20 percent of cutaneous anthrax infections are fatal, but with treatment the fatality rate is less than 1 percent (CDC, 2000c). A recent case report describes bioterrorist-related cutaneous anthrax in an infant (Freedman et al., 2002).

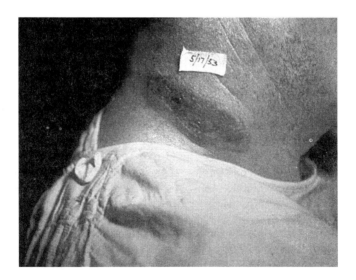

FIGURE 2-1 Cutaneous anthrax lesion.
SOURCE: Public Health Image Library, CDC.

Gastrointestinal Anthrax

Eating meat contaminated with anthrax spores can result in gastrointestinal or oropharyngeal infection. Pathological examinations show ulcerations with edema and mucosal necrosis in the affected area (Dixon et al., 1999). A gastrointestinal infection initially produces nausea, vomiting, and fever, followed by often severe abdominal pain, bloody diarrhea, and ascites. As these symptoms are common to other acute abdominal conditions, gastrointestinal anthrax can be difficult to identify. Blood loss and fluid and electrolyte imbalances can lead to shock, and death may follow intestinal perforation or anthrax toxemia (Dixon et al., 1999). From 25 to 75 percent of cases may be fatal (Brachman and Friedlander, 1999). An oropharyngeal infection, which is milder than the gastrointestinal form, produces fever, visible ulcers, and local edema and swollen lymph glands that can interfere with swallowing and breathing (Dixon et al., 1999).

Inhalational Anthrax

Inhalational anthrax has been a rare disease because there are limited circumstances when spores whose particle sizes are sufficiently small (less than 5 micrometers [μm]) to be inhaled deep into the lung are suspended in air. When anthrax spores are inhaled, they are deposited in the alveolar spaces, where they are taken up by macrophages and transported to the mediastinal and peribronchial lymph nodes. In the lymph nodes, spores germinate to become vegetative, multiply, and cause hemorrhagic mediastinitis. They also move into the bloodstream and spread throughout the body. At Sverdlovsk, the modal incubation period from exposure to the onset of symptoms was 10 days, but some cases developed up to 6 weeks after the reported exposure (Dixon et al., 1999; Inglesby et al., 1999; Meselson et al., 1994).

The initial symptoms of inhalational anthrax, which resemble those of influenza and other common upper respiratory infections, include malaise, fatigue, and cough. In days, severe respiratory distress develops, with dyspnea, cyanosis, and strident cough. Other symptoms may include fever, chills, and subcutaneous edema of the chest and neck (Brachman and Friedlander, 1999). Radiographic examination of the chest usually shows a characteristic widening of the mediastinum and pleural effusions (see Figure 2-2). Shock may develop, and hemorrhagic meningitis (see Figure 2-3) may occur in about 50 percent of cases (Brachman and Friedlander, 1999). Death usually occurs within 24 hours following the onset of acute symptoms. At Sverdlovsk, the mean interval from the onset of initial symptoms to death was 3 days (Dixon et al., 1999). On the basis of previously limited observations, inhalational anthrax was fatal in 80 to 90 percent of cases

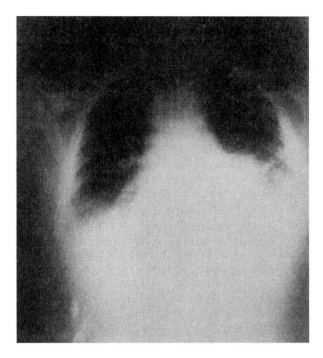

FIGURE 2-2 Chest radiograph characteristic of inhalational anthrax.
SOURCE: Public Health Image Library, CDC.

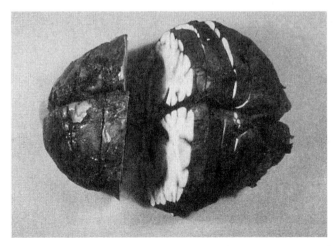

FIGURE 2-3 Hemorrhagic meningitis caused by anthrax.
SOURCE: Public Health Image Library, CDC.

(CDC, 2000c). Aggressive treatment early enough in the course of the disease appears to improve the rate of survival.

A review of the first 10 reported patients with inhalational anthrax resulting from the bioterrorism release of anthrax spores in the autumn of 2001 indicated that all 10 had abnormal chest X rays (Jernigan et al., 2001). Abnormalities included infiltrates, pleural effusion, and mediastinal widening. Mediastinal lymphadenopathy was observed in seven patients. Extensive sweating was a prominent feature in these 10 patients, although it had not been emphasized in reports of earlier cases. A brief period of improvement after the earliest symptoms noted in earlier cases was not seen in these patients. The median incubation period from exposure to the onset of symptoms was 4 days in the six patients for whom the time of exposure was known. Six of the 10 patients described in the paper survived with multidrug antibiotic regimens and aggressive supportive care (e.g., drainage of pleural effusions). Additional case reports describe clinical features of the tenth and eleventh cases of bioterrorism-related inhalational anthrax (Barakat et al., 2002; Mina et al., 2002).

Treatment

Penicillin, doxycycline, and ciprofloxacin are the primary antibiotics recommended for treatment of all forms of anthrax (CDC, 2000c), although there are no formal studies of clinical treatment of inhalational anthrax in humans (Inglesby et al., 1999). Both doxycycline and ciprofloxacin were recommended as initial therapy for infections associated with the recent bioterrorist attack in the United States (CDC, 2001c). Mild cutaneous cases can be treated effectively with oral medication, but treatment does not alter the course of the skin lesion. Other forms of anthrax and more serious cutaneous cases must be treated with intravenous antibiotics. Additional supportive therapy may be needed to prevent septic shock, to maintain fluid and electrolyte balance, and to maintain a patent airway. If inhalational exposure to anthrax spores is known or suspected but symptoms have not developed, the Centers for Disease Control and Prevention (CDC) recommends a 60-day course of antibiotic treatment to protect against delayed germination of spores (CDC, 2001b). If available, at least three doses of anthrax vaccine can be administered.

Pathogenesis

When anthrax spores are introduced into the body by any route, they are taken up by macrophages and germinate into vegetative bacteria with an antiphagocytic capsule that deters the host's immune response to the organism. The vegetative bacteria multiply and secrete toxins that produce local edema and necrosis. If bacteria are carried to regional lymph nodes, they multiply further and produce additional edema and necrosis and enter the bloodstream to produce a systemic infection (Brachman and Friedlander, 1999; Dixon et al., 1999).

The virulence of B. *anthracis* derives from the production of three toxin proteins and the capsule. The toxin proteins, encoded on the pXO1 plasmid, are protective antigen (PA), edema factor (EF), and lethal factor (LF). To produce active toxins, PA must bind to cellular receptors and then bind with either EF or LF (see Figure 2-4). The human cellular receptor for PA has recently been identified and characterized and named anthrax toxin receptor (Bradley et al., 2001). The resulting edema toxin or lethal toxin can then enter the cell. The effects of edema toxin appear to result from EF, an adenylate cyclase that increases intracellular levels of cyclic adenosine monophosphate, which upsets water homeostasis (Dixon et al., 1999). Edema toxin may also impair neutrophil function. LF is a zinc metalloprotease that cleaves two mitogen-activated protein kinase kinases. The mechanism by which it leads to death of the host remains unknown but

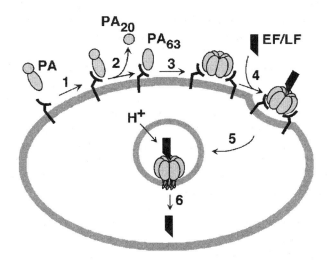

FIGURE 2-4 Model of anthrax toxin action. (1) PA binds to cellular receptor. (2–3) The protein is cleaved and activated to form a heptameric prepore. (4) LF, EF, or both bind to the heptamer, and the resulting complex is taken into an acidic compartment in the cell through endocytosis. (5–6) The acidic pH initiates the heptamer to pierce the membrane of the cell and translocate LF, EF, or both into the cytosol, where the toxins lead to damage. [Reprinted, with permission, from *Biochemistry* 38:10432–10441 (1999). Copyright 1999 by American Chemical Society.]

may involve suppression of the inflammatory response (Pellizzari et al., 1999, Erwin et al., 2001).

A second plasmid, pXO2, contains a gene that encodes the synthesis of a polyglutamyl capsule that inhibits phagocytosis of the vegetative bacteria.

Full virulence requires both plasmids. Attenuated spore vaccines have been developed with bacterial strains missing one or both plasmids. The livestock vaccine currently in use in the United States and other countries, known as the Sterne vaccine, is derived from a noncapsulated *B. anthracis* variant that lacks the pXO2 plasmid. The vaccine currently licensed for human use in the United States, AVA, however, is a cell-free filtrate containing PA as the principal immunogen.

ANTHRAX VACCINE DEVELOPMENT

Early work on the development of a vaccine against anthrax in animals was carried out in the 1880s by W. S. Greenfield and by Louis Pasteur (Turnbull, 1991). What became known as Pasteur's vaccine used an encapsulating nontoxigenic strain of *B. anthracis* administered to animals in two doses that differed in their degrees of heat attenuation (Turnbull, 1991, 2000). A live spore vaccine developed by Sterne in the 1930s eventually supplanted Pasteur's vaccine and remains in use for livestock in many parts of the world. It is credited with marked reductions in the incidence of anthrax cases or in the absence of anthrax cases in vaccinated herds, reducing the devastating impact of the disease in both animals and humans in areas where vaccination is carried out. Analogous vaccines were developed in the former Soviet Union and China, where they are used for humans as well as in animals (Turnbull, 2000). Limited data regarding the safety and efficacy of the vaccine used in humans in the former Soviet Union have been reported (Demicheli et al., 1998; Shlyakhov and Rubenstein, 1994).

Live spore vaccines, such as the Sterne vaccine, have been associated with residual virulence that leads to occasional casualties in livestock and thus have not been considered appropriate for human use in the West. Therefore, when interest in the potential use of anthrax as a biological warfare agent arose after World War II, work to develop inactivated vaccines began in both the United States, at Fort Detrick, Maryland, and the United Kingdom, at Porton Down (Turnbull, 2000).

In the United States, the research to develop an anthrax vaccine used *B. anthracis* cultures in synthetic medium without proteins or other macromolecules (Turnbull, 2000). A production system was described in 1954 (Wright et al., 1954), including a chemically defined growth medium and a method of concentrating, stabilizing, and partially purifying protective antigen by precipitation. The safety and efficacy of this vaccine were evaluated in a controlled trial conducted between 1955 and 1959 at goat hair-processing mills in the eastern United States (Brachman et al., 1962). The initial production method was soon modified for scale-up, with changes in the culture conditions, product purification method, and strain of the organism used (Auerbach and Wright, 1955; Puziss and Wright, 1963; Wright and Puziss, 1957; Wright et al., 1962).

The current vaccine, AVA,[1] was licensed in 1970 for manufacture by the Michigan Department of Public Health. Both the production plant and the product line were eventually sold to a private company, BioPort, which at the time of this report was the sole U.S. manufacturer of an anthrax vaccine. The product license for AVA calls for subcutaneous administration of a basic series of six doses of 0.5 milliliters each. After administration of the initial dose, subsequent doses are administered at 2 weeks, 4 weeks, 6 months, 12 months, and 18 months. Annual booster doses are required.

USE OF ANTHRAX VACCINE

As was noted above, *B. anthracis* is a widespread organism, and anthrax disease has long been endemic in many agricultural areas. The disease was not, until quite recently, considered threatening outside certain industrial or agricultural settings that allowed exposure. The licensed anthrax vaccine had routinely been administered to the limited population of U.S. workers with occupational exposure to anthrax bacteria or spores. It is estimated that 68,000 doses of AVA were distributed between 1974 and 1989 (Ellenberg, 1999).

In the United States in recent years, however, AVA has been used primarily by the military to protect troops from weaponized *B. anthracis* (Brachman and Friedlander, 1999; Mazzuchi et al., 2000). At the time of the Gulf War, there were fears that Iraq had produced weapons containing anthrax spores. More than 300,000 doses of AVA were distributed during Operation Desert Storm, probably to more than 150,000 service members (Army Information Paper, 1991).

Although no biological weapons were used against U.S. or other coalition forces during the Gulf War, subsequent inspections of Iraq in 1995 and 1996 by the United Nations Special Commission and the International Atomic Energy Agency revealed that 8,000 liters of anthrax spore suspension had been produced and that during the Gulf War in 1991 Iraq had 200 bombs and 25 ballistic missiles containing biological agents (Henderson, 1999; Zilinskas, 1997). More recent information indicates that Iraq has

---

[1]The anthrax vaccine is adsorbed to aluminum hydroxide (Alhydrogel), which acts as an adjuvant. An adjuvant is a component that augments the immune response. Many vaccines require adjuvants for efficient elicitation of an immune response.

been renovating biological, chemical, and nuclear warfare research sites 3 years after barring international inspectors (Bohlen, 2001). In 1997, as a result of the concerns about biological weapons, then Secretary of Defense William Cohen initiated a plan to vaccinate all U.S. service members against anthrax. Immunizations began in March 1998 under DoD's Anthrax Vaccine Immunization Program (AVIP). As of November 29, 2001, 522,529 service members had received 2,098,544 of doses of AVA (http://www.anthrax.osd.mil/Flash_interface/default.html, accessed January 11, 2002).

Implementation of AVIP has been slowed by a limited supply of vaccine. Renovations were begun at the manufacturing plant in 1998, and BioPort, the sole manufacturer, did not receive approval from the Food and Drug Administration (FDA) for release of newly manufactured vaccine until January 31, 2002. DoD has been able to continue immunizations, despite the limited supply of vaccine, but not at the rate first planned. In July 2000, in November 2000, and again in June 2001, DoD slowed the anthrax immunization program, focusing only on troops thought to be at greatest potential risk (http://www.anthrax.osd.mil, accessed September 5, 2000; Marshall, 2000).

In the autumn of 2001, more than 30,000 civilians were potentially exposed to anthrax in bioterrorist incidents involving the distribution of highly infectious spores through the U.S. mail (CDC, 2001d,e). Beginning in December 2001, CDC began offering vaccination with AVA as a treatment option for selected exposed civilians. This therapeutic use of the vaccine following exposure was not included under the official vaccine license and is being monitored under the provisions of an Investigational New Drug application. As of February 25, 2002, the latest data available at the time that this report was completed, 192 people had begun receiving doses of AVA (Ashford, 2002).

The committee emphasizes that this report is addressed to DoD and focuses on the licensed use of AVA for immunization before exposure to anthrax spores.

CONCERNS ABOUT USE OF AVA

AVIP and the product AVA have become focal points of great concern on the part of at least segments of the military and interested public. A few service members have refused the vaccine, at the risk of court-martial, because of their perception that it is particularly dangerous.[2] Among the

---

[2]Studies of service member's knowledge, attitudes, and beliefs regarding the anthrax vaccine are being planned by CDC to help DoD to better understand and respond to such concerns.

concerns are complaints among Gulf War veterans of chronic multisystem clinical conditions that still lack a definable relationship to the anthrax vaccine or to other events in their Gulf War experiences (IOM, 2000b).

The U.S. Congress has responded to these concerns, and hearings have been held in the U.S. House of Representatives and the U.S. Senate.[3] The hearings typically included several current or former service members (or family members of service personnel) who had raised concerns about the adverse events that they had experienced or observed or about the responses of military health care providers to these concerns. The witness list usually also included officials from DoD or a branch of the military service, FDA, and sometimes the manufacturer of AVA. As noted in Appendix C, the IOM Committee to Assess the Safety and Efficacy of the Anthrax Vaccine also held a public hearing to gather information from people with concerns about the vaccine. The IOM committee benefited from the perspective provided by the speakers, many of whom also provided testimony during congressional hearings. The witnesses described persistent and debilitating symptoms ranging from fever, headache, and malaise to swelling, joint pain, and tinnitus, which they ascribed to the anthrax vaccine. Several witnesses also described specific serious conditions including hypogonadism; Stevens-Johnson syndrome, which affected their vision as well as their skin; and aplastic anemia, which proved fatal. In addition, many witnesses observed that when they reported their symptoms to medical personnel, the health care providers seemed to be unaware of the Vaccine Adverse Event Reporting System (VAERS) or unwilling to file a report with VAERS and often seemed to doubt that the vaccine could have caused their symptoms.

AVAILABLE DATA ON AVA

In its letter report of March 2000, *An Assessment of the Safety of the Anthrax Vaccine*, the IOM Committee on Health Effects Associated with Exposures During the Gulf War expressed regret over the lack of information about the vaccine in the peer-reviewed published literature (IOM,

---

[3]Christopher Shays, chair of the Subcommittee on National Security, Veterans Affairs, and International Relations of the Committee on Government Reform and Oversight convened a series of hearings in 1999 and 2000 on AVIP and on allegations that adverse event reporting to the Vaccine Adverse Event Reporting System does not adequately reflect the actual rate of adverse events. Congressman Steve Buyer, chair of the Subcommittee on Military Personnel of the House Committee on Armed Services, also held a hearing on AVIP, and the Committee on Appropriations chaired by Ted Stevens held a hearing on Gulf War illnesses, as had Congressman Shays. The Senate Committee on Armed Services, chaired by Senator John Warner, also held 3 days of hearings in 2000. Those hearings were on AVIP and DoD's antibiological warfare agent vaccine acquisition program.

2000a). It listed an array of studies that were unpublished or ongoing that could contribute to the body of information on which conclusions regarding health effects could be based.

As the study presented in this report began, representatives of DoD provided assurances to IOM that all relevant information from DoD would be made readily available to the committee and that efforts would be made to publish the data from completed studies. DoD and its investigators have followed through on these assurances. Most of the studies that have been carried out by DoD investigators to assess the safety and efficacy of the anthrax vaccine have now been written up as manuscripts and submitted for publication. Additional studies have been published since the letter report was released (e.g., CDC, 2000a; Gunzenhauser et al., 2001; Pittman et al., 2001, 2002; Rehme et al., 2002). In addition, one of the most important contributions to the committee's evaluation was in the form of analyses of data from military databases carried out at the committee's request. In accordance with its charge, the earlier IOM committee (Committee on Health Effects Associated with Exposures During the Gulf War) reviewed only the published, peer-reviewed literature to reach its conclusions about safety. The current committee had a different purpose and as a result chose to review all the studies it was aware of and for which adequate descriptions of the study methods, data analyses, and results were made available. These studies are systematically reviewed in the chapters that follow.

Several previous IOM committees evaluating possible causal associations between vaccines or other exposures and specific health outcomes have chosen to describe their findings with a weight-of-evidence approach (IOM, 1991, 1994, 2000b). Their findings placed associations between the exposure of interest and the health outcome into categories such as sufficient evidence of a causal relationship, sufficient evidence of an association, limited or suggestive evidence of an association, inadequate or insufficient evidence to determine whether an association does or does not exist, and limited or suggestive evidence of no association. The current committee chose not to use that approach because it was not asked to evaluate exposure to AVA as a cause of specific health outcomes. Rather, the committee was asked to provide an overall evaluation of the anthrax vaccine's safety. In addition, its charge included addressing various aspects of the efficacy of AVA, as well as manufacturing issues, two topics for which a weight-of-evidence approach is not readily applicable.

REFERENCES

Army Information Paper (from an Army staff officer). 1991. Numbers of service members vaccinated during Operation Desert Storm. [Online]. Available: http://www.gulflink.osd.mil/va/va_refs/n46en087/0215_027_0000001.htm [accessed January 18, 2002].

Ashford D. 2002. Information on the number of participants enrolled in vaccine IND application. E-mail to Joellenbeck L, Institute of Medicine, Washington, D.C., February 25.

Auerbach BA, Wright GG. 1955. Studies on immunity in anthrax. VI. Immunizing activity of protective antigen against various strains of *Bacillus anthracis*. *Journal of Immunology* 75:129–133.

Barakat LA, Quentzel HL, Jernigan JA, Kirschke DL, Griffith K, Spear SM, Kelley K, Barden D, Mayo D, Stephens DS, Popovic T, Marston C, Zaki SR, Guarner J, Shieh WJ, Carver HW 2nd, Meyer RF, Swerdlow DL, Mast EE, Hadler JL. 2002. Fatal inhalational anthrax in a 94-year-old Connecticut woman. *JAMA* 287(7):863–868.

Bohlen C. 2001, December 20. Vanishing Taliban, a British force on deck, spilled Iraqi secrets. *New York Times*. p. B1.

Brachman PS, Friedlander AM. 1999. Anthrax. In: Plotkin SA, Orenstein WA, eds. *Vaccines*, 3rd ed. Philadelphia, Pa.: W. B. Saunders Co. Pp. 629–637.

Brachman PS, Gold H, Plotkin S, Fekety FR, Werrin M, Ingraham NR. 1962. Field evaluation of a human anthrax vaccine. *American Journal of Public Health* 52:632–645.

Bradley KA, Mogridge J, Mourez M, Collier RJ, Young JA. 2001. Identification of the cellular receptor for anthrax toxin. *Nature* 414(6860):225–229.

Brown K. 2001. Anthrax: a "sure killer" yields to medicine. *Science* 294(5548):1813–1814.

CDC (Centers for Disease Control and Prevention). 2000a. Surveillance for adverse events associated with anthrax vaccination—U.S. Department of Defense, 1998–2000. *MMWR (Morbidity and Mortality Weekly Report)* 49(16):341–345.

CDC. 2000b. Human ingestion of *Bacillus anthracis*–contaminated meat—Minnesota, August 2000. *MMWR (Morbidity and Mortality Weekly Report)* 49(36):813–816.

CDC. 2000c. Use of anthrax vaccine in the United States: recommendations of the Advisory Committee on Immunization Practices (ACIP). *MMWR (Morbidity and Mortality Weekly Report)* 49(RR-15):1–20.

CDC. 2001a. Human anthrax associated with an epizootic among livestock—North Dakota, 2000. *MMWR (Morbidity and Mortality Weekly Report)* 50(32):677–680.

CDC. 2001b. Update: investigation of bioterrorism-related anthrax and interim guidelines for exposure management and antimicrobial therapy, October 2001. *MMWR (Morbidity and Mortality Weekly Report)* 50(42):909–919.

CDC. 2001c. CDC health advisory: updated information about how to recognize and handle a suspicious package or envelope. [Online]. Available: http://www.bt.cdc.gov/DocumentsApp/Anthrax/10312001/han50.asp [accessed January 18, 2002].

CDC. 2001d. Update: investigation of bioterrorism-related anthrax and adverse events from antimicrobial prophylaxis. *MMWR (Morbidity and Mortality Weekly Report)* 50(44):973–976.

CDC. 2001e. Update: investigation of bioterrorism-related inhalational anthrax—Connecticut, 2001. *MMWR (Morbidity and Mortality Weekly Report)* 50(47):1049–1051.

Dixon TC, Meselson M, Guillemin J, Hanna PC. 1999. Anthrax. *New England Journal of Medicine* 341(11):815–826.

Demicheli V, Rivetti D, Deeks JJ, Jefferson T, Pratt M. 1998. The effectiveness and safety of vaccines against human anthrax: a systematic review. *Vaccine* 16(9-10):880–884.

Ellenberg SS. 1999. *Vaccine Adverse Events Reporting System*. Statement at the July 21, 1999, Hearing of the Subcommittee on National Security, Veterans Affairs, and International Relations, Committee on Government Reform, U.S. House of Representatives, Washington, D.C.

Erwin JL, DaSilva LM, Bavari S, Little SF, Friedlander AM, Chanh TC. 2001. Macrophage-derived cell lines do not express proinflammatory cytokines after exposure to *Bacillus anthracis* lethal toxin. *Infection and Immunity* 69(2):1175–1177.
Freedman A, Afonja O, Chang MW, Mostashari F, Blaser M, Perez-Perez G, Lazarus H, Schacht R, Guttenberg J, Traister M, Borkowsky W. 2002. Cutaneous anthrax associated with microangiopathic hemolytic anemia and coagulopathy in a 7-month-old infant. *JAMA* 287(7):869–874.
Friedlander AM. 2000. Anthrax: clinical features, pathogenesis, and potential biological warfare threat. *Current Clinical Topics in Infectious Diseases* 20:335–349.
Gallagher TC, Strober BE. 2001. Cutaneous *Bacillus anthracis* infection. *New England Journal of Medicine* 345(22):1646–1647.
Gunzenhauser JD, Cook JE, Parker ME, Wright I. 2001. Acute side effects of anthrax vaccine in ROTC cadets participating in advanced camp, Fort Lewis, 2000. *MSMR (Medical Surveillance Monthly Report)* 7(5):4–14.
Henderson DA. 1999. The looming threat of bioterrorism. *Science* 283(5406):1279–1282.
Inglesby TV, Henderson DA, Bartlett JG, Ascher MS, Eitzen E, Friedlander AM, Hauer J, McDade J, Osterholm MT, O'Toole T, Parker G, Perl TM, Russell PK, Tonat K. 1999. Anthrax as a biological weapon: medical and public health management. *JAMA* 281(18):1735–1745.
IOM (Institute of Medicine). 1991. Howson CP, Howe CJ, Fineberg HV, eds. *Adverse Effects of Pertussis and Rubella Vaccines.* Washington, D.C.: National Academy Press.
IOM. 1994. Stratton KE, Howe CJ, Johnston RB, eds. *Adverse Events Associated with Childhood Vaccines: Evidence Bearing on Causality.* Washington, D.C.: National Academy Press.
IOM. 2000a. *An Assessment of the Safety of the Anthrax Vaccine: A Letter Report.* Washington, D.C.: National Academy Press.
IOM. Fulco CE, Liverman CT, Sox HC, eds. 2000b. *Gulf War and Health.* Washington, D.C.: National Academy Press.
Jernigan JA, Stephens DS, Ashford DA, Omenaca C, Topiel MS, Galbraith M, Tapper M, Fisk TL, Zaki S, Popovic T, Meyer RF, Quinn CP, Harper SA, Fridkin SK, Sejvar JJ, Shepard CW, McConnell M, Guarner J, Shieh WJ, Malecki JM, Gerberding JL, Hughes JM, Perkins BA. 2001. Bioterrorism-related inhalational anthrax: the first 10 cases reported in the United States. *Emerging Infectious Diseases* 7(6):933–944.
Marshall E. 2000. Bioterrorism. DOD retreats on plan for anthrax vaccine. *Science* 289(5478):382–383.
Mazzuchi JF, Claypool RG, Hyams KC, Trump D, Riddle J, Patterson RE, Bailey S. 2000. Protecting the health of U.S. military forces: a national obligation. *Aviation, Space, and Environmental Medicine* 71(3):260–265.
Meselson M, Guillemin J, Hugh-Jones M, Langmuir A, Popova I, Shelokov A, Yampolskaya O. 1994. The Sverdlovsk anthrax outbreak of 1979. *Science* 266(5188):1202–1208.
Mina B, Dym JP, Kuepper F, Tso R, Arrastia C, Kaplounova I, Faraj H, Kwapniewski A, Krol CM, Grosser M, Glick J, Fochios S, Remolina A, Vasovic L, Moses J, Robin T, DeVita M, Tapper ML. 2002. Fatal inhalational anthrax with unknown source of exposure in a 61-year-old woman in New York City. *JAMA* 287(7):858–862.
Pellizzari R, Guidi-Rontani C, Vitale G, Mock M, Montecucco C. 1999. Anthrax lethal factor cleaves MKK3 in macrophages and inhibits the LPS/IFN gamma-induced release of NO and TNFalpha. *FEBS Letters* 462(1-2):199–204.
Pittman PR, Gibbs PH, Cannon TL, Friedlander AM. 2001. Anthrax vaccine: short-term safety experience in humans. *Vaccine* 20(5–6):972–978.

Pittman PR, Kim-Ahn G, Pifat DY, Coon K, Gibbs P, Little S, Pace-Templeton J, Myers R, Parker GW, Friedlander AM. 2002. Anthrax vaccine: safety and immunogenicity of a dose-reduction, route comparison study in humans. *Vaccine* 20(9–10):1412–1420.

Plotkin SA, Brachman PS, Utell M, Bumford FH, Atchison MM. 1960. An epidemic of inhalation anthrax, the first in the twentieth century. *American Journal of Medicine* 29:992–1001.

Puziss M, Wright GG. 1963. Studies on immunity in anthrax. X. Gel adsorbed protective antigen for immunization of man. *Journal of Bacteriology* 85:230–236.

Rehme PA, Wiliams R, Grabenstein JD. 2002. Ambulatory medical visits among anthrax vaccinated and unvaccinated personnel after return from Southwest Asia. *Military Medicine* 167:205–210.

Roche KJ, Chang MW, Lazarus H. 2001. Cutaneous anthrax infection. *New England Journal of Medicine* 345(22):1611.

Shlyakhov EN, Rubinstein E. 1994. Human live anthrax vaccine in the former USSR. *Vaccine* 12(8):727–730.

Turnbull PC. 1991. Anthrax vaccines: past, present and future. *Vaccine* 9(8):533–539.

Turnbull PCB. 2000. Current status of immunization against anthrax: old vaccines may be here to stay for a while. *Current Opinion in Infectious Diseases* 13(2):113–120.

Wright GG, Puziss M. 1957. Elaboration of protective antigen of *Bacillus anthracis* under anaerobic conditions. *Nature* 179:916–917.

Wright GG, Hedberg MA, Slein JB. 1954. Studies on immunity in anthrax. III. Elaboration of protective antigen in a chemically-defined, non-protein medium. *Journal of Immunology* 72:263–269.

Wright GG, Puziss M, Neely WB. 1962. Studies on immunity in anthrax. IX. Effect of variations in cultural conditions on elaboration of protective antigen by strains of *Bacillus anthracis*. *Journal of Immunology* 83:515–522.

Zilinskas RA. 1997. Iraq's biological weapons: the past as future? *JAMA* 278(5):418–424.

3

Anthrax Vaccine Efficacy

Evaluating the efficacy of the Anthrax Vaccine Adsorbed (AVA), particularly against inhalational exposure to anthrax, was a crucial part of this committee's charge. The charge specifically calls for evaluation of (1) the efficacy of the anthrax vaccine (AVA) in protecting humans from inhalational anthrax, (2) the efficacy of AVA against all known strains of *Bacillus anthracis*, and (3) the correlation of the effectiveness of the vaccine in animal models to its ability to protect humans. This chapter presents the committee's observations and findings regarding the efficacy of AVA against inhalational anthrax and all known strains. The committee also examines what is known and what must still be established regarding the correlation of immune protection in animal models with immune protection in humans.

The term *efficacy* generally refers to the ability of a product to achieve its desired effect under ideal conditions, such as a controlled clinical trial in which the product is consistently administered as prescribed. The *effectiveness* of a product is its ability to achieve the desired effect under real-world conditions. The charge to the committee uses both terms, and in many situations the terms are used interchangeably, with the context showing whether the effects were observed under laboratory-controlled or real-world conditions. In this report the committee is concerned primarily with evaluating efficacy.

It is important to note that efficacy is relative, not absolute. A variety of factors can play a role in determining the degree of protection from a vaccine, which can include the size of the inoculum of exposure, the strain of the pathogen, and the host response. Even a vaccine considered highly effective may fail to protect some individuals under some circumstances.

EVALUATING EFFICACY OF AVA FOR INHALATIONAL ANTHRAX

The data used to evaluate the efficacy of AVA come from three sources. Studies with textile mill workers tested the efficacy of AVA and a related vaccine against occupational exposures to anthrax spores. Serological studies with humans tested the ability of AVA to elicit antibodies to protective antigen (PA), an indication of an immune response to the vaccine. Studies with animals tested the efficacy of the vaccine in protecting the animals from inhalational exposure to anthrax spores.

Human Efficacy Trials

Brachman and colleagues (1962) conducted the only randomized, placebo-controlled trial of the efficacy of a PA-containing anthrax vaccine. Although the safety information that it provides is reported separately in Chapter 6, here the committee describes the information on vaccine efficacy provided in that study. The vaccine studied was not AVA but was an earlier formulation produced from the R1-NP mutant of the Vollum strain of anthrax manufactured by Merck (see Chapter 7 for more details). The study was carried out from January 1955 through March 1959 in four textile mills in the northeastern United States that processed raw, imported goat hair for production into the interlinings of suit coats. The goat hair was typically contaminated with anthrax spores, and workers were exposed during handling of this material. Before receiving the vaccine, the average annual incidence of cutaneous anthrax among workers at these four mills ranged from 0.6 to 1.8 cases per 100 workers.

The worker population eligible for the study included 1,249 men and women with no history of prior anthrax infection. Approximately 47 percent of employees worked in high-risk areas within the mills, and about one-half of the eligible study subjects came from one of the four mills (Mill A). Rates of refusal to participate in the study among the four mills ranged from <1 to 45 percent, and refusals were approximately equally distributed between the placebo and vaccine groups.

Participating workers were randomly allocated by length of employment, age, department, and job to receive either vaccine or placebo. Inoculations of 0.5 milliliters (ml) of either vaccine or placebo (0.1 percent alum) were given; the first three inoculations were administered at 2-week intervals, followed by three injections at 6-month intervals and annual boosters thereafter. Those referred to as "complete" inoculees received at least the first three injections and subsequent inoculations on schedule (personal communication, S. A. Plotkin, consultant to the Institute of Medicine Committee to Assess the Safety and Efficacy of the Anthrax Vaccine, January 29, 2001). Otherwise, the inoculees were referred to as "incomplete." There were 379 complete vaccine recipients and 414 complete placebo recipients. Only data for those designated complete inoculees were included in the calculation of efficacy. Routine visits and environmental sampling were conducted throughout the study to confirm exposure and identify cases of anthrax.

Over the course of the study, 26 cases of anthrax occurred, including an outbreak of 9 cases over a 10-week period at one of the mills (Mill A). Twenty-one of the 26 cases were cutaneous anthrax and 5 were cases of inhalational anthrax, all of which occurred during the outbreak at Mill A. Of the 26 cases, 3 occurred among vaccine recipients (1 complete and 2 incomplete inoculees), 17 occurred among individuals in the placebo group (15 complete and 2 incomplete inoculees), and 6 cases occurred among individuals who were not inoculated with the vaccine or the placebo. None of the cases of inhalational anthrax occurred in persons who had received the vaccine.

The overall effectiveness of the vaccine against anthrax infection generally was 92.5 percent (lower 95 percent confidence interval = 65 percent): 91.4 percent in the high-risk group of workers and 100 percent in the low-risk group of workers. It was not possible to evaluate the efficacy of the vaccine against inhalational anthrax separately because of the small number of cases. (Given the definition of "complete" vaccination in the published paper, one of the cases counted in the incomplete vaccination group should have been included in the complete vaccination group. Doing so would have reduced the reported effectiveness somewhat. It is not possible to calculate the effectiveness after the addition of this case to the complete vaccination group since the necessary information is not provided in the paper.)

As part of another effort, the Centers for Disease Control and Prevention (CDC) collected observational data on the occurrence of anthrax in industrial settings like textile mills between 1962 and 1974 (FDA, 1985). During this period, both the Merck vaccine and AVA, produced by the Michigan Department of Public Health, were used and 27 cases of cutaneous anthrax were identified. No cases occurred in those who had received the full course of immunizations. Three cases occurred in persons who worked in or near mills but who were not mill employees and who were not vaccinated. The remaining 24 cases occurred among mill employees; 3 of these had received one or two doses of the vaccine, and the remaining 21 persons were unvaccinated. Thus, of the 27 cases observed, 2 occurred in persons who had received two doses of vaccine, 1 occurred in a person who had received one dose of the vaccine, and the other 24 occurred in persons who were completely unvaccinated.

Finding: The randomized field study carried out by Brachman and colleagues (1962) provides solid evidence indicating the efficacy of a vaccine similar to AVA against *B. anthracis* infection. The subsequent CDC data are supportive. However, the small number of inhalational cases in those studies provides insufficient information to allow a conclusion to be made about the vaccine's efficacy against inhalational infection.

Human Antibody Response to AVA

Information regarding the ability of AVA to elicit antibodies in human vaccinees is available from five studies.

An indirect hemagglutination assay and an enzyme-linked immunosorbent assay (ELISA) for antibodies to PA were carried out with serum specimens from 190 vaccinees (Johnson-Winegar, 1984). Serum samples were obtained 2 weeks after the third immunization in the vaccination series. By the indirect hemagglutination assay, 83 percent of vaccinees seroconverted (titer of 1:8 or above). Other data indicated that at 2 weeks after an annual booster immunization that follows the six-dose regimen, all 85 vaccinees evaluated had seroconverted.

Two retrospective serological studies evaluating the effect of the dosing interval on the human antibody response (Pittman et al., 2000) served as preliminary studies for the larger prospective study described later (Pittman et al., 2002). Increasing the interval between the first and second doses of vaccine from 2 to 4 weeks resulted in a statistically significant three- to fourfold increase in the geometric mean anti-PA immunoglobulin G (IgG) antibody titer measured several weeks after the administration of the second dose.

Data on the human antibody response to AVA were also provided by a study of volunteers from Ft. Bragg, North Carolina. Pittman and colleagues (Pittman, 2001; Pittman et al., 1997, in press) conducted a study to assess the persistence of antibodies against *B. anthracis* 18 to 24 months after initial vaccination during Operations Desert Shield and Desert Storm and to assess the safety and immunogenicity of a vaccine booster dose. Study participants were recruited from among active-duty personnel at Fort Bragg in 1992 and 1994. The study population consisted of 495 male Desert Shield or Desert Storm veterans who received one to three primary doses of AVA in 1990 or 1991. Serological analyses were performed for a subset of participants (20 participants who had received AVA only and 259 participants who had received both AVA and pentavalent botulinum toxoid) whose blood had been drawn prior to and 24 to 36 days after receipt of booster doses of vaccine.

Evaluation of anti-PA IgG levels indicated that roughly 2 years after their initial vaccinations, the proportion of volunteers (20 to 50 percent) with detectable anti-*B. anthracis* antibodies was low, and among those with detectable antibodies, persisting antibody levels were low. After receipt of booster doses, all but two volunteers had detectable anti-PA antibody responses. The geometric mean titers (ELISA) in those with detectable antibody responses ranged from roughly 4,500 in those who had received only one initial dose to 10,000 in those who had received three priming doses. Data on reactogenicity are reported in Chapter 6.

A pilot study carried out at the U.S. Army Medical Research Institute of Infectious Diseases examined immune responses to alternative AVA dosing schedules and routes of administration (Pittman et al., 2002). In that study, 173 U.S. military and civilian volunteers (109 men and 64 women) were randomized to one of seven groups, defined on the basis of dosing schedule and route of administration. Three experimental dosing schedules were tested: a single injection on day 0, injections on days 0 and 14, and injections on days 0 and 28. For each experimental dosing schedule, two groups were established: one group was inoculated subcutaneously and the other group was inoculated intramuscularly. A control group was administered AVA by the licensed six-dose schedule and subcutaneous administration.

The anti-PA IgG concentrations measured 2 weeks after the administration of two doses of AVA 4 weeks apart (either intramuscularly or subcutaneously) were comparable to those measured 2 weeks after the administration of three doses (given subcutaneously) 2 weeks apart (the licensed dosing schedule). The distribution of peak anti-PA IgG antibody concentration did not differ among those who received two doses (either intramuscularly or subcutaneously) 4 weeks apart and those who received three doses (subcutaneously) 2 weeks apart. Antibody response rates (>25 micrograms per milliliter [μg/ml]) for these groups were 96 to 100 percent (the reasons for the insensitivity of the ELISA described in that study were unclear to the committee). Similar results were obtained by a toxin neutralization antibody (TNA) assay. A single dose of AVA was not sufficient to elicit peak anti-PA antibody concentrations or seroconversion rates comparable to those achieved by the licensed dosing schedule.

These findings indicate that AVA administered by its licensed dosing schedule as well as by schedules that omit the dose administered at 2 weeks generates substantial antibody responses (at least 25 μg/ml) in 96 to 100 percent of recipients. CDC plans to conduct a larger randomized, controlled, multicenter trial to test the immunogenicity of AVA using a reduced number of doses administered intramuscularly.

The data presented above regarding the antibody responses generated by AVA in humans will be useful when future studies (passive protection studies, discussed later in this chapter) determine a likely protective level of anti-PA antibody on the basis of the results obtained from animal studies.

Efficacy Data from Animal Models

Extrapolation of Results from Animal Studies to Humans

Food and Drug Administration (FDA) regulations spell out the criteria required to prove "effectiveness" (meaning efficacy in the context of this report) through controlled clinical investigations and field trials.[1] However, for potentially lethal exposures such as inhalational exposure to anthrax spores, there is a serious problem in meeting these criteria. Field studies that rely on natural exposure to disease are not feasible as a means of evaluating the efficacy of the anthrax vaccine because inhalational anthrax is very rare, even in areas where anthrax occurs naturally or where it is an occupational hazard. Moreover, the particular concern regarding inhalational anthrax is exposure to anthrax spores processed for use as biological weapons. Controlled trials in which subjects are exposed to potentially lethal agents such as anthrax spores are simply not ethical. They would involve the administration of a potentially lethal substance to healthy human volunteers without a proven treatment that could be used if the vaccine or some other protective agent being tested failed.

Recognizing the need to provide for circumstances in which efficacy studies with humans cannot be ethically conducted, FDA published a proposed rule in October 1999 regarding the use of data from animal studies (FDA, 1999). In it FDA recommended the evidence needed to demonstrate the efficacy of new drugs for use against lethal or permanently disabling toxic substances. Although AVA is already a licensed vaccine, noting FDA's proposed requirements for the approval of such vaccines in the future can be helpful in evaluations of data from animal studies regarding the efficacy of AVA.[2] At the time this report was completed, the proposed rule for using data from animal studies had not yet been finalized. The committee

---

[1]The regulations are described in (a) Review Procedures to Determine that Licensed Biological Products Are Safe, Effective, and Not Misbranded Under Prescribed, Recommended, or Suggested Conditions of Use (21 C.F.R. § 601.25 [2001]) and (b) FDA Action on Applications and Abbreviated Applications: Adequate and Well-Controlled Studies (21 C.F.R. § 314.126 [2001]).

[2]In its proposed rule, FDA proposed that evidence from studies with animals be relied upon when controlled trials with humans cannot ethically be carried out. It would do so, however, only when "there is a reasonably well-understood pathophysiological mechanism of the toxicity of the substance and its prevention or substantial reduction by the product; the

hopes that all parties involved continue to work toward finalization of the rule as quickly as possible.

Finding: Because additional clinical trials to test the efficacy of AVA in humans are not feasible and challenge trials with volunteers are unethical, by necessity animal models represent the only sources of the supplementary data needed to evaluate AVA's efficacy.

Choice Among Animal Models of Human Disease

Animal models inevitably have different strengths and weaknesses in representing human disease and immunity. Therefore, different models may be appropriate for different applications. Animal models with pathological and immunological characteristics similar to those of humans could be considered the most appropriate ones for evaluations of vaccine efficacy. This is not to say that other animal models might not be appropriate for certain screening purposes, but it is important to weigh the data obtained with those models accordingly. The sections below review and compare the pathological and immunological features of different animal models in relation to human anthrax disease and immunity.

Comparison of Anthrax Pathology in Humans and Animals

As described in Chapter 2, anthrax is a zoonotic disease (a disease in which the same organism infects and causes disease in both humans and animals) caused by *B. anthracis*. *B. anthracis* most commonly infects grazing animals, as *B. anthracis* spores are stable for long periods in soil and grazing animals are the most readily available hosts. Humans can also be infected, however, generally from contact with the products of infected animals such as hides, hair or wool, meat, or by-products. Also, as discussed earlier in this report, the same organism produces diseases with different clinical manifestations (cutaneous, gastrointestinal, or inhalational), depending on the site of exposure and infection.

Pathology of Inhalational Anthrax in Humans As discussed in Chapter 2, inhaled anthrax spores are phagocytosed (taken up) by macrophages and transported from the lungs to the nearby peribronchial and mediastinal

---

effect is independently substantiated in multiple animal species, including species expected to react with a response predictive for humans; the animal study endpoint is clearly related to the desired benefit in humans, generally the enhancement of survival or prevention of major morbidity; and the data or information on the kinetics and pharmacodynamics of the product or other relevant data or information, in animals and humans, allows selection of an effective dose in humans."

lymph nodes (Albrink, 1961; Ross, 1957). The spores germinate in the lymph nodes and produce the three toxin components: PA, edema factor (EF), and lethal factor (LF). The toxins damage the lymph nodes, with subsequent dissemination via the bloodstream to many distant sites.

Information about the characteristic features of inhalational anthrax has primarily been gained from autopsy studies. In 1957, five cases of inhalational anthrax occurred at a goat hair-processing mill in New Hampshire. Four cases were fatal, and three of these were examined by autopsy. Pathology findings in the three cases included hemorrhagic edema in the mediastinum, hemorrhagic lymph nodes, and pleural effusions (leaking of fluid from the lining of the lungs). Two of the three cases demonstrated enlarged spleen, and microscopic hemorrhages and inflammation of the meninges (the lining of the brain; Albrink et al., 1960; Plotkin et al., 1960).

In a 1966 case of human inhalational anthrax, the patient also had a hemorrhagic edematous mediastinum and mediastinal lymph nodes, as well as a pleural effusion. The outer membrane of the brain had microscopic hemorrhages and inflammation (LaForce et al., 1969). In a case of anthrax described in a weaver in 1978, the patient similarly had pleural effusion, hemorrhagic mediastinitis, and leptomeningitis, as well as an enlarged spleen (Suffin et al., 1978).

The 1979 release of anthrax spores from a military facility in the town of Sverdlovsk in the former USSR led to 68 deaths (Guillemin, 1999). Necropsies were performed and tissue samples and microscopic slides were preserved for 42 cases, providing a wealth of additional information demonstrating the pathological changes in human tissue that occur as a result of inhalational exposure to anthrax spores.

The most striking pathological features in the anthrax cases from Sverdlovsk were prominent and consistent lesions of hemorrhagic thoracic lymphadenitis and hemorrhagic mediastinitis (Abramova et al., 1993; Walker, 2001). These consist of bloody, inflamed lymph nodes in the chest and bleeding and inflammation of the tissues in the area between the lungs. In addition, disseminated infection was often noted, with bacteremia, meningitis, and involvement of the submucosa of the gastrointestinal tract, particularly the small intestine, stomach, and colon. Another noteworthy aspect was edema, particularly in the lungs, mediastinum, pleurae (lining of the lung), and brain. The vascular damage that led to the edema was thought to be consistent with the effects of the toxins secreted by *B. anthracis* (Abramova et al., 1993; Walker, 2001).

As noted in Chapter 2, review of the first 10 reported cases of inhalational anthrax resulting from the bioterrorism release of anthrax spores in the autumn of 2001 indicated that all 10 patients had abnormal chest X rays (Jernigan et al., 2001). Abnormalities included infiltrates, pleural effusion, and mediastinal widening. Mediastinal lymphadenopathy was observed in seven patients.

Pathophysiology of Anthrax in Potential Animal Models The pathophysiology of anthrax infections varies in different animal models, making the disease in some species more similar than that in others to the disease in humans. Also, the organism characteristics associated with virulence in various animal species differ.

Mice and Rats Mice are considered among the laboratory animals most susceptible to infection with B. anthracis. However, inbred mouse strains differ in their susceptibilities to lethal infection with different strains of B. anthracis. In contrast to humans, the pathophysiology of anthrax in mice depends upon the encapsulation of the bacillus rather than the toxins (Welkos, 1991). The degree of virulence in the mouse model is correlated with the presence of the polyglutamic acid capsule on the bacillus (Welkos, 1991). In contrast, rats are extremely sensitive to the effects of the toxins but are relatively resistant to infection (Young et al., 1946). Thus, neither mice nor rats are considered good models of human anthrax.

Guinea Pigs Guinea pigs are also highly sensitive to anthrax and have been used for many years to study the pathogenesis of B. anthracis infection (Ross, 1957). The pathological changes observed in guinea pigs after inhalational exposure to B. anthracis are characterized by widespread edema and hemorrhage, particularly in the spleen, lungs, and lymph nodes. As seen in other animal models, the cellular inflammatory response observed after inhalational exposure is limited, consistent with a fulminating septicemia rather than a primary pulmonary infection (Albrink and Goodlow, 1959; Ross, 1957).

Rabbits In rabbits the effects observed from inhalational infection with B. anthracis are similar to those seen in humans and rhesus monkeys. Substantial pathological lesions are consistently observed in the spleen, lymph nodes, lungs, gastrointestinal tract, and adrenal glands (Zaucha et al., 1998). Inflammation, hemorrhage, and edema are frequently observed in the mediastinum and the intrathoracic lymph nodes. Hemorrhage and edema are sometimes found in the meninges of the brain, but with less inflammation than that seen in humans and rhesus monkeys (Zaucha, 2001). Other differences between rabbits and humans or rhesus monkeys include milder mediastinal lesions and a lower incidence of lung lesions. The weaker inflammatory response in rabbits may be the result of the shorter observed survival time, limiting development of leukocytic infiltration (Zaucha et al.,

1998). Primary pneumonic foci were not observed in rabbits, although they have been observed in humans, perhaps as the result of preexisting pulmonary disease.

Nonhuman Primates

Chimpanzees. At least one paper describes the effects of experimentally induced inhalational anthrax in chimpanzees (Albrink and Goodlow, 1959). Two of the four test animals in that study survived, despite evident bacteremia. They were later rechallenged with anthrax spore aerosols (only one animal survived rechallenge with a larger dose). The pathological changes resembled those observed in guinea pigs, mice, and monkeys, with widespread edema and hemorrhage, particularly in the spleen, lungs, and lymph nodes. Death appeared to result from fulminating sepsis rather than a primary pulmonary infection.

Rhesus monkeys. Most information about the pathology of inhalational anthrax in nonhuman primates is gleaned from studies carried out with rhesus monkeys (*Macaca mulatta*; also called macaques). The pathophysiology of anthrax in rhesus monkeys is similar to that in humans. Several studies have reported on the gross pathological changes observed in rhesus monkeys exposed to inhaled aerosolized anthrax spores (Berdjis et al., 1962; Fritz et al., 1995; Gleiser et al., 1963). Berdjis and colleagues (1962) described their findings from serial postmortem observation of young *M. mulatta* monkeys exposed to low and high doses of inhaled spores. They observed edema, hemorrhage, necrosis, and inflammatory infiltrates in the lungs, lymph nodes, spleen, and liver. Two autopsy studies of animals that died from inhalational exposure to anthrax (Fritz et al., 1995; Gleiser et al., 1963) had somewhat different findings. Both reported edema, hemorrhage, and necrosis of the lymph nodes in the monkeys; but in the first study (Gleiser et al., 1963), the affected lymph nodes were predominantly intrathoracic (hilar, mediastinal, and tracheobronchial), whereas in the more recent study (Fritz et al., 1995) the mesenteric lymph nodes were more commonly involved. Enlargement of the spleen was common in the study by Gleiser and colleagues but not in the study by Fritz and colleagues. Hemorrhagic meningitis was observed in a third of the animals in the study by Gleiser and colleagues and in half of the animals in the study by Fritz and colleagues. In addition, Dalldorf and colleagues (1971) described similar pathological effects of inhalational anthrax on cynomolgus monkeys (*Macaca fascicularis*), another type of macaque. Dalldorf and colleagues observed involvement of the mediastinal lymph nodes in all infected subjects, which led to edema and hemorrhage and which was accompanied by bacteremia.

Conclusion

From what is known and from the information described above, it appears that the pathology of anthrax in nonhuman primates such as macaques best mimics that seen in humans after inhalational exposure to *B. anthracis*. However, nonhuman primates are available in only limited numbers and are very costly to study. Although guinea pigs and, to some extent, rabbits are more susceptible to the disease than monkeys and humans, they are much more readily available and therefore may be helpful for use in the screening of various interventions.

Efficacy of AVA Against Anthrax in Animal Models

Mice

It is difficult to immunize mice against anthrax. Different strains of mice differ dramatically in their susceptibilities to different *B. anthracis* strains and in the protection from challenge afforded by AVA and other anthrax vaccines (Welkos and Friedlander, 1988). In fact, the bacterial capsule rather than the toxin appears to be the primary virulence factor for mice, so that vaccines such as AVA based on the PA aspect of anthrax toxins (LF or EF) are of reduced efficacy (Welkos, 1991; Welkos et al., 1993). Only when PA was combined with a potent adjuvant was protection conferred (Welkos et al., 1990). Protection against strains fully virulent in the mouse may involve mechanisms in addition to humoral immunity (Welkos and Friedlander, 1988).

Hamsters

Few data describing the efficacy of AVA in hamsters are available. However, Fellows and colleagues (2002) have demonstrated that AVA failed to protect Golden Syrian hamsters against parenteral challenge with virulent *B. anthracis* spores.

Guinea Pigs

Guinea pigs have been used extensively in anthrax vaccine development and serve as the standard test system for evaluations of anthrax vaccine potency. In the potency test, guinea pigs are immunized parenterally and are challenged with 1,000 spores of the Vollum strain administered subcutaneously (FDA, 1973).

However, guinea pigs are difficult to protect by immunization with human anthrax vaccines. The guinea pig is considered susceptible to spore infection but relatively resistant to anthrax toxins (Lincoln et al., 1967). Several studies in which guinea pigs were administered anthrax spores intramuscularly have indicated that the anti-PA antibodies stimulated by AVA are not sufficient to protect guinea pigs from intramuscular challenge with all strains of *B. anthracis* (Fellows et al., 2001; Ivins et al., 1994; Little and Knudson, 1986; Turnbull et al., 1986). An intramuscular challenge of guinea pigs with 10,000 spores of 33 different strains of *B. anthracis* showed that AVA provided only limited or minimal protection against most of the strains (Fellows et al., 2001). Similarly, guinea pigs challenged with anthrax spore aerosols were not well protected (survival rate, 20 to 26 percent) by AVA (Ivins et al., 1995). In contrast, guinea pigs were protected from several challenge strains when they were given live vaccines, although these vaccines often induced lower titers of antibodies to PA than cell-free preparations did (Little and Knudson, 1986; Turnbull et al., 1986). These data suggest that antigens in addition to PA or antibodies to PA epitopes other than those elicited by exposure to the human vaccines play a role in guinea pig immunity.

Aluminum hydroxide (used in AVA) appears to drive the helper T cell 2 humoral response with little or no enhancement of the helper T cell 1 cellular response. When guinea pigs were administered PA vaccines in conjunction with certain adjuvants known to enhance the helper T cell 1-mediated immune response as well as the humoral immune response, the animals were substantially protected (up to 100 percent) from an intramuscular challenge (Ivins et al., 1992) and an aerosol challenge (Ivins et al., 1995) with spores of the Ames strain. Augmentation of protection by addition of adjuvants was also seen with the PA vaccine produced in the United Kingdom (Jones et al., 1996; Turnbull et al., 1988). These findings suggest that the relevant epitopes for induction of a protective immune response in the guinea pig are present in AVA but that the vaccine may not stimulate the full complement of immune mechanisms needed for protection in this animal model (Ivins et al., 1994; Turnbull et al., 1988).

Rabbits

Studies of immunization of rabbits with AVA have recently shown that rabbits may show promise for use in the development of a correlate of protection from aerosol challenge with anthrax spores. Rabbits were given two doses of various dilutions of AVA and were then challenged with a lethal dose (roughly 1×10^7 spores, or 100 times the amount expected to kill half of the animals) of spores of the Ames strain of *B. anthracis*. Survival was correlated with the levels of anti-PA IgG and with TNA at the time of the peak antibody response and at the time of challenge (Pitt, 2001;

Pitt et al., 1999, 2001). These results were confirmed with a second lot of AVA (Pitt, 2001; Pitt et al., 2001). Pitt and colleagues (2001) also found that two human doses of AVA (0.5 ml) from three different lots of the vaccine provided rabbits with substantial protection (survival rates of 90 to 100 percent) from both subcutaneous and aerosol exposures to the Ames strain. In another study, AVA was found to completely protect rabbits from four of six anthrax isolates[3] of diverse geographical origin found to be highly virulent in guinea pigs and protected 90 percent of the animals from the other two isolates (Fellows et al., 2001).

Nonhuman Primates (Macaques)

Several studies have evaluated the efficacy of AVA against aerosol challenge with anthrax spores in rhesus monkeys. In one study, all monkeys given two 0.5-ml doses (the same dose licensed for use in humans) of AVA intramuscularly survived challenge with spores of the Ames strain (roughly 1×10^7 to 4×10^7 spores, or 255 to 760 times the amount expected to kill half of the animals, respectively) at 8 or 38 weeks after vaccination, whereas 88 percent survived challenge after 100 weeks (Ivins et al., 1996). In another study, all 10 monkeys that received two 0.5-ml doses of AVA intramuscularly survived challenge with a lethal dose of spores of the Ames strain (899 times the amount expected to kill half of the animals) 3 months after immunization (Pitt et al., 1996). In a third study, a single 0.5-ml intramuscular dose of AVA protected all 10 monkeys from aerosol challenge with spores of the Ames strain (approximately 5×10^6 spores, or 93 times the amount expected to kill half of the animals) at 6 weeks. Two of the animals (20 percent) demonstrated transient bacteremia for 1 day (Ivins et al., 1998). A study challenging 10 monkeys each with large doses (400-1,000 times the amount expected to kill half of the animals) of two isolates virulent in guinea pigs and rabbits found AVA to provide complete protection from one isolate and 80 percent protection from the other (Fellows et al., 2001).

Conclusions on the Efficacy of AVA Against Anthrax in Animal Models

From what is known and described above about the immune protection against infection with *B. anthracis* offered by AVA in humans and animals, it appears that AVA is effective in protecting both macaques and rabbits

---

[3]An isolate is a living bacterium now in culture that has been isolated from a specific patient or other source. Other than its source, no other information may be available. A number of isolates may belong to a single strain.

from inhalational exposure to the strains of anthrax tested. It affords incomplete protection in mice and guinea pigs.

As described earlier, the pathophysiology of anthrax in nonhuman primates most resembles that in humans. Among the smaller and more available laboratory animals, rabbits most closely resemble nonhuman primates in terms of the pathology of anthrax and their response to the anthrax vaccine. The guinea pig does not appear to be a good model because its response to the vaccine differs from that of the nonhuman primate. Although monkeys are consistently protected from anthrax challenge by a vaccine containing PA and alum, the protection of guinea pigs varies with the anthrax strain. For certain strains, protection in guinea pigs is enhanced by particular adjuvants known to stimulate cell-mediated immunity, although such adjuvants do not appear to be necessary for the protection of primates.

Finding: The macaque and the rabbit are adequate animal models for evaluation of the efficacy of AVA for the prevention of inhalational anthrax.

EFFICACY OF AVA AGAINST ALL KNOWN *B. ANTHRACIS* STRAINS

A variety of different *B. anthracis* strains are found in nature worldwide (Fellows et al., 2001; Keim et al., 2000), and the tissue samples analyzed from victims of the Sverdlovsk outbreak in 1979 that resulted from the release of spores from the Soviet biological weapons facility indicated the presence of several strains of *B. anthracis* (Grinberg et al., 2001; Jackson et al., 1998). It is important to establish whether AVA can afford protection against the full range of naturally occurring and engineered *B. anthracis* strains. This section reviews the evidence on the efficacy of AVA against all known anthrax strains.

Auerbach and Wright (1955) showed that rabbits immunized with protective antigen precipitated with alum from the R1-NP mutant of the Vollum strain of *B. anthracis* were protected against subcutaneous injections with 33 different virulent strains of *B. anthracis*. They similarly evaluated guinea pigs using 10 different challenge strains. The guinea pigs were protected from most strains, although they were partially susceptible to three of them.

Little and Knudson (1986) also showed that guinea pigs immunized with AVA are protected from many (18 out of 27), although not all, strains. Better protection was afforded by the live Sterne vaccine. (Live vaccines are not considered sufficiently safe for human use in the United States.) Turnbull and colleagues (1986) similarly found better protection from live spore vaccines but found AVA to provide very little (17 percent) protection against three strains other than Vollum. Ivins and colleagues (1994) confirmed that the level of protection afforded by AVA in guinea pigs differs depending on the challenge strain, although, in contrast to Turnbull's findings, in the majority of cases they found that protection was afforded against even the more vaccine-resistant strains. Fellows and colleagues (2001) also showed that the level of protection afforded by AVA in guinea pigs varied according to the *B. anthracis* isolate. Survival rates after intramuscular challenge with the spores of 33 geographically diverse *B. anthracis* isolates ranged from 6 to 100 percent.

The same study, however, established convincingly the efficacy of AVA in protecting macaques and rabbits from aerosol challenge with the spores of several virulent *B. anthracis* isolates shown to be lethal in AVA-immunized guinea pigs. Since macaques and rabbits appear to be the best available animal models of inhalational anthrax in humans, as discussed earlier in this chapter, the efficacy of AVA in protecting these species from aerosol challenge with a variety of virulent isolates is noteworthy. However, the relative virulence of strains does not necessarily correlate across species. Nonetheless, no AVA-resistant isolates have been demonstrated in nonhuman primates.

Observational data from human studies also support the efficacy of AVA against a variety of strains. The participants in the previously described study by Brachman and colleagues (1962), in which the Merck vaccine was effective against *B. anthracis* infection, were exposed to animal products from diverse geographical locations that had presumably been contaminated with multiple strains of *B. anthracis*. Similarly, the vaccinated participants in the CDC observational study were also at risk for exposure to a broad spectrum of *B. anthracis* strains. In neither instance, however, were the exposure strains evaluated.

A 1997 study published by Pomerantsev and colleagues proposed that novel strains of anthrax might be bioengineered to evade protection from current anthrax vaccines. However, the committee found serious flaws in the study. For example, the investigators provided no information regarding the levels of anti-PA antibody achieved following immunization. Hamsters were used as the challenge model, but little is known about them as an animal model. In addition, the engineered strains of *B. anthracis* used were poorly characterized genetically (i.e., it is not known how many copies of the cereolysin gene were inserted, where they were located in the genome, and whether polar effects were possible), which makes it difficult to interpret the results of the study. Recent news reports describe efforts of U.S. scientists to obtain samples of the strain described by Pomerantsev and colleagues (1997) and possible plans on the part of U.S. scientists to engineer a similar strain (Loeb, 2001). These efforts reflect concerns that AVA could be defeated by such engineered strains. For the reasons elaborated below, the committee believes that AVA should be effective against natural and plausible engineered strains of *B. anthracis*.

AVA is primarily a PA-based vaccine. The efficacy of AVA against a broad spectrum of *B. anthracis* strains is consistent with the critical role of PA in the pathogenesis of anthrax (Bhatnagar and Batra, 2001; Cataldi et al., 1990; Smith and Keppie, 1954). As described in Chapter 2, PA is necessary for the anthrax toxins to enter cells and cause damage. As shown in Figure 2-4, PA binds to a special cellular receptor and is activated to form heptamers at the cell surface. The heptamers bind to toxin proteins (EF and LF), and the resulting complexes are brought into an acidic compartment in the cell. In this acidic environment the PA heptamer inserts into the membrane and mediates the translocation of EF and LF into the cytosol, where the toxins do their damage. Therefore, for the anthrax toxins to create injury in the body, PA must be competent to carry out multiple complicated tasks: it must bind to its receptor, form a heptamer, and bring EF and LF into the cell. However, there is evidence that the ability of PA to perform these complex tasks is not robust. The quaternary structure of PA (see Petosa et al. [1997] for the crystallographic structure) is complex, requiring assembly of a heptamer, as noted above. Sellman and colleagues (2001; see also Mogridge et al. [2001]) have shown that the presence of even a few mutant subunits within a heptamer deactivates the ability of the heptamer to function. A deactivated heptamer likely would not be able to deliver EF and LF to the cytosol. The committee considers it highly unlikely that a mutant PA could be constructed at this time that would retain its function in these multiple steps yet escape protective antibodies directed against the wild-type PA, such as those generated by AVA.

Further evidence that it is difficult for changed versions of PA to function is found in the degree to which it has been conserved in nature. Recent research has established that the *B. anthracis* genome is highly conserved among strains isolated across a wide geographical area (Jackson, 2001; Keim et al., 1997). Furthermore, data presented at the 2001 International Anthrax Meeting show that PA is also very highly conserved (Jackson, 2001; Price et al., 1999). Because PA is critical to virulence and because its structure is so highly conserved, it appears likely that changing its structure would alter and thus eliminate its toxic action.

Finding: It is unlikely that either naturally occurring or anthrax strains with bioengineered protective antigen could both evade AVA and cause the toxicity associated with anthrax.

CORRELATION OF PROTECTION: ANIMAL MODELS AND HUMAN IMMUNITY

Establishing Animal Model Correlates of Anthrax Vaccine Efficacy

Reuveny and colleagues (2001) recently published findings from studies with guinea pigs evaluating anti-PA antibody and TNA as correlates of protection from *B. anthracis*. Guinea pigs were immunized with single injections of various dilutions of PA vaccine or with PA vaccine inactivated to various extents by heat and were then challenged with an intradermal injection of Vollum strain *B. anthracis* spores. An additional study used passive immunization of the guinea pigs with various amounts of hyperimmune sera before challenge. The investigators reported associations between percent survival of the guinea pigs and both anti-PA IgG antibody titers and TNA titers. However, the TNA titers appeared to be a better correlate of protection in this model system, whereas the anti-PA IgG antibody titers determined by ELISA had a limited value in predicting protective immunity. The passive transfer studies showed similar results, and the fact that hyperimmune sera could protect the animals indicates that a humoral response alone may be sufficient to confer protection.

It must be noted that immunity to *B. anthracis* is complex. While anti-PA antibodies have been shown to be necessary and sufficient for protection in the studies reviewed below, other studies, while confirming the central role of anti-PA antibodies, suggest that other antigens may also contribute to the ability to confer protection from the disease in some animal models (Brossier et al., 2002; Cohen et al., 2000; Pezard et al., 1995). Indeed several studies indicate difficulty in establishing a direct correlation between PA-specific antibody titers and protection (Ivins et al., 1990, 1995; Turnbull, 1991; Turnbull et al., 1986, 1988) whereas others have succeeded (see Reuveny et al. [2001] discussed above and Barnard and Friedlander [1999] discussed below).

Efficacy studies have indicated that PA must be present in a cell-free anthrax vaccine or produced by a live vaccine to achieve protection (Ivins et al., 1986, 1992, 1998). Little and colleagues (1997) showed by passive transfer between guinea pigs that the serum of animals immunized against PA was protective for naïve recipients (but that anti-EF and anti-LF antibodies were not). McBride and colleagues (1998) showed that recombinant PA administered with an appropriate adjuvant would protect guinea pigs from aerosol challenge. Barnard and Friedlander (1999) demonstrated that the protective efficacy of recombinant PA vaccines correlated with the anti-PA antibody titers they elicited in vivo and the level of PA they produced in vitro. Beedham and colleagues (2001) showed that several susceptible strains of mice could be protected from challenge by immunization with recombinant PA with adjuvant. Furthermore, their study indicated that protection resulted from circulating antibody, as passively transferred lymphocytes were not protective.

As described earlier, Pitt and colleagues (2001) reported serological correlates of immunity against inhalational anthrax in rabbits. The animals were immunized with AVA, and the levels of antibody to PA and TNA associated with protection were quantified. The levels of either antibody at 6 and 10 weeks after immunization proved to be predictive of survival.

Efforts have been made to evaluate the relationship between levels of anti-PA antibody and protection from *B. anthracis* challenge in nonhuman primates. A study by Ivins and colleagues (1998) indicated that rhesus monkeys have a strong immune response to PA, as evidenced by high titers of antibody to PA and high TNA titers. A single dose of AVA protected the monkeys from aerosol challenge with anthrax spores (roughly 5×10^6 spores). The high level of protection provided made it difficult to correlate anti-PA IgG antibody titers or other measures with levels of protection. Fellows and colleagues (2001) showed that rhesus monkeys had strong anti-PA antibody responses to two doses of 0.5 ml of AVA and were protected (80 to 100 percent survival) from aerosol challenge with spores from two virulent isolates.

Finding: The available data indicate that immunity to anthrax is associated with the presence of antibody to protective antigen.

The information reviewed by the committee shows that humans and certain laboratory animals both manifest the same disease after infection with *B. anthracis* and that both are protected by immunization with AVA, which elicits the production of antibodies to PA. This information establishes a *qualitative* correlation between antibodies to PA and protection in animal models and in humans. To move forward with research on the current anthrax vaccine or any new vaccines, however, a *quantitative* correlation of the protective levels of antibodies in animals with the antibody titers obtained after full immunization in humans is needed. Those correlates in animal models can then be used to test new vaccines for efficacy with confidence that the data from animal studies will be predictive of the clinical results obtained with immunized humans.

Correlating the protective level of antibody can, in principle, be accomplished either by active immunization or by passive immunization. In the first instance, animals would be vaccinated with various doses of vaccine and their antibody levels would be measured. They would then be challenged to determine the level of circulating antibody at which protection would no longer be reliable.

For passive immunization studies, it is necessary to immunize animals of the model species, collect the serum of the immunized animals, and administer different concentrations of that antibody-containing serum to naïve animal hosts. The latter procedure provides passive immunity to the hosts. The hosts must then be challenged with aerosolized *B. anthracis* spores to determine which animals survive during the period of observation and hence what concentration of antibody must be present to protect the host. The period of observation of the animals will need to be limited (on the order of 2 weeks after challenge), in keeping with the half-life of immunoglobulin. It would be useful to determine a correlation between the inoculum size (the number of spores) and the antibody level associated with protection. An inoculum size sufficient to simulate or exceed the quantity of spores likely to be encountered during exposure must be established.

After the intraspecies passive transfer assay in animal models, the next step extends to the human vaccinee. Here, appropriate laboratory animals would receive different concentrations of antibody-containing serum from humans vaccinated with anthrax vaccine. Again, the passively immunized animals would be challenged with aerosolized spores of an appropriate inoculum size to determine the extent of survival.

In the case of immunity to anthrax, the concentration of antibody to PA is of particular interest because PA is necessary for the virulence of the different strains in both humans and animal models. A similar strategy might be applied by using toxin neutralization. The TNA assay is a functional test that evaluates the amount of antibody needed to inactivate the lethal *B. anthracis* toxin complex of LF and PA (together, lethal toxin). The ability of test serum samples to neutralize lethal toxin in vitro is compared with that of a standard serum sample by using cytotoxicity as the endpoint of the assay (Pittman et al., 2002). Antibodies to either protein might be expected to neutralize cytotoxicity, but the assay is principally used to quantify antibody to PA.

Once quantitative correlates (the amount of antibody or toxin neutralization activity necessary for full protection from *B. anthracis* challenge) are established, a new vaccine could be administered to naïve animals over a range of concentrations to determine the dose required to obtain a level of antibody known to be protective. Finally, the investigational product could be administered to healthy human volunteers to determine its ability to stimulate production of comparable quantities of antibody and thereby choose the appropriate dose regimen required for protection. Furthermore, the resulting human antibody would be collected and the serum would be administered to additional naïve laboratory animals to confirm transferable passive immunity by showing that the antibodies produced would protect the host animal.

The data from studies with animals already developed suggest that serological correlates of human immunity can be developed in appropriate animal models. The committee commends this work and encourages its further development.

> Recommendation: Additional passive protection studies with rabbits and monkeys, including the transfer of animal and human sera, are urgently needed to quantify the protective levels of antibody in vivo against different challenge doses of anthrax spores.

> Recommendation: Additional active protection studies should be conducted or supported to develop data that describe the relationship between immunity and both specific and functional quantitative antibody levels, including studies of
>
> - the relationship between the vaccine dose and the resulting level of antibody in the blood of test animals that protects the animals from challenge;
> - the relationship between the level of antibody that protects animals from challenge and the level of antibody present in humans vaccinated by the regimen currently recommended for the licensed product; and
> - the vaccine dose that results in a level of antibody in the blood of human volunteers similar to that in the blood of protected animals.

Measurements of anti-PA antibody titers will be crucial to the success of the research described above. Progress will be hampered if assay results are not comparable across laboratories.

> Recommendation: The Department of Defense should support efforts to standardize an assay for quantitation of antibody levels that can be used across laboratories carrying out research on anthrax vaccines.

POSTEXPOSURE USE OF ANTHRAX VACCINE

Evidence that postal workers and congressional staff were exposed to aerosolized anthrax spores from anthrax-laden letters sent through the U.S. mail in the autumn of 2001 resulted in questions about the efficacy of AVA in protecting people from infection when the vaccine is administered after exposure to anthrax spores. No data from studies with humans are available to evaluate the efficacy of AVA in these circumstances. However, two papers provide information from studies with rhesus monkeys.

Henderson and colleagues (1956) carried out studies in which penicillin, immune serum, and a PA-based vaccine (a predecessor of AVA) were administered after animals had been exposed to aerosolized anthrax spores. Their findings suggested that postexposure vaccination together with penicillin successfully protected animals after challenge with roughly 7.5×10^5

spores (15 times the amount expected to kill half of the animals), whereas penicillin given alone for 5 or 10 days did not. Postexposure vaccination alone was not evaluated. The investigators estimated that 15 to 50 percent of the spores were still in the lungs of the animals 42 days after exposure and that traces of the spores remained even 100 days after exposure.

Friedlander and colleagues (1993) carried out similar studies with penicillin, ciprofloxacin, doxycycline, and AVA. Rhesus monkeys were exposed by inhalation to an initial challenge of roughly 4×10^5 spores. Animals given vaccine alone were not protected. Animals given antibiotics for 30 days were well protected during the time of treatment, but after antibiotics were discontinued in the group receiving antibiotics alone, 10 to 30 percent of the animals succumbed to anthrax. None of the animals treated with doxycycline for 30 days plus vaccination died of anthrax. The surviving animals treated with antibiotics alone did not have evidence of an antibody response to PA, whereas vaccinated animals made antibodies.

The survivors from the first experiment were rechallenged with roughly 3×10^6 spores (about 50 times the amount expected to kill half of the animals). Only those that had been vaccinated were significantly protected.

Administration of antibiotics for 30 days after exposure to aerosolized spores provided protection (70 to 90 percent survival) after antibiotics were discontinued. However, the data also indicated that spores can persist for long periods (up to 58 days in one animal). The protection offered by use of the combination of vaccination and antibiotics was complete but was not statistically different from that offered by the use of antibiotics only.

Taken together, these limited data suggest that the use of vaccine in combination with an appropriate antibiotic for 30 days could provide excellent postexposure protection against inhalational anthrax. Although the additional benefit from receiving the vaccine after a prolonged period of antibiotic use is not proven, reliance on the vaccine alone after exposure is clearly insufficient, as some protection is needed during the time required for an immune response to develop. Additional studies on the postexposure use of AVA with antibiotics are needed.

> **Recommendation:** The Department of Defense should pursue or support additional research with laboratory animals on the efficacy of AVA in combination with antibiotics administered following inhalational exposure to anthrax spores. Studies should focus on establishment of an appropriate duration for antibiotic prophylaxis after vaccine administration.

CONCLUSIONS REGARDING EFFICACY

A vaccine similar to the licensed vaccine, AVA, was shown to be effective against cutaneous anthrax in humans in the field trial supporting the original application for licensure of AVA (Brachman et al., 1962). Although that study had too few cases to evaluate the vaccine's efficacy for the prevention of inhalational disease, the five inhalational cases observed occurred only among nonvaccinated or placebo recipients, whereas none occurred among vaccinated workers. Data from CDC on cases reported between 1962 and 1974 also indicated that the vaccine offered protection against the cutaneous form of the disease (FDA, 1985). Furthermore, laboratory experiments indicate that AVA provides effective protection against inhalational challenge in rabbits and macaques, the animal models in which the disease is most reflective of the disease in humans (Fellows et al., 2001; Ivins et al., 1996, 1998; Pitt et al., 2001).

Again, such efficacy is relative. When macaques were exposed experimentally to doses of up to about 900 times the amount expected to kill half of the animals, 88 to 100 percent of the animals were protected, as described earlier. This can be considered very effective protection. However, simulation studies conducted by Canadian researchers suggest that a person opening a letter filled with anthrax spores and standing over it for 10 minutes could inhale up to 3,000 times, and perhaps as much as 9,000 times, the amount of spores expected to kill half of a group of exposed people (Brown, 2001, 2002). Exposures to anthrax spores released in public places or in most military encounters might be expected to be lower. Without experimental data from extremely high challenge doses, it is difficult to anticipate the potential limits of the vaccine's efficacy. For this reason the committee has recommended studies of vaccine protection as a function of challenge dose.

Because PA is critical to the virulence of *B. anthracis* and because PA's structure is so highly conserved, it appears likely that changing its structure would alter and thus eliminate its toxic action. Thus, it is unlikely that either naturally occurring anthrax strains or strains with bioengineered PA could both evade AVA and cause the toxicity associated with anthrax. Data from studies with animals suggest that AVA will offer protection against strains with PA-based toxicity. Finally, the available data indicate that immunity to anthrax is associated with the presence of antibodies to PA, such as those stimulated by the anthrax vaccine.

> **Finding: The committee finds that the available evidence from studies with humans and animals, coupled with reasonable assumptions of analogy, shows that AVA as licensed is an effective vaccine for the protection of humans against anthrax, including inhalational anthrax, caused by any known or plausible engineered strains of *B. anthracis*.**

REFERENCES

Abramova FA, Grinberg LM, Yampolskaya OV, Walker DH. 1993. Pathology of inhalational anthrax in 42 cases from the Sverdlovsk outbreak of 1979. *Proceedings of the National Academy of Sciences USA* 90(6):2291–2294.

Albrink WS. 1961. Pathogenesis of inhalation anthrax. *Bacteriological Reviews* 25:268–273.

Albrink WS, Goodlow RJ. 1959. Experimental inhalation anthrax in the chimpanzee. *American Journal of Pathology* 35(5):1055–1065.

Albrink WS, Brooks SM, Biron RE, Kopel M. 1960. Human inhalation anthrax: a report of three fatal cases. *American Journal of Pathology* 36(4):457–468.

Auerbach BA, Wright GG. 1955. Studies on immunity in anthrax. VI. Immunizing activity of protective antigen against various strains of *Bacillus anthracis*. *Journal of Immunology* 75:129–133.

Barnard JP, Friedlander AM. 1999. Vaccination against anthrax with attenuated recombinant strains of *Bacillus anthracis* that produce protective antigen. *Infection and Immunity* 67(2):562–567.

Beedham RJ, Turnbull PC, Williamson ED. 2001. Passive transfer of protection against *Bacillus anthracis* infection in a murine model. *Vaccine* 19(31):4409–4416.

Berdjis CC, Gleiser CA, Hartman HA, Kuehne RW, Gochenour WS. 1962. Pathogenesis of respiratory anthrax in *Macaca mulatta*. *British Journal of Experimental Pathology* 43:515–524.

Bhatnagar R, Batra S. 2001. Anthrax toxin. *Critical Reviews in Microbiology* 27(3):167–200.

Brachman PS, Gold H, Plotkin S, Fekety FR, Werrin M, Ingraham NR. 1962. Field evaluation of a human anthrax vaccine. *American Journal of Public Health* 52:632–645.

Brossier F, Levy M, Mock M. 2002. Anthrax spores make an essential contribution to vaccine efficacy. *Infection and Immunity* 70(2):661–664.

Brown D. 2001, December 12. Canadian study shows anthrax's easy spread: one letter could cause many deaths. *Washington Post*. p. A27.

Brown D. 2002, February 11. Agency with most need didn't get anthrax data: CDC unaware of Canadian study before attacks. *Washington Post*. p. A3.

Cataldi A, Labruyere E, Mock M. 1990. Construction and characterization of a protective antigen-deficient *Bacillus anthracis* strain. *Molecular Microbiology* 4(7):1111–1117.

Cohen S, Mendelson I, Altboum Z, Kobiler D, Elhanany E, Bino T, Leitner M, Inbar I, Rosenberg H, Gozes Y, Barak R, Fisher M, Kronman C, Velan B, Shafferman A. 2000. Attenuated nontoxinogenic and nonencapsulated recombinant *Bacillus anthracis* spore vaccines protect against anthrax. *Infection and Immunity* 68(8):4549–4558.

Dalldorf FG, Kaufmann AF, Brachman PS. 1971. Woolsorters' disease. An experimental model. *Archives of Pathology* 92(6):418–426.

FDA (Food and Drug Administration). 1973. Subpart C—Anthrax Vaccine, Adsorbed. *Federal Register* 38(223):32067–32068.

FDA. 1985. Biological products: bacterial vaccines and toxoids: implementation of efficacy review. Proposed rule. *Federal Register* 50(240):51002–51117.

FDA. 1999. New drug and biological drug products; evidence needed to demonstrate efficacy of new drugs for use against lethal or permanently disabling toxic substances when efficacy studies in humans ethically cannot be conducted. *Federal Register* 64(192):53960–53970.

Fellows PF, Linscott MK, Ivins BE, Pitt ML, Rossi CA, Gibbs PH, Friedlander AM. 2001. Efficacy of a human anthrax vaccine in guinea pigs, rabbits, and rhesus macaques against challenge by *Bacillus anthracis* isolates of diverse geographical origin. *Vaccine* 19(23–24):3241–3247.

Fellows PF, Linscott MK, Little SF, Gibbs P, Ivins BE. 2002. Anthrax vaccine efficacy in golden Syrian hamsters. *Vaccine* 20(9–10):1421–1424.

Friedlander AM, Welkos SL, Pitt ML, Ezzell JW, Worsham PL, Rose KJ, Ivins BE, Lowe JR, Howe GB, Mikesell P, Lawrence WB. 1993. Postexposure prophylaxis against experimental inhalation anthrax. *Journal of Infectious Diseases* 167(5):1239–1243.

Fritz DL, Jaax NK, Lawrence WB, Davis KJ, Pitt ML, Ezzell JW, Friedlander AM. 1995. Pathology of experimental inhalation anthrax in the rhesus monkey. *Laboratory Investigation; a Journal of Technical Methods and Pathology* 73(5):691–702.

Gleiser CA, Berdjis CC, Hartman HA, Gochenour WS. 1963. Pathology of experimental respiratory anthrax in *Macaca mulatta*. *British Journal of Experimental Pathology* 44:416–426.

Grinberg LM, Abramova FA, Yampolskaya OV, Walker DH, Smith JH. 2001. Quantitative pathology of inhalational anthrax. I. Quantitative microscopic findings. *Modern Pathology* 14(5):482–495.

Guillemin J. 1999. *Anthrax: the Investigation of a Deadly Outbreak*. Berkeley and Los Angeles, Calif.: University of California Press.

Henderson DW, Peacock S, Belton FC. 1956. Observations on the prophylaxis of experimental pulmonary anthrax in the monkey. *Journal of Hygiene* 54:28–36.

Ivins BE, Ezzell JW Jr, Jemski J, Hedlund KW, Ristroph JD, Leppla SH. 1986. Immunization studies with attenuated strains of *Bacillus anthracis*. *Infection and Immunity* 52(2):454–458.

Ivins BE, Welkos SL, Knudson GB, Little SF. 1990. Immunization against anthrax with aromatic compound-dependent (aro⁻) mutants of *Bacillus anthracis* and with recombinant strains of *Bacillus subtilis* that produce anthrax protective antigen. *Infection and Immunity* 58(2):303–308.

Ivins BE, Welkos SL, Little SF, Crumrine MH, Nelson GO. 1992. Immunization against anthrax with *Bacillus anthracis* protective antigen combined with adjuvants. *Infection and Immunity* 60(2):662–668.

Ivins BE, Fellows PF, Nelson GO. 1994. Efficacy of a standard human anthrax vaccine against *Bacillus anthracis* spore challenge in guinea pigs. *Vaccine* 12(10):872–874.

Ivins B, Fellows P, Pitt L, Estep J, Farchaus J, Friedlander A, Gibbs P. 1995. Experimental anthrax vaccines: efficacy of adjuvants combined with protective antigen against an aerosol *Bacillus anthracis* spore challenge in guinea pigs. *Vaccine* 13(18):1779–1784.

Ivins BE, Fellows PF, Pitt MLM, Estep JE, Welkos SL, Worsham PL, Friedlander AM. 1996. Efficacy of a standard human anthrax vaccine against *Bacillus anthracis* aerosol spore challenge in rhesus monkeys. *Salisbury Medical Bulletin* 87(Suppl):125–126.

Ivins BE, Pitt ML, Fellows PF, Farchaus JW, Benner GE, Waag DM, Little SF, Anderson GW Jr, Gibbs PH, Friedlander AM. 1998. Comparative efficacy of experimental anthrax vaccine candidates against inhalation anthrax in rhesus macaques. *Vaccine* 16(11–12):1141–1148.

Jackson PJ. 2001. Genetic diversity in *B. anthracis*. Presentation to the Institute of Medicine Committee to Assess the Safety and Efficacy of the Anthrax Vaccine, Meeting III, Washington, D.C.

Jackson PJ, Hugh-Jones ME, Adair DM, Green G, Hill KK, Kuske CR, Grinberg LM, Abramova FA, Keim P. 1998. PCR analysis of tissue samples from the 1979 Sverdlovsk anthrax victims: the presence of multiple *Bacillus anthracis* strains in different victims. *Proceedings of the National Academy of Sciences USA* 95(3):1224–1229.

Jernigan JA, Stephens DS, Ashford DA, Omenaca C, Topiel MS, Galbraith M, Tapper M, Fisk TL, Zaki S, Popovic T, Meyer RF, Quinn CP, Harper SA, Fridkin SK, Sejvar JJ, Shepard CW, McConnell M, Guarner J, Shieh WJ, Malecki JM, Gerberding JL, Hughes JM, Perkins BA. 2001. Bioterrorism-related inhalational anthrax: the first 10 cases reported in the United States. *Emerging Infectious Diseases* 7(6):933–944.

Johnson-Winegar A. 1984. Comparison of enzyme-linked immunosorbent and indirect hemagglutination assays for determining anthrax antibodies. *Journal of Clinical Microbiology* 20(3):357–361.

Jones MN, Beedham RJ, Turnbull PCB, Fitzgeorge RB, Manchee RJ. 1996. Efficacy of the UK human anthrax vaccine in guinea pigs against aerosolised spores of *Bacillus anthracis*. *Salisbury Medical Bulletin* 87(Suppl):123–124.

Keim P, Kalif A, Schupp J, Hill K, Travis SE, Richmond K, Adair DM, Hugh-Jones M, Kuske CR, Jackson P. 1997. Molecular evolution and diversity in *Bacillus anthracis* as detected by amplified fragment length polymorphism markers. *Journal of Bacteriology* 179(3):818–824.

Keim P, Price LB, Klevytska AM, Smith KL, Schupp JM, Okinaka R, Jackson PJ, Hugh-Jones ME. 2000. Multiple-locus variable-number tandem repeat analysis reveals genetic relationships within *Bacillus anthracis*. *Journal of Bacteriology* 182(10):2928–2936.

LaForce FM, Bumford FH, Feeley JC, Stokes SL, Snow DB. 1969. Epidemiologic study of a fatal case of inhalation anthrax. *Archives of Environmental Health* 18(5):798–805.

Lincoln RE, Walker JS, Klein F, Rosenwald AJ, Jones WI. 1967. Value of field data for extrapolation in anthrax. *Federation Proceedings* 26(5):1558–1562.

Little SF, Knudson GB. 1986. Comparative efficacy of *Bacillus anthracis* live spore vaccine and protective antigen vaccine against anthrax in the guinea pig. *Infection and Immunity* 52(2):509–512.

Little SF, Ivins BE, Fellows PF, Friedlander AM. 1997. Passive protection by polyclonal antibodies against *Bacillus anthracis* infection in guinea pigs. *Infection and Immunity* 65(12):5171–5175.

Loeb V. 2001, September 5. U.S. seeks duplicate of Russian anthrax: microbe to be used to check vaccine. *Washington Post*. p. A16.

McBride BW, Mogg A, Telfer JL, Lever MS, Miller J, Turnbull PC, Baillie L. 1998. Protective efficacy of a recombinant protective antigen against *Bacillus anthracis* challenge and assessment of immunological markers. *Vaccine* 16(8):810–817.

Mogridge J, Mourez M, Lacy B, Collier RJ. 2001. Role of protective antigen oligomerization in anthrax toxin action. In: *Program and Abstracts of the Fourth Annual Conference on Anthrax*. Washington, D.C.: American Society for Microbiology.

Petosa C, Collier RJ, Klimpel KR, Leppla SH, Liddington RC. 1997. Crystal structure of the anthrax toxin protective antigen. *Nature* 385(6619):833–838.

Pezard C, Weber M, Sirard JC, Berche P, Mock M. 1995. Protective immunity induced by *Bacillus anthracis* toxin-deficient strains. *Infection and Immunity* 63(4):1369–1372.

Pitt MLM. 2001. Animal models for anthrax vaccine efficacy. Presentation to the Institute of Medicine Committee to Assess the Safety and Efficacy of the Anthrax Vaccine, Meeting III, Washington, D.C.

Pitt MLM, Ivins BE, Estep JE, Farchaus J, Friedlander AM. 1996. Comparison of the efficacy of purified protective antigen and MDPH to protect non-human primates from inhalation anthrax. *Salisbury Medical Bulletin* 87(Suppl):130.

Pitt ML, Little S, Ivins BE, Fellows P, Boles J, Barth J, Hewetson J, Friedlander AM. 1999. In vitro correlate of immunity in an animal model of inhalational anthrax. *Journal of Applied Microbiology* 87(2):304.

Pitt ML, Little SF, Ivins BE, Fellows P, Barth J, Hewetson J, Gibbs P, Dertzbaugh M, Friedlander AM. 2001. In vitro correlate of immunity in a rabbit model of inhalational anthrax. *Vaccine* 19(32):4768–4773.

Pittman PR. 2001. Anthrax vaccine: the Fort Bragg Booster Study. Presentation to the Institute of Medicine Committee to Assess the Safety and Efficacy of the Anthrax Vaccine, Meeting II, Washington, D.C.

Pittman PR, Sjogren MH, Hack D, Franz D, Makuch RS, Arthur JS. 1997. *Serologic Response to Anthrax and Botulinum Vaccines*. Protocol No. FY92-5, M109, Log No. A-5747. Final report to the Food and Drug Administration. Fort Detrick, Md.: U.S. Army Medical Research Institute of Infectious Diseases.

Pittman PR, Mangiafico JA, Rossi CA, Cannon TL, Gibbs PH, Parker GW, Friedlander AM. 2000. Anthrax vaccine: increasing intervals between the first two doses enhances antibody response in humans. *Vaccine* 19(2–3):213–216.

Pittman PR, Kim-Ahn G, Pifat DY, Coon K, Gibbs P, Little S, Pace-Templeton J, Myers R, Parker GW, Friedlander AM. 2002. Anthrax vaccine: safety and immunogenicity of a dose-reduction, route comparison study in humans. *Vaccine* 20(9–10):1412–1420.

Pittman PR, Hack D, Mangiafico J, Gibbs P, McKee KT, Jr, Friedlander AM, Sjogren MH. In press. Antibody response to a delayed booster dose of anthrax vaccine and botulinum toxoid. *Vaccine*.

Plotkin SA, Brachman PS, Utell M, Bumford FH, Atchison MM. 1960. An epidemic of inhalation anthrax, the first in the twentieth century. *American Journal of Medicine* 29:992–1001.

Pomerantsev AP, Staritsin NA, Mockov YuV, Marinin LI. 1997. Expression of cereolysine AB genes in *Bacillus anthracis* vaccine strain ensures protection against experimental hemolytic anthrax infection. *Vaccine* 15(17–18):1846–1850.

Price LB, Hugh-Jones M, Jackson PJ, Keim P. 1999. Genetic diversity in the protective antigen gene of *Bacillus anthracis*. *Journal of Bacteriology* 181(8):2358–2362.

Reuveny S, White MD, Adar YY, Kafri Y, Altboum Z, Gozes Y, Kobiler D, Shafferman A, Velan B. 2001. Search for correlates of protective immunity conferred by anthrax vaccine. *Infection and Immunity* 69(5):2888–2893.

Ross JM. 1957. The pathogenesis of anthrax following the administration of spores by the respiratory route. *Journal of Pathology and Bacteriology* 73:485–494.

Sellman BR, Mourez M, Collier RJ. 2001. Dominant-negative mutants of a toxin subunit: an approach to therapy of anthrax. *Science* 292(5517):695–697.

Smith H, Keppie J. 1954. Observations on experimental anthrax: demonstration of a specific lethal factor produced in vivo by *Bacillus anthracis*. *Nature* 173:869.

Suffin SC, Carnes WH, Kaufmann AF. 1978. Inhalation anthrax in a home craftsman. *Human Pathology* 9(5):594–597.

Turnbull PC. 1991. Anthrax vaccines: past, present and future. *Vaccine* 9(8):533–539.

Turnbull PC, Broster MG, Carman JA, Manchee RJ, Melling J. 1986. Development of antibodies to protective antigen and lethal factor components of anthrax toxin in humans and guinea pigs and their relevance to protective immunity. *Infection and Immunity* 52(2):356–363.

Turnbull PC, Leppla SH, Broster MG, Quinn CP, Melling J. 1988. Antibodies to anthrax toxin in humans and guinea pigs and their relevance to protective immunity. *Medical Microbiology and Immunology* 177(5):293–303.

Walker D. 2001. Quantitative pathology of inhalational anthrax. Presentation to the Institute of Medicine Committee to Assess the Safety and Efficacy of the Anthrax Vaccine, Meeting III, Washington, D.C.

Welkos SL. 1991. Plasmid-associated virulence factors of non-toxigenic (pX01⁻) *Bacillus anthracis*. *Microbial Pathogenesis* 10(3):183–198.

Welkos SL, Friedlander AM. 1988. Comparative safety and efficacy against *Bacillus anthracis* of protective antigen and live vaccines in mice. *Microbial Pathogenesis* 5(2):127–139.

Welkos S, Becker D, Friedlander A, Trotter R. 1990. Pathogenesis and host resistance to *Bacillus anthracis*: a mouse model. *Salisbury Medical Bulletin* 63(Suppl):49–52.

Welkos SL, Vietri NJ, Gibbs PH. 1993. Non-toxigenic derivatives of the Ames strain of *Bacillus anthracis* are fully virulent for mice: role of plasmid pX02 and chromosome in strain-dependent virulence. *Microbial Pathogenesis* 14(5):381–388.

Young GA Jr, Zelle MR, Lincoln RE. 1946. Respiratory pathogenicity of *Bacillus anthracis* spores. I. Methods of study and observations on pathogenesis. *Journal of Infectious Diseases* 79:233–246.

Zaucha GM. 2001. The pathology of experimental inhalational anthrax in rabbits and rhesus monkeys. Presentation to the Institute of Medicine Committee to Assess the Safety and Efficacy of the Anthrax Vaccine, Meeting III, Washington, D.C.

Zaucha GM, Pitt LM, Estep J, Ivins BE, Friedlander AM. 1998. The pathology of experimental anthrax in rabbits exposed by inhalation and subcutaneous inoculation. *Archives of Pathology and Laboratory Medicine* 122(11):982–992.

4

Safety: Introduction

Vaccines are important tools for the prevention of serious infectious diseases. Through vaccination programs, naturally occurring smallpox has been eradicated globally and the incidence of other diseases including diphtheria, measles, mumps, pertussis, polio, and rubella has declined substantially in the United States and many other countries. As with any pharmaceutical product or medical procedure, however, the use of vaccines carries a risk of adverse health effects that must be weighed against the expected health benefit. Expectations for the safety of vaccines are especially high because, in contrast to therapeutic agents, which are given when a disease is known to be present (or at least suspected), vaccines are usually given to healthy people to protect them against a disease that they may not be exposed to in the future.

Until 1990, Anthrax Vaccine Adsorbed (AVA) had been administered primarily to a small population of workers—veterinarians, processors of animal hair and hides, and laboratory personnel—with a high risk of exposure to anthrax. Administration of AVA to U.S. military personnel during the Gulf War and more recently under the Anthrax Vaccine Immunization Program (AVIP) substantially increased the numbers of persons vaccinated and produced concerns among some that the vaccine might be responsible for serious adverse health effects.

As with efficacy, it is important to note that safety is relative, not absolute. In general, the term *safety* reflects expectations of relative freedom from, but not necessarily the complete absence of, harmful effects when a product is used prudently, considering the condition of the recipient and the health risk the product is directed against.[1] No single set of criteria defines acceptable limits on the frequency and severity of harmful effects. For this report the committee was charged with assessing the safety of AVA in terms of the frequency, types, and severities of adverse reactions, including differences in those reactions by sex, and long-term health implications of AVA vaccination.

This chapter reviews the concerns about the safety of AVA that have been raised and discusses issues related to the identification of vaccine-related adverse events. The types of information examined by the committee regarding the safety of AVA are summarized as well. The details of the available data and the committee's findings and recommendations regarding the safety of AVA and further safety monitoring are presented in the subsequent two chapters, with Chapter 5 reviewing the findings that have emerged from case reports of adverse reactions to AVA and Chapter 6 reviewing the results of formal epidemiologic studies.

SAFETY CONCERNS ABOUT THE ANTHRAX VACCINE

AVA was originally licensed in 1970. A Food and Drug Administration (FDA) review completed in 1975 classified AVA as safe and effective and found that use of AVA is indicated "only for certain occupational groups with a risk of uncontrollable or unavoidable exposure to the organism. It is recommended for individuals in industrial settings who come in contact with imported animal hides, furs, wool hair (especially goat hair, bristles, and bone meal, as well as in laboratory workers involved in ongoing studies on the organism" (FDA, 1985, p. 51058). More widespread use of the vaccine during the Gulf War and as part of AVIP, however, has resulted in new concerns about its possible association with serious acute and chronic health problems. Some have proposed that vaccination with AVA could have contributed to the chronic multisystem health complaints of some Gulf War veterans (GAO, 1999b,c; Nicolson et al., 2000). With the expansion of mandatory vaccination under AVIP, there have also been concerns that the health impact of vaccination with AVA was being missed because adverse events were underreported to military health care providers and to the Vaccine Adverse Event Reporting System (VAERS), operated by the Centers for Disease Control and Prevention and FDA (GAO, 1999d; Rovet,

---

[1]The definition of safety used by FDA is "the relative freedom from harmful effect to persons affected, directly or indirectly, by a product when prudently administered, taking into consideration the character of the product in relation to the condition of the recipient at the time" (21 C.F.R. § 600.3 [1999]).

1999). More than 400 members of the military who refused to accept vaccination with AVA have left military service voluntarily or involuntarily (Weiss, 2001), and mandatory vaccination against anthrax is reported to have been an important factor to some Air National Guard and Air Force Reserve personnel when making their decision to leave military service or move to inactive status (GAO, 2000).

As described in Chapter 2, the symptoms associated with vaccination against anthrax reported by witnesses at congressional hearings and directly to this Institute of Medicine (IOM) committee included fever, headache, malaise, swelling, joint pain, and tinnitus. Several witnesses also reported conditions that they ascribed to receipt of the anthrax vaccine, including hypogonadism; Stevens-Johnson syndrome, which affected their vision as well as their skin; and fatal aplastic anemia.

Recent reports from an IOM committee examining the potential health effects of agents to which Gulf War veterans may have been exposed concluded that receipt of AVA was associated with transient acute local and systemic effects (e.g., redness, swelling, and fever) but that the available evidence was "inadequate/insufficient" to determine whether any association with long-term adverse health effects exists (IOM, 2000a,b). That committee restricted its review, however, to the limited number of published studies. Since those IOM reports were completed, results of new Department of Defense (DoD) studies of health effects following vaccination with AVA have become available. The present report examines these new findings and reviews the older data.

IDENTIFYING VACCINE-RELATED ADVERSE EVENTS

An *adverse event* is an undesirable health outcome that follows a given exposure, as to a vaccine, but for which a causal relationship with the exposure may or may not have been established. If a causal relationship can be determined, adverse events can also be referred to as *adverse effects* or *adverse reactions*.

Determining whether receipt of a vaccine has caused a subsequent adverse event can be difficult (Chen, 2000; Ellenberg and Chen, 1997; IOM, 1997). Several IOM committees have had the task of evaluating evidence regarding suspected links between various vaccines and particular adverse events (IOM, 1991, 1994a,b, 2000b, 2001). The available data indicate that some vaccines are associated with rare but serious adverse effects (IOM, 1991, 1994a). In other cases, however, the available evidence does not support the hypothesized associations between adverse events and vaccination (IOM, 1994a, 2001). Several factors involved in assessment of whether a vaccine is associated with adverse events are reviewed here.

Characterizing Adverse Events

Adverse events can be characterized in terms of their extent, severity, duration, and timing of onset. The extent of adverse events can be either *local* or *systemic*. Local events, such as redness or soreness, affect a single area of the body, typically in the area of the injection. Systemic events, such as fever or malaise, have a more generalized effect on the body. The severity of adverse events is usually categorized as mild, moderate, or severe, and definitions of these categories vary.[2] The duration of events can be characterized as *acute* or *chronic*, with acute events having a relatively short course and chronic events having a lingering, perhaps permanent, effect on health status. *Immediate-onset* events are ones that have an observed onset within minutes, hours, or days following vaccination, whereas *later-onset* events are ones that arise months or years after vaccination. The characterization of events as "short term" and "long term" has been avoided in this report because these terms can be confusing; sometimes they refer to the duration of the event (standing for "acute" and "chronic," respectively), and other times they refer to the timing of onset (standing for "immediate" and "later," respectively).

Active Versus Passive Surveillance

Surveillance to detect adverse events can be either active or passive. *Active surveillance* requires direct, systematic follow-up of all vaccinated individuals to determine the presence or absence of adverse events. Information is usually collected at specified time intervals. Active surveillance is used as part of the extensive clinical testing that must be conducted to establish the safety and efficacy of a vaccine before it is licensed for use. The resource demands of active surveillance generally make it practical only for formal research studies. In contrast to the routine checks made by active surveillance to ensure complete and uniform reporting, with *passive surveillance* one waits for medical personnel or vaccinees to provide reports (Noah, 1997). Such reports are inherently incomplete, and this is well recognized as a major limitation of passive surveillance.

The information reviewed by the committee regarding the safety of vaccination with AVA is derived from both active and passive surveillance.

---

[2]The committee notes that the term *serious* has a regulatory definition. A serious event is one that results in death, a life-threatening adverse experience, or an intervention to prevent inevitable development of a life-threatening experience, hospitalization or prolongation of hospitalization, or a congenital anomaly or birth defect (Postmarketing Reporting of Adverse Drug Experiences. 21 C.F.R. § 314.80 [2000]). Thus, adverse events described as severe nonetheless may not be considered serious from a regulatory perspective.

A passive spontaneous surveillance system, VAERS, is the principal tool used in the United States for the routine monitoring of adverse events that may occur following any vaccination. VAERS and the VAERS data related to AVA are discussed in Chapter 5. DoD has also used data from formal epidemiologic studies, both ad hoc studies and analyses of the data in the Defense Medical Surveillance System (DMSS), to look for evidence of an association between vaccination with AVA and adverse events. These methods and results are discussed in Chapter 6.

Difficulties in Assessing Vaccine Safety

Several factors are known to make it difficult to assess the safety of vaccines (IOM, 1997, 2000b).

Small Study Populations

The number of people who are included in clinical trials conducted before vaccine licensure is relatively small compared with the number of people who will receive a vaccine once it is in general use. These studies can detect frequent reactions that disqualify a product as unsafe or that are considered acceptable given the expected benefit and intended use of the product. Premarketing studies are too small to reliably detect rare events that may be observed only when a vaccine is used by a much larger population. Instead, postmarketing surveillance efforts, such as those that are conducted by vaccine manufacturers and through VAERS (see Chapter 5) and that include formal epidemiologic studies of the type described in Chapter 6, are used to help identify less common adverse events after a vaccine is marketed and used by larger numbers of individuals.

Lack of Long-Term Follow-up

Prospective vaccine studies are usually designed to monitor subjects for only a few weeks or months and so typically provide no evidence regarding adverse events that might occur in the future.

Multiple Exposures

In vaccine trials it is possible to establish some control over other clinical and environmental exposures that a study population may experience. Those controls help increase the likelihood that observed events can be attributed to the vaccine. For vaccines in routine use, however, vaccinees are often exposed to many other factors that might affect their health, including other vaccines (administered simultaneously in the same injection, at the same site, or at a distant location), making it difficult to isolate any effect of the vaccine in question.

Lack of Unique Symptoms

No unique set of symptoms or clinical test results establishes a diagnosis of a vaccine-related adverse event. Many symptoms that follow vaccination (e.g., fever and itching) can arise from various sources, and the fact that the symptom follows vaccination may be a coincidental rather than a causal relationship.

Means of Data Collection

As noted above, routine monitoring for adverse events following vaccination depends primarily on spontaneous reports of cases of adverse events. Such reports can signal possible vaccine-related problems but cannot be used to determine incidence rates of adverse events. Because such reporting is mostly voluntary, the data collected are typically incomplete and unrepresentative of the overall experience of the population of vaccine recipients. Reporting can be affected by factors such as the seriousness of the event, the time that has elapsed since vaccination, and levels of awareness or suspicion of an association between a particular adverse event and vaccination.

Active surveillance also has limitations for assessment of vaccine safety. When conducted by a hands-on approach like ad hoc data collection, active surveillance can suffer from multiple potential sources of error in data collection, ranging from imbalanced respondent recall to respondent non-cooperation. Even when active surveillance is conducted with powerful tools like automated linked data systems, described in detail in this report because of the unique usefulness of the military's DMSS, the data from such systems have important limitations (described in Chapter 6). Furthermore, the organization, analysis, and interpretation of the data in such massive data sets also pose many challenges, including lack of a current methodology to address the many thousands of possible simultaneous comparisons, problems with data quality and validation, and limitations in the nature of the medical care and other experiences being captured in the data sets.

GAINING PERSPECTIVE ON ADVERSE EVENTS FOLLOWING VACCINATION

Studies of the adverse events observed following vaccination with the other vaccines routinely administered to adults can provide some perspective on reports of adverse events following vaccination with AVA. The committee commissioned a review of published peer-reviewed reports from prospective vaccine studies that included active surveillance of adverse events (Treanor, 2001). That review included an examination of data on sex differences in reports of adverse events. To identify studies for review, Treanor searched the Medline database for English-language reports on pertussis, Lyme disease, pneumococcal polysaccharide, meningococcal polysaccharide A and C, typhoid fever, influenza, hepatitis A, hepatitis B, and rabies vaccines and on diphtheria and tetanus (Td) toxoids, published from 1966 through 2000. Treanor also examined unpublished reports from a few directly relevant studies. All of the reports reviewed were limited to the acute events observed during limited follow-up periods.

The rates of local and systemic reactions are summarized in Table 4-1. As with AVA, local effects observed included injection site pain or arm soreness, erythema, swelling, induration, and pruritis. For some vaccines, such local effects were common. For example, erythema or swelling was reported by 22 to 35 percent of recipients of Td toxoids (Halperin et al., 2000a; Macko and Powell, 1985; Middaugh, 1979; Van der Wielen et al., 2000) and by 11 to 21 percent of recipients of influenza vaccine (al-Mazrou et al., 1991; Banzhoff et al., 2000; Halperin et al., 1998; Scheifele et al., 1990). Local pain of any degree was reported by 50 percent or more of recipients of acellular pertussis vaccine (Englund et al., 1992; Halperin et al., 2000a,b; Keitel et al., 1999; Van der Wielen et al., 2000), Td toxoids (Halperin et al., 2000b; Macko and Powell, 1985; Van der Wielen et al., 2000), influenza vaccine (al-Mazrou, 1991; Aoki et al., 1993; Jackson et al., 1999; Nichol et al., 1996; Scheifele et al., 1990), Lyme disease vaccine (Keller et al., 1994), and meningococcal polysaccharide vaccine (Diez-Domingo et al., 1998). In other studies, however, pain was reported by less than 20 percent of recipients of recombinant hepatitis B vaccine (Rustgi et al., 1995; Schiff et al., 1995; Tron et al., 1989) and rabies vaccine (Anderson et al., 1980). Rates of moderate to severe pain were low.

Reported systemic reactions included fever, malaise, fatigue, and joint pain. Such reactions affected less than 35 percent of vaccine recipients, with the highest rates observed in studies of influenza vaccine (al-Mazrou et al., 1991; Nichol et al., 1996). Rates of moderate to severe systemic reactions were generally less than 5 percent. Reports of fever ranged from none in studies of acellular pertussis vaccine recipients (Halperin et al., 2000b) and hepatitis A vaccine recipients (Czeschinski et al., 2000; Westblom et al., 1994) to 18 percent in studies of rabies vaccine recipients (Chutivongse et al., 1995); in most studies, fever was observed in less than 10 percent of vaccine recipients.

Sex differences in reactions to AVA vaccination are a source of concern, but data from studies of other vaccines are limited because most have not reported separate results for men and women. When such data are available, they generally show higher rates of local pain for women. For

TABLE 4-1 Local and Systemic Event Rates Reported in Selected Prospective Vaccine Trials

Vaccine	Reference	Number of Subjects	Fever
Acellular pertussis	Van der Wielen et al., 2000	96	4
	Halperin et al., 2000a	126	0
	Halperin et al., 2000b	149	7
Hepatitis A	Scheifele and Bjornson, 1993	64	3
	Westblom et al., 1994	186	0
	Hoke et al., 1995	91	3
	Czeschinski et al., 2000	75	0
Hepatitis B	Halliday et al., 1990	594	1
	Schiff et al., 1995	382	0.3
	Czeschinski et al., 2000	75	4
Influenza	Schiefele et al., 1990	266	13
	al-Mazrou et al., 1991	330	9
	Aoki et al., 1993	76	2
	Nichol et al., 1996	418	6
	Banzhoff et al., 2000	61	2
	Banzhoff et al., 2000	61	1
	Halperin et al., 1998		1
Rabies	Anderson et al., 1980	234	3
	Chutivongse et al., 1995	202	18
	Jaiiaroensup et al., 1998	599	2
	Fritzell et al., 1992	46	—
Tetanus-diphtheria	Middaugh, 1979	697	—
	Macko and Powell, 1985	100	7
	Van der Wielen et al., 2000	98	9
	Halperin et al., 2000a	126	0.8

[a]Systemic side effects include malaise, fatigue, and decreased energy, but headache was not included.

[b]In studies in which the category "any" was not reported, the rate of the most frequent systemic side effect is used.

Percent of Subjects Reporting the Following Side Effects Following Vaccination

	Systemic[a]	Erythema or Swelling		Pain		
Any[b]	Moderate or Severe	Any	Moderate or Severe	Any	Moderate or Severe	Any Disability
27	1[c]	12	1[c]	72	0[c]	—[d]
17	8	15	3	51	7	—
29	10	13	10[e]	77	11	—
16	—	8	—	52	—	—
22	—	5	—	47	—	—
4	—	4	—	40	—	—
14	0	40	2	41	1	—
—	—	9	—	16	—	—
—	—	0.5	—	11	—	—
10	7	99	3	43	6	—
—	—	20	—	86	—	—
33	—	18	—	24	—	1
17	—	—	—	61	—	—
34	—	—	—	64	21	6
18	4	21	0	28	2	—
18	4	21	0	28	2	—
11	1[c]	11	8[c]	35	3[c]	—
3	—	18	—	14	—	—
—	—	—	—	4	—	—
—	—	1	—	20	—	—
—	—	13	—	52	—	—
—	—	35	—	43	—	—
—	—	30	—	75	27	—
17	1[c]	35	6[c]	83	0[c]	—
26	8	22	11[e]	85	15	—

[c]In these studies, the descriptor "clinically significant" was used in place of "moderate or severe" or "greater than moderate."
[d]Not reported.
[e]In these studies, local reactions were dichotomized as >10 mm or <10 mm in diameter.

SOURCE: Treanor (2001).

influenza vaccine, for example, rates of arm soreness were 34 percent for men and 49 percent for women, but rates of systemic effects were similar (Nichol et al., 1996). An analysis of 14 unpublished studies of influenza vaccine given to young adults also found that women had significantly higher rates of six of seven local effects and of two of five systemic effects (Beyer et al., 1996). The pooled odds ratio for any local symptom for men compared with that for women was 0.32 (95 percent confidence interval [CI] = 0.26 to 0.40), and the pooled odds ratio for any systemic symptom was 0.51 (95 percent CI = 0.39 to 0.67). An unpublished comparison based on acellular pertussis and hepatitis A vaccines found that for either vaccine women had higher rates of local reactions (redness, lumps, and swelling) than men and that women and men had similar (and low) rates of systemic reactions, including fever, chills, muscle aches, and decreased activity (Ward, 2001). An unpublished study of higher and lower doses of influenza vaccine also found a significantly higher rate of local pain among women who received the lower vaccine dose (Treanor, 2001).

AVA differs from many vaccines in that it is licensed for subcutaneous rather than intramuscular administration, but few studies of any vaccine have compared the effects following administration of the vaccine by these two routes. For the hepatitis B (Yamamoto et al., 1986) and rabies (Selimov et al., 1988) vaccines, similar rates of local and systemic effects have been observed when the vaccine is administered by either route. For the meningococcal polysaccharide vaccine, local erythema was more common when it was administered by the subcutaneous route (Ruben et al., 2001). Also, a study of rabies vaccine found that intradermal administration was associated with lower rates of local pain (3 percent) compared with the rates after intramuscular administration (19 percent) but higher rates of local pruritis (29 versus 3 percent; Jaiiaroensup et al., 1998). Unpublished data from a pilot study of an adjuvanted pneumococcal vaccine show higher rates of local erythema and induration with subcutaneous administration but higher rates of pain on injection with intramuscular administration (Treanor, 2001). While a number of commonly used and well-tolerated vaccines are administered subcutaneously (e.g., inactivated poliovirus, measles-mumps-rubella, varicella, and meningococcal vaccines), they differ from AVA in that they are not inactivated bacterial vaccines.

The findings from the studies that were reviewed are subject to limitations, many of which also apply to studies of AVA. In particular, the observed effects are linked to a vaccine because they are observed following administration of the vaccine but are not necessarily linked through other evidence of causality. In a few studies, comparisons with placebo controls help strengthen or weaken the observed association with those effects. For example, recipients of influenza vaccine reported substantially higher rates of arm soreness (64 percent) compared with recipients of a placebo (24 percent), but rates of fever were the same in vaccine and placebo recipients (6 percent; Nichol et al., 1996). In addition, because of the small sample sizes of most of these studies, the studies could not reliably detect rare events. Finally, most vaccine studies are conducted to assess efficacy rather than adverse effects. The lack of a standard set of adverse effects to be reported and the lack of standard definitions of such effects or of their severity can make it difficult to interpret or compare the results and data from different reports.

SOURCES OF INFORMATION REGARDING THE SAFETY OF AVA

To assess the safety of the anthrax vaccine, the committee examined information from individual case reports and from published and unpublished epidemiologic studies conducted with human populations. Individual case reports and case series provide information about illnesses that individuals or clinicians suspect may be linked with a specific exposure. Such reports can help to generate hypotheses about possible associations but are rarely helpful in confirming such associations. The case reports relating to AVA come from VAERS (see Chapter 5). The committee also heard personal testimony regarding adverse events following vaccination with AVA. These statements, some of which concerned cases reported to VAERS, added valuable insight into the conditions that some military personnel are experiencing.

Epidemiologic studies, which examine relationships between exposures (e.g., vaccination) and health outcomes in defined populations, provide a stronger basis for assessing causality than case reports. Most of the information reviewed by the committee came from such sources. Data are available from two randomized controlled clinical trials (Brachman et al., 1962; Pittman et al., 2002) and from several observational studies. Some of the observational studies include control groups, which make it possible to compare rates of adverse events in those with and without vaccination. The studies are mixed in their use of active and passive surveillance for adverse events. The key features and findings of each study are presented in Chapter 6. The committee did not include various studies that have sought to identify risk factors for the health problems reported by some Gulf War veterans. Although some of these studies have suggested an association between veterans' health problems and vaccinations (e.g., Cherry et al., 2001; Hotopf et al., 2000), they were not designed to study the effects of vaccine exposure. In addition, the analyses and the interpretation of their results are hindered by the veterans' exposure to multiple vaccines, incomplete vaccination records, and the need to rely on self-reports of vaccine exposure.

Results from animal and in vitro studies were also considered. However, most animal studies of vaccination with AVA do not present information regarding the presence or absence of reactions. The few studies that do comment on reactions (Darlow et al., 1956; IOM, 2000a; Ivins et al., 1998; Wright et al., 1954) report no vaccine-related adverse effects. Two laboratory assessments of possible vaccine contaminants are discussed at the end of this chapter. However, although animal and laboratory studies can, in some instances, elucidate the biological plausibility of a possible association between vaccination and an adverse event, they cannot provide direct evidence of causality in humans.

AVA contains aluminum hydroxide as an adjuvant. Aluminum has been used in vaccines for nearly 70 years in the form of the salts aluminum hydroxide, aluminum phosphate, and alum (Malakoff, 2000). Some have expressed concerns about the safety of aluminum adjuvants (e.g., Gherardi et al., 1998). For its assessment of the safety of AVA, the committee focused on data from studies of the complete vaccine product. This approach captures the contribution that aluminum might make to any vaccine-related adverse health effects associated with AVA, although it does not make it possible to attribute any effects to aluminum per se.

Reviews such as this one are often restricted to reports published in the peer-reviewed literature because the peer-review process provides some assurance that a study meets essential standards of quality. The committee decided, however, to consider unpublished epidemiologic analyses conducted by DoD and other researchers, because such studies offered the best available and most direct analyses of the possible association between AVA and various health outcomes. Many of the manuscripts describing these studies were under review or were being prepared for submission to a journal at the time they were presented to the committee. Committee members heard presentations from the researchers who conducted these studies and had an opportunity to question them about their study methodologies and analyses as well as to review draft manuscripts.[3] In some cases, the researchers conducted additional analyses in response to requests from the committee. Thus, sufficient information was available in these instances to judge the quality of the research and determine the degree to which results should contribute to conclusions about vaccine safety.

The committee reviewed all safety-related information that was brought to its attention and weighed the scientific merits of each element in arriving at conclusions regarding the safety of AVA. As indicated above, individual case reports and case series are useful for raising concerns or stimulating further research but are rarely conclusive in establishing causal associa-

---

[3]Documents and overheads provided to the committee are available to the public through the Public Access Records Office, National Academy of Sciences.

tions. Controlled epidemiologic studies provide the best evidence for the examination of associations of vaccination and subsequent adverse events. In evaluations of the studies presented to the committee, additional weight was given to those that (1) used active surveillance rather than self-reports of postimmunization events; (2) included sufficiently large numbers of subjects; (3) had clearly specified, objective criteria for the definition of adverse events; and (4) had sufficiently long postimmunization follow-up intervals to allow identification of later-onset events. Those studies that included a suitable unimmunized comparison group or in which evaluators were blinded to the subjects' vaccination status were especially useful to the committee.

TESTING FOR VACCINE CONTAMINATION

Among the concerns that have been raised about the anthrax vaccine is that contaminants in the vaccine product are producing adverse health outcomes. Laboratory analyses have been conducted to test for the presence of two suggested contaminants, mycoplasma and squalene.

Mycoplasma

Mycoplasma contamination of the anthrax vaccine has been suggested as a possible cause of illness among Gulf War veterans (Nicolson et al., 2000). Mycoplasmas are a distinctive type of bacteria that lack cell walls (Baseman and Tully, 1997). Many mycoplasma species appear to be harmless constituents of the normal human microbial flora, but others are associated with various diseases, including atypical pneumonia, genitourinary infections, joint diseases, and opportunistic infections in persons with compromised immune systems. Mycoplasma contamination is considered possible in vaccines produced in cell cultures, and FDA requires testing to demonstrate the absence of such contamination (Hart et al., 2002). For vaccines like AVA that are not derived from cell cultures, contamination is considered unlikely. However, to respond to the concerns about AVA, DoD commissioned two nonmilitary laboratories to conduct studies with samples from five AVA lots. The samples were obtained from eight different DoD vaccination clinics.

Hart and colleagues (2002) have reported on the results of those tests. Tests for the presence of live organisms were conducted at the National Cancer Institute's Mycoplasma Laboratory, which is located in Frederick, Maryland, and operated by Science Applications International Corporation. No mycoplasma colonies could be cultivated from the vaccine samples tested. In addition, tests of a vaccine sample deliberately inoculated with mycoplasma showed no presence of viable organisms after 24 hours. Separate tests by polymerase chain reaction assay, conducted at Charles River Tektagen, a commercial facility, showed no presence of mycoplasma DNA in any of the samples.

Squalene

Some Gulf War veterans and others have expressed concerns about whether squalene might be present in the anthrax vaccine and whether it has the potential to cause health effects. Squalene is a hydrocarbon compound found in many natural sources, including olive oil and the human body. In humans it is a precursor in the synthesis of cholesterol and is also found in oils of the skin (Kelly, 1999; Final Report, 1982). In the 1970s the average dietary intake of squalene was calculated to be 24 milligrams (mg) per day in a 2,000-calorie diet (Liu et al., 1976). Among people whose diets include more olive oil, squalene consumption can range from 200 to 400 mg/day (Smith, 2000). Roughly 60 percent of the squalene consumed in the diet is absorbed through the gastrointestinal tract; much of what is absorbed is converted into cholesterol (Strandberg et al., 1990).

The IOM Committee on Health Effects Associated with Exposures During the Gulf War (IOM, 2000b) examined in detail evidence regarding the potential health effects of squalene, including those that might be related to its use as a vaccine adjuvant. In the United States, it has been tested in animal studies of anthrax vaccine and in human studies of other vaccines (GAO, 1999a; Ivins et al., 1995; Ott et al., 1995), but it is not used in any human vaccine currently in use in the United States. An influenza vaccine with squalene as an adjuvant has been approved and distributed in Europe and has not been associated with adverse health events. The prior IOM (2000b) review resulted in the conclusion that, in certain animals and under selected conditions, squalene has been found to produce arthritis and neuropathology, but it also resulted in the conclusion that the relevance of toxicity findings for animals to humans is uncertain, in part because humans absorb squalene differently from animals. The human studies testing a squalene-containing adjuvant in other vaccines found only transient acute effects.

DoD sponsored a study by SRI International, a private company, to assay AVA and other pharmaceuticals for squalene at the level of parts per billion. The study report, dated August 14, 2001, found that 1 lot of over 30 lots tested contained measurable levels of squalene. Three samples from that lot contained squalene at 7, 9, and approximately 1 parts per billion, respectively. Use of vaccine from that lot has not been associated with elevated rates of adverse events (see the discussion of the Special Immunizations Program in Chapter 6).

Conclusion

Because the available data demonstrate the absence of mycoplasma contamination and demonstrate that the presence of trace amounts of squalene is not associated with an increase in the rates of adverse events following vaccination with AVA, the committee concludes that further investigation of possible AVA contamination is not warranted at this time.

REFERENCES

al-Mazrou A, Scheifele DW, Soong T, Bjornson G. 1991. Comparison of adverse reactions to whole-virion and split-virion influenza vaccines in hospital personnel. *Canadian Medical Association Journal* 145(3):213–218.

Anderson LJ, Winkler WG, Hafkin B, Keenlyside RA, D'Angelo LJ, Deitch MW. 1980. Clinical experience with a human diploid cell rabies vaccine. *JAMA* 244(8):781–784.

Aoki FY, Yassi A, Cheang M, Murdzak C, Hammond GW, Sekla LH, Wright B. 1993. Effects of acetaminophen on adverse effects of influenza vaccination in health care workers. *Canadian Medical Association Journal* 149(10):1425–1430.

Banzhoff A, Schwenke C, Febbraro S. 2000. Preservative-free influenza vaccine. *Immunology Letters* 71(2):91–96.

Baseman JB, Tully JG. 1997. Mycoplasmas: sophisticated, reemerging, and burdened by their notoriety. *Emerging Infectious Diseases* 3(1):21–32.

Beyer WE, Palache AM, Kerstens R, Masurel N. 1996. Gender differences in local and systemic reactions to inactivated influenza vaccine, established by a meta-analysis of fourteen independent studies. *European Journal of Clinical Microbiology and Infectious Diseases* 15(1):65–70.

Brachman PS, Gold H, Plotkin S, Fekety FR, Werrin M, Ingraham NR. 1962. Field evaluation of a human anthrax vaccine. *American Journal of Public Health* 52:632–645.

Chen RT. 2000. Special methodological issues in pharmacoepidemiology studies of vaccine safety. In: Strom BL, ed. *Pharmacoepidemiology*. 3rd ed. West Sussex, England: John Wiley & Sons, Ltd. Pp. 707–732.

Cherry N, Creed F, Silman A, Dunn G, Baxter D, Smedley J, Taylor S, Macfarlane GJ. 2001. Health and exposures of United Kingdom Gulf War veterans. Part II. The relation of health to exposure. *Occupational and Environmental Medicine* 58(5):299–306.

Chutivongse S, Wilde H, Benjavongkulchai M, Chomchey P, Punthawong S. 1995. Postexposure rabies vaccination during pregnancy: effect on 202 women and their infants. *Clinical Infectious Diseases* 20(4):818–820.

Czeschinski PA, Binding N, Witting U. 2000. Hepatitis A and hepatitis B vaccinations: immunogenicity of combined vaccine and of simultaneously or separately applied single vaccines. *Vaccine* 18(11–12):1074–1080.

Darlow HM, Belton FC, Henderson DW. 1956. The use of anthrax antigen to immunize man and monkey. *Lancet* ii(Sept 8):476–479.

Diez-Domingo J, Albert A, Valdivieso C, Ballester A, Diez LV, Morant A. 1998. Adverse events after polysaccharide meningococcal A&C vaccine. *Scandinavian Journal of Infectious Diseases* 30(6):636–638.

Ellenberg SS, Chen RT. 1997. The complicated task of monitoring vaccine safety. *Public Health Reports* 112(1):10–20.

Englund JA, Glezen WP, Barreto L. 1992. Controlled study of a new five-component acellular pertussis vaccine in adults and young children. *Journal of Infectious Diseases* 166(6): 1436–1441.

FDA (Food and Drug Administration). 1985. Biological products: bacterial vaccines and toxoids: implementation of efficacy review. Proposed rule. *Federal Register* 50(240): 51002–51117.

Final Report. 1982. Final report on the safety assessment of squalane and squalene. *Journal of the American College of Toxicology* 1(2):37–56.

Fritzell C, Rollin PE, Touir M, Sureau P, Teulieres L. 1992. Safety and immunogenicity of combined rabies and typhoid fever immunization. *Vaccine* 10(5):299–300.

GAO (General Accounting Office). 1999a. *Gulf War Illnesses: Questions About the Presence of Squalene Antibodies in Veterans Can Be Resolved*. GAO/NSIAD-99-5. Washington, D.C.: GAO.

GAO. 1999b. *Medical Readiness: Safety and Efficacy of the Anthrax Vaccine*. GAO/T-NSIAD-99-148. Washington, D.C.: GAO.

GAO. 1999c. *Anthrax Vaccine: Safety and Efficacy Issues*. GAO/T-NSAID-00-48. Washington, D.C.: GAO.

GAO. 1999d. *Medical Readiness: DoD Faces Challenges in Implementing Its Anthrax Vaccine Immunization Program*. GAO/NSIAD-00-36. Washington, D.C.: GAO.

GAO. 2000. *Anthrax Vaccine: Preliminary Results of GAO's Survey of Guard/Reserve Pilots and Aircrew Members*. GAO-01-92T. Washington, D.C.: GAO.

Gherardi RK, Coquet M, Cherin P, Authier FJ, Laforet P, Belec L, Figarella-Branger D, Mussini JM, Pellissier JF, Fardeau M. 1998. Macrophagic myofasciitis: an emerging entity. Groupe d'Etudes et Recherche sur les Maladies Musculaires Acquises et Dysimmunitaires (GERMMAD) de l'Association Francaise contre les Myopathies (AFM). *Lancet* 352(9125):347–352.

Halliday ML, Rankin JG, Bristow NJ, Coates RA, Corey PN, Strickler AC. 1990. A randomized double-blind clinical trial of a mammalian cell-derived recombinant DNA hepatitis B vaccine compared with a plasma-derived vaccine. *Archives of Internal Medicine* 150(6): 1195–1200.

Halperin SA, Nestruck AC, Eastwood BJ. 1998. Safety and immunogenicity of a new influenza vaccine grown in mammalian cell culture. *Vaccine* 16(13):1331–1335.

Halperin SA, Smith B, Russell M, Hasselback P, Guasparini R, Skowronski D, Meekison W, Parker R, Lavigne P, Barreto L. 2000a. An adult formulation of a five-component acellular pertussis vaccine combined with diphtheria and tetanus toxoids is safe and immunogenic in adolescents and adults. *Vaccine* 18(14):1312–1319.

Halperin SA, Smith B, Russell M, Scheifele D, Mills E, Hasselback P, Pim C, Meekison W, Parker R, Lavigne P, Barreto L. 2000b. Adult formulation of a five component acellular pertussis vaccine combined with diphtheria and tetanus toxoids and inactivated poliovirus vaccine is safe and immunogenic in adolescents and adults. *Pediatric Infectious Disease Journal* 19(4):276–283.

Hart MK, DelGiudice RA, Korch GW. 2002. Absence of mycoplasma contamination in anthrax vaccine. *Emerging Infectious Diseases* 8(1):94–96.

Hoke CH Jr, Egan JE, Sjogren MH, Sanchez J, DeFraites RF, MacArthy PO, Binn LN, Rice R, Burke A, Hill J, et al. 1995. Administration of hepatitis A vaccine to a military population by needle and jet injector and with hepatitis B vaccine. *Journal of Infectious Diseases* 171(Suppl 1):S53–S60.

Hotopf M, David A, Hull L, Ismail K, Unwin C, Wessely S. 2000. Role of vaccinations as risk factors for ill health in veterans of the Gulf War: cross sectional study. *British Medical Journal* 320(7246):1363–1367.

IOM (Institute of Medicine). Howson CP, Howe CJ, Fineberg HV, eds. 1991. *Adverse Effects of Pertussis and Rubella Vaccines*. Washington, D.C.: National Academy Press.

IOM. 1994a. Stratton KR, Howe CJ, Johnston RB Jr, eds. *Adverse Events Associated with Childhood Vaccines: Evidence Bearing on Causality.* Washington, D.C.: National Academy Press.

IOM. 1994b. Stratton KR, Howe CJ, Johnston RB Jr, eds. *Research Strategies for Assessing Adverse Events Associated with Vaccines: a Workshop Summary.* Washington, D.C.: National Academy Press.

IOM. 1997. *Vaccine Safety Forum: Summaries of Two Workshops.* Washington, D.C.: National Academy Press.

IOM. 2000a. *An Assessment of the Safety of the Anthrax Vaccine: A Letter Report.* Washington, D.C.: National Academy Press.

IOM. 2000b. Fulco CE, Liverman CT, Sox HC, eds. *Gulf War and Health.* Washington, D.C.: National Academy Press.

IOM. 2001. Stratton K, Gable A, Shetty P, McCormick M, eds. *Immunization Safety Review: Measles-Mumps-Rubella Vaccine and Autism.* Washington, D.C.: National Academy Press.

Ivins B, Fellows P, Pitt L, Estep J, Farchaus J, Friedlander A, Gibbs P. 1995. Experimental anthrax vaccines: efficacy of adjuvants combined with protective antigen against an aerosol *Bacillus anthracis* spore challenge in guinea pigs. *Vaccine* 13(18):1779–1784.

Ivins BE, Pitt ML, Fellows PF, Farchaus JW, Benner GE, Waag DM, Little SF, Anderson GW Jr, Gibbs PH, Friedlander AM. 1998. Comparative efficacy of experimental anthrax vaccine candidates against inhalation anthrax in rhesus macaques. *Vaccine* 16(11–12): 1141–1148.

Jackson LA, Benson P, Sneller VP, Butler JC, Thompson RS, Chen RT, Lewis LS, Carlone G, DeStefano F, Holder P, Lezhava T, Williams WW. 1999. Safety of revaccination with pneumococcal polysaccharide vaccine. *JAMA* 281(3):243–248.

Jaiiaroensup W, Lang J, Thipkong P, Wimalaratne O, Samranwataya P, Saikasem A, Chareonwai S, Yenmuang W, Prakongsri S, Sitprija V, Wilde H. 1998. Safety and efficacy of purified Vero cell rabies vaccine given intramuscularly and intradermally. (Results of a prospective randomized trial). *Vaccine* 16(16):1559–1562.

Keitel WA, Muenz LR, Decker MD, Englund JA, Mink CM, Blumberg DA, Edwards KM. 1999. A randomized clinical trial of acellular pertussis vaccines in healthy adults: dose-response comparisons of 5 vaccines and implications for booster immunization. *Journal of Infectious Diseases* 180(2):397–403.

Keller D, Koster FT, Marks DH, Hosbach P, Erdile LF, Mays JP. 1994. Safety and immunogenicity of a recombinant outer surface protein A Lyme vaccine. *JAMA* 271(22):1764–1768.

Kelly GS. 1999. Squalene and its potential clinical uses. *Alternative Medicine Review* 4(1):29–36.

Liu GC, Ahrens EH Jr, Schreibman PH, Crouse JR. 1976. Measurement of squalene in human tissues and plasma: validation and application. *Journal of Lipid Research* 17(1):38–45.

Macko MB, Powell CE. 1985. Comparison of the morbidity of tetanus toxoid boosters with tetanus-diphtheria toxoid boosters. *Annals of Emergency Medicine* 14(1):33–35.

Malakoff D. 2000. Public health: aluminum is put on trial as a vaccine booster. *Science* 288(5470):1323–1324.

Middaugh JP. 1979. Side effects of diphtheria-tetanus toxoid in adults. *American Journal of Public Health* 69(3):246–249.

Nichol KL, Margolis KL, Lind A, Murdoch M, McFadden R, Hauge M, Magnan S, Drake M. 1996. Side effects associated with influenza vaccination in healthy working adults. A randomized, placebo-controlled trial. *Archives of Internal Medicine* 156(14):1546–1550.

Nicolson GL, Nass M, Nicolson N. 2000. Anthrax vaccine: controversy over safety and efficacy. *Antimicrobics and Infectious Disease Newsletter* 18:1–6.

Noah DN. 1997. Microbiology. In: Detels R, Holland WW, McEwen J, Omenn GS, eds. *Oxford Textbook of Public Health*. Vol. 2. *The Methods of Public Health*. 3rd ed. New York, N.Y.: Oxford University Press Inc. Pp. 929–949.

Ott G, Barchfeld GL, Chernoff D, Radhakrishmnan R, van Hoogevest P, Van Nest G. 1995. Design and evaluation of a safe and potent adjuvant for human vaccines. In: Powell MF, Newman MJ, Burdman JR, eds. *Vaccine Design: The Subunit and Adjuvant Approach*. New York, N.Y.: Plenum Press. Pp. 227–296.

Pittman PR, Kim-Ahn G, Pifat DY, Coon K, Gibbs P, Little S, Pace-Templeton J, Myers R, Parker GW, Friedlander AM. 2002. Anthrax vaccine: safety and immunogenicity of a dose-reduction, route comparison study in humans. *Vaccine* 20(9–10):1412–1420.

Rovet RJ, Lieutenant, U.S. Air Force. 1999. *Anthrax Vaccine Adverse Event Reporting*. Statement at the July 21, 1999, hearing of the Subcommittee on National Security, Veterans Affairs and International Relations, Committee on Government Reform, U.S. House of Representatives, Washington, D.C.

Ruben FL, Froeschle JE, Meschievitz C, Chen K, George J, Reeves-Hoche MK, Pietrobon P, Bybel M, Livingood WC, Woodhouse L. 2001. Choosing a route of administration for quadrivalent meningococcal polysaccharide vaccine: intramuscular versus subcutaneous. *Clinical Infectious Diseases* 32(1):170–172.

Rustgi VK, Schleupner CJ, Krause DS. 1995. Comparative study of the immunogenicity and safety of Engerix-B administered at 0, 1, 2, and 12 months and Recombivax HB administered at 0, 1, and 6 months in healthy adults. *Vaccine* 13(17):1665–1668.

Scheifele DW, Bjornson G, Johnston J. 1990. Evaluation of adverse events after influenza vaccination in hospital personnel. *Canadian Medical Association Journal* 142(2):127–130.

Scheifele DW, Bjornson GJ. 1993. Evaluation of inactivated hepatitis A vaccine in Canadians 40 years of age or more. *Canadian Medical Association Journal* 148(4):551–555.

Schiff GM, Sherwood JR, Zeldis JB, Krause DS. 1995. Comparative study of the immunogenicity and safety of two doses of recombinant hepatitis B vaccine in healthy adolescents. *Journal of Adolescent Health* 16(1):12–17.

Selimov MA, Toigombaeva VS, Zgurskaya GN, Kulikova LG, Kodkind GK. 1988. Specific activity of tissue culture antirabic vaccine Rabivak-Vnukovo-32 with short intramuscular vaccination schedule. *Acta Virologica* 32(3):217–226.

Smith TJ. 2000. Squalene: potential chemopreventive agent. *Expert Opinion on Investigational Drugs* 9(8):1841–1848.

Strandberg TE, Tilvis RS, Miettinen TA. 1990. Metabolic variables of cholesterol during squalene feeding in humans: comparison with cholestyramine treatment. *Journal of Lipid Research* 31(9):1637–1643.

Treanor JJ. 2001. Adverse reactions following vaccination of adults. Commissioned paper. Committee to Assess the Safety and Efficacy of the Anthrax Vaccine, Institute of Medicine, Washington, D.C.

Tron F, Degos F, Brechot C, Courouce AM, Goudeau A, Marie FN, Adamowicz P, Saliou P, Laplanche A, Benhamou JP, et al. 1989. Randomized dose range study of a recombinant hepatitis B vaccine produced in mammalian cells and containing the S and PreS2 sequences. *Journal of Infectious Diseases* 160(2):199–204.

Van der Wielen M, Van Damme P, Joossens E, Francois G, Meurice F, Ramalho A. 2000. A randomised controlled trial with a diphtheria-tetanus-acellular pertussis (dTpa) vaccine in adults. *Vaccine* 18(20):2075–2082.

Ward J. 2001. APERT study: systemic and local reactions. E-mail to Edwards K, Joellenbeck L, Institute of Medicine Committee to Assess the Safety and Efficacy of the Anthrax Vaccine, Washington, D.C., February 8.

Weiss R. 2001, September 29. Demand growing for anthrax vaccine: fear of bioterrorism attack spurs requests for controversial shot. *Washington Post.* p. A16.

Westblom TU, Gudipati S, DeRousse C, Midkiff BR, Belshe RB. 1994. Safety and immunogenicity of an inactivated hepatitis A vaccine: effect of dose and vaccination schedule. *Journal of Infectious Diseases* 169(5):996–1001.

Wright GG, Green TW, Kanode RG Jr. 1954. Studies on immunity in anthrax. V. Immunizing activity of alum-precipitated protective antigen. *Journal of Immunology* 73:387–391.

Yamamoto S, Kuroki T, Kurai K, Iino S. 1986. Comparison of results for phase I studies with recombinant and plasma-derived hepatitis B vaccines, and controlled study comparing intramuscular and subcutaneous injections of recombinant hepatitis B vaccine. *Journal of Infection* 13(Suppl A):53–60.

5

Safety: Case Reports

During the course of the committee's deliberations, it heard and received in writing considerable testimony from individuals describing adverse events that occurred to them or their family members following vaccination against anthrax. Reports of adverse events have also been featured in newspaper reports and congressional testimony. Some of these events were quite severe, and the committee sympathizes with the presenters and understands their concerns about their illnesses.

These statements and stories in the media are examples of a broader category of information, that is, case reports of adverse events following the use of a vaccine. The committee identified two published case reports related to Anthrax Vaccine Adsorbed (AVA; Kerrison et al., 2002; Swanson-Biearman and Krenzelok, 2001). The most extensive collection of case reports of adverse events following vaccination is contained in the Vaccine Adverse Event Reporting System (VAERS), and the committee focused its attention there. Many of the experiences described to the committee directly were also reported to VAERS. This chapter reviews the characteristics of VAERS and the manner in which VAERS data related to the anthrax vaccine are used by responsible agencies. A summary of the VAERS reports and the committee's interpretation of this information are also presented.

VACCINE ADVERSE EVENT REPORTING SYSTEM

VAERS is a passive surveillance system begun in 1990 as part of the response to the National Childhood Vaccine Injury Act of 1986.[1] It is the nation's principal system for the collection of reports on adverse events following the use of any vaccine licensed in the United States. The system is coadministered by two federal agencies, the Centers for Disease Control and Prevention (CDC) and the Food and Drug Administration (FDA), which previously operated two separate surveillance systems. VAERS objectives include the following: (1) detecting previously unrecognized adverse events following the use of licensed vaccines; (2) detecting unusual increases in previously reported events; (3) detecting preexisting conditions that may promote adverse events and contraindicate additional vaccine doses; (4) detecting vaccine lots for which unusual numbers and unusual types of events are reported; (5) serving as a registry for rare vaccine-related adverse events; and (6) providing national data on the numbers of reported adverse events by vaccine type and recipient age (Singleton et al., 1999). It is also intended to trigger further clinical, epidemiologic, or laboratory studies of vaccine safety (Chen, 2000; Mootrey, 2000).

VAERS Reporting Process

VAERS receives spontaneous reports of adverse events following vaccination. From 1990, when VAERS began, through December 2001, VAERS received more than 126,000 reports on events associated with vaccines of all types (Iskander, 2002). Anyone can submit a report to VAERS, including vaccine recipients or their family members, and more than one report can be submitted about the same adverse event. Reporting is encouraged for any clinically significant event following vaccination, but health care providers are required to report any event listed by the manufacturer as a contraindication to the administration of additional doses of the vaccine as well as certain other specified events (VAERS, 2001). Most reports are submitted by health care providers directly (30 percent) or through the vaccine manufacturer (42 percent; Iskander, 2001b). Figure 5-1 illustrates the flow of information into and through VAERS.

Each year, reporting forms along with instructions and a cover letter encouraging reporting are mailed to about 200,000 health care providers (Iskander, 2001a). The forms are also available on the Internet (http://www.vaers.org/, http://www.fda.gov/cber/vaers/vaers.htm, http://www.cdc.gov/nip/). A VAERS report form includes spaces for the reporter to provide demographic information about the vaccine recipient and an open-ended description of the adverse event(s), treatment, outcome, relevant laboratory or diagnostic information, timing of the vaccination and the adverse event,

---
[1]National Childhood Vaccine Injury Act of 1986. P. L. No. 99-660 (1986).

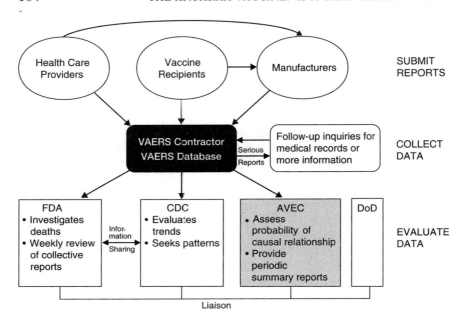

FIGURE 5-1 VAERS information flowchart. AVEC is unique to the anthrax vaccine.

vaccine type and lot number, and preexisting conditions. (See Appendix E for a copy of the form.)

Reports can be submitted by mail or fax, or the information can be provided over the telephone. Reports are submitted to the VAERS contractor, who acknowledges their receipt with a letter to the reporter (Chen et al., 1994; Singleton et al., 1999). The contractor assigns a unique identifier to each report, assigns codes to the adverse events reported, and enters the data into a computer database. Duplicate reports are removed or linked if the different reports provide different information (Iskander, 2001a).

Certain adverse events are classified as serious[2]: a death, a life-threatening illness, or an illness that results in a permanent disability, hospitalization, or prolongation of a hospital stay (Singleton et al., 1999). Manufacturers are also required to report "other medically important conditions" (Iskander, 2001b). Within 5 days of the receipt of a report of a serious event, nurses working for the VAERS contractor initiate follow-up inquiries to the vaccine recipient or reporter to gather more information, including medical or autopsy records, if they are available (E. Miller, CDC,

---

[2]Postmarketing Reporting of Adverse Drug Experiences. 21 C.F.R. § 314.80 (2000).

personal communication, May 24, 2001). As a result of the additional information, the medical coding of the event may be changed.

Review of VAERS Data by FDA and CDC

Both FDA and CDC regularly review data from VAERS reports for patterns in the data that suggest the possibility of previously unrecognized adverse events. For regulatory purposes, FDA reviews individual reports to assess whether the reported events are adequately reflected in product labeling (FDA, 2001). FDA also reviews all reports of serious adverse events soon after receipt by the VAERS contractor and may occasionally investigate other events as well. All reports of deaths are investigated to determine the official cause of death and to obtain any autopsy information. FDA staff examine VAERS data to look for unusual or unexpected patterns or trends associated with a vaccine or a vaccine lot and meet weekly to discuss any newly identified patterns observed. FDA does not attempt to evaluate whether the reported events have a causal association with the vaccine in question, but the agency is empowered to recall any vaccine or vaccine lot found to be associated with an unacceptably high rate of reports of adverse events (FDA, 2001). VAERS reports are routinely reviewed carefully after a vaccine has been on the market for a few years and data based on experience with the vaccine have been collected. The accumulated VAERS reports are also summarized and discussed in journal articles. FDA does not have a priori thresholds or numbers of reports of a particular adverse event that trigger additional follow-up but instead relies on a constellation of data including, among other factors, the seriousness of the reports, the similarities of case descriptions, and the size of the vaccine lot in question. In the case of the anthrax vaccine, data on the number of doses administered are available from the Department of Defense's (DoD's) Defense Medical Surveillance System (DMSS) and inform FDA's interpretation of the adverse events reports.

CDC focuses on collective reports and attempts to determine unusual epidemiologic trends and associations (FDA, 2001). For each vaccine, aggregated data from VAERS reports are evaluated weekly for unusual numbers of cases, types of adverse events, or other unexpected features. CDC also receives information about cases flagged during FDA's weekly review of reports. As at FDA, CDC analysts generally rely on clinical judgment rather than specific quantitative thresholds of adverse events to initiate additional follow-up. If VAERS reports raise concerns, studies are undertaken to develop more definitive information.

Limitations of VAERS

As the only system for the collection of information on adverse events reported in association with the use of all U.S. licensed vaccines after they are marketed, VAERS is an essential resource for the monitoring of vaccine safety. An unexpected increase in the numbers of reports about a product or a series of reports of an unexpected or unusual adverse event can catalyze additional information gathering and investigation. However, VAERS also has certain critical limitations (Chen, 2000; Ellenberg and Chen, 1997; IOM, 1994a,b). Adverse events that occur soon after a vaccination may be reported to VAERS whether or not they are causally related to the vaccination. Duplicate reports of the same case may be submitted, and the medical information provided may be incorrect or incomplete. The complexity of the information that comes into the system (e.g., multiple exposures and multiple outcomes) also makes analysis difficult. In addition, VAERS provides no information on the incidence of similar events among persons who have not been vaccinated.

Because VAERS is a passive system that relies on spontaneous reporting, adverse events are likely to be underreported to an unknown extent, and underreporting may also vary over time and among various kinds of adverse events. One analysis found that the "reporting efficiency" of VAERS ranged from 68 percent for vaccine-associated poliomyelitis following administration of oral polio vaccine to <1 percent for rash following administration of the measles-mumps-rubella vaccine (Rosenthal and Chen, 1995). Moreover, for most vaccines there are no data about the number of doses actually administered, although there may be data from other sources on the number of doses distributed. As a result of these limitations, it is nearly impossible to calculate accurate rates of adverse events from VAERS data. A numerator based on the number of reports can be assumed to differ from the true number of events, and there are no data on the total number of doses administered for the denominator (Mootrey, 2000; Singleton et al., 1999; Tilson, 1992).

In the case of AVA, however, DoD has maintained records on vaccine doses administered since the start of the Anthrax Vaccine Immunization Program (AVIP) in 1998. This information provides a denominator that is useful in the interpretation of changes in the frequencies of conditions reported to VAERS. In addition, the availability of data from DMSS on diagnoses for hospitalizations and outpatient visits (see Chapter 6) gives DoD a unique opportunity to evaluate the completeness of reporting to VAERS. Adverse events for which medical attention was received can be systematically identified within DMSS, and efforts can be made to determine whether those events are included in VAERS.

However, it is important to recognize that increased reporting is not a goal in and of itself. For VAERS, like any other spontaneous reporting system, there is no expectation or possibility of complete reporting. This inherent characteristic of spontaneous reporting systems must be recognized to properly interpret the data that they produce. Only in the context of an extremely organized health care system, such as that administered by DoD, can exposures be truly quantified and outcomes more completely reported. Even then, determination of true rates of reactions requires formal epidemiologic studies that provide complete ascertainment of numerators and denominators (see Chapter 6). For spontaneous reporting systems, then, the goal should be not simply more complete reporting but more detailed and insightful reporting, including more clinical data on each case and the selective reporting of cases that are novel, serious, or both. Increasing the numbers of reports of poorly documented events is unlikely to be helpful in determining which events are truly vaccine related.

> **Finding:** The presence or absence of VAERS reports (or other case reports) cannot be considered in and of itself to provide adequate evidence of causal association or its absence. Reports may suggest hypotheses for further investigation, but it must be borne in mind that many different factors beyond the presence of health symptoms can influence whether a report is filed.

DoD AND VAERS

Because most recipients of the anthrax vaccine are U.S. military personnel, DoD has two roles in connection with VAERS. First, military health care providers who administer AVA and other vaccines also prepare and submit VAERS reports on adverse events that follow vaccinations. Second, DoD has an interest in learning from VAERS data of any signals of possible safety concerns. "Signals" are the earliest indication of a possible causal relationship between an exposure and a health event. Such signals can come from the anecdotal experiences of patients suffering an adverse event following the exposure or from preliminary analyses of data. A signal does not mean that a causal relationship exists, as there may be other explanations for the apparent association. Instead, a signal is merely an indication that further investigation is needed. For AVA, DoD has also sought a special independent mechanism for review of VAERS reports, the Anthrax Vaccine Expert Committee (AVEC).

Submission of VAERS Reports

DoD, which administers most of the anthrax vaccine used in the United States, has a central role in the reporting of any adverse events that occur following vaccination. Since 1995, DoD policy has required submission of

VAERS reports for any adverse event that results in the loss of time from duty of more than 24 hours or any period of hospitalization (Department of the Air Force, 1995). This requirement has been reiterated with specific emphasis for the anthrax vaccine:

> [A] Form VAERS-1 must be completed and submitted using Service reporting procedures for those events resulting in a hospital admission or time lost from duty for greater than 24 hours or for those events suspected to have resulted from contamination of a vaccine lot. Further, health care providers are encouraged to report other adverse events that in the provider's professional judgment appear to be unexpected in nature or severity. In addition, the patient or a health care provider may submit a Form VAERS-1 directly to the Food and Drug Administration (FDA) for any possible adverse event. (Bailey, 1999, p. 1)

Reports from Navy and Air Force health care providers are to be submitted directly to VAERS, whereas reports from Army health care providers are to be submitted through a military treatment facility's Pharmacy and Therapeutics Committee, which forwards them to VAERS. Copies of VAERS reports must also be submitted to a service's reportable disease officer within 7 days of an adverse event.

Concerns About Reporting to VAERS

Some service members have expressed concern that they have been discouraged from submitting VAERS reports regarding the anthrax vaccine. According to service member testimony to the U.S. Congress as well as statements made to this Institute of Medicine (IOM) committee, reporting to VAERS has at times "met reluctance" or taken place only after delays (U.S. Congress, House of Representatives, Committee on Government Reform, 2000, p. 36; Irelan, 2000; Nietupski, 2001). In at least one Air Force squadron there is a perception that seeking care for symptoms of unknown origin or filing a VAERS report carries the risk of being labeled as a malingerer or as depressed or could jeopardize a service member's flight status (Tanner, 2001; U.S. Congress, House of Representatives, Committee on Government Reform, 2000, p. 39). In a General Accounting Office survey of National Guard and Air Force Reserve pilots and aircrew members (GAO, 2000), 60 percent of those who reported experiencing reactions that they attributed to the anthrax vaccine had not discussed those reactions with military health care personnel or their supervisors. In addition, 71 percent of those surveyed were unaware of VAERS, representing a substantial opportunity for underreporting. (The level of awareness of VAERS among the general public is not known.) Testimony to the committee indicated that at the start of AVIP at least some military physicians had little knowledge of VAERS and VAERS reporting procedures (Buck, 2001).

In response to such concerns, the acting assistant secretary of defense for health affairs requested in October 2000 that the surgeons general of the services remind medical personnel of the need for high-quality, empathetic medical care for vaccinees and of policies for submission of VAERS reports (Clinton, 2000). The surgeon general of the Army's memorandum of October 27, 2000 (Peake, 2000) noted that DoD policy for reporting to VAERS (Bailey, 1999; Department of the Air Force, 1995) set the *minimum* requirements for submissions of reports (i.e., if vaccine-related reactions result in hospitalization or the loss of time from duty of more than 24 hours or if contaminated or dangerous lots are suspected). The memorandum also urged submission of reports "for any event that may be related to a vaccination. If a patient wants to submit a VAERS report, help him or her submit one" (Peake, 2000). Memoranda to Navy and Air Force medical personnel provided similar messages, noting that it is not the provider's responsibility to determine the causality of the adverse event (Carlton, 2000; Surgeon General of the Navy, 2000).

A potential additional step to facilitate reporting to VAERS was described to the committee in July 2001. Plans were noted to provide new guidelines for military health care providers for coding a health event as vaccine related.

> Finding: Concerns of service members that reporting to VAERS is sometimes discouraged within the military setting have been responded to appropriately with reminders to physicians that DoD policy requires submission of a VAERS report for postvaccination health events that result in hospitalization or the loss of time from duty of more than 24 hours. Additional steps, however, are possible to facilitate reporting to VAERS, including improvements in the coding of health care visits that are potentially vaccine related.

> Recommendation: DoD should develop and implement a system to automate the generation of VAERS reports within the military health care system, using codes to identify from automated records those health care visits that are potentially vaccine related. Use of these codes should generate an automatic filing of a VAERS report that includes the specific diagnoses for the clinical event(s) that prompted the health care visit. However, the submission of reports to VAERS should not be restricted to visits assigned codes that identify them as potentially vaccine related.

DoD Access to and Use of VAERS Data

The AVIP Agency, which is part of DoD, monitors VAERS reports related to the use of AVA. The Army Medical Surveillance Activity produces weekly summaries from the copies of VAERS reports that DoD health care providers submit to the services' disease reporting systems. Monthly cross-checks with VAERS managers ensure that the AVIP Agency learns, in a redacted manner, of reports sent directly to VAERS without a report through military channels (Grabenstein, 2001b). DoD also receives information about VAERS reports through AVEC, a committee of civilian experts convened to review VAERS reports related to AVA (see below for a further discussion of AVEC). As a liaison member of AVEC, the AVIP Agency receives copies of all AVA-related VAERS reports (with identifiers removed) and of the additional records sought by AVEC for a substantial fraction of cases (Grabenstein, 2001c). In addition, DoD has access to the redacted information in the AVEC database. A contractor to the AVIP Agency maintains this database and codes and enters data for use by AVEC (Grabenstein, 2001c). An AVEC medical reviewer audits the accuracy of the data entered. DoD may not disclose information from individual reports because the data belong to AVEC and because of the restrictions that are part of the Privacy Act (Grabenstein, 2001b).

Anthrax Vaccine Expert Committee

The Department of Health and Human Services (DHHS) convened AVEC in 1998 in response to a request from the Army surgeon general (Sever et al., in press). It is a committee of civilian physicians and scientists and was formed to provide ongoing independent expert medical review of VAERS reports related to anthrax vaccination. DHHS recruited the committee members through the Expert Witness Program of the Vaccine Injury Compensation Program (http://bhpr.hrsa.gov/vicp/INDEX.HTM). Committee members have expertise in neurology, infectious diseases, rheumatology, epidemiology, and statistics, as well as experience and interest in vaccine-related adverse events. The committee includes liaison members from DoD's AVIP Agency, FDA's Center for Biologics Evaluation and Research, and CDC's National Immunization Program. AVEC has staff support from the DHHS National Vaccine Injury Compensation Program. DoD provides DHHS with funding to support the activities of the committee, but the agreement between the two departments gives DHHS full independence in the selection of AVEC members and in all activities of the committee (Grabenstein, 2001c; Sever et al., in press).

AVEC reviews AVA-related VAERS reports individually to assess the probability of a causal relationship between the reported adverse event and the anthrax vaccine and in aggregate to determine if any patterns are evident from the reports. AVEC and its procedures were modeled after the Advisory Committee on Causality Assessment (ACCA), an expert advisory group convened by the Canadian government in 1994 to review all reports of serious and unusual vaccine-associated adverse events from both active and passive monitoring systems in Canada (Collet et al., 2000). Both ACCA and AVEC use the criteria of the World Health Organization to assign categories of "very likely/certain," "probable," "possible," "unlikely," "unrelated," or "unclassifiable" to the likelihood of a causal relationship between the adverse event and the vaccine (Caserta, 2000; Collet et al., 2000; Sever et al., in press).

The review of individual reports begins when the VAERS contractor provides redacted copies of reports to AVEC as they are received. A single AVEC member makes a preliminary review and assessment of each case using a case assessment form (Appendix F). Additional medical records are sought as needed through VAERS to provide more information on the adverse event and its resolution or longer-term outcome. At intervals of 3 to 6 weeks, batches of the reports with preliminary assessments are sent to the full committee and a teleconference is held to discuss each case (Weibel, 2001). On the basis of that discussion, the committee may modify the preliminary categorization of a case or decide to seek additional information. Information from the case assessment form, including the conclusions of the committee, is entered into an AVEC database (Caserta, 2000). Further evaluation takes place as part of the preparation of manuscripts for publication. The causality assessments involve only the medically qualified civilian members of AVEC. The nonmedical members, liaison members from government agencies, and other support personnel play no role in the process (Grabenstein, 2001c; Sever et al., in press).

The aggregate review is an ongoing process operating in parallel with the case reviews. The statistician and epidemiologist on AVEC compile and analyze information from the database in an effort to discern any patterns that relate to specific symptoms, severity, lot numbers, or other factors. They also use information available from DMSS to estimate the number of vaccine doses administered during the time period in question. This added information provides some ability to look at trends in reporting rates for adverse events. AVEC gives additional scrutiny to adverse events that appear in 1 percent or more of the reports it receives and particularly to any repeated serious and "other medically important" adverse events, taking into account the committee's previous classifications of the likelihood of a causal association between the particular adverse event and the vaccine. No formal protocols have been established to determine the number of reports of a given adverse event over a specified period of time that would initiate additional action.

To date, AVEC has not observed a cluster of events that it believed warranted concerns about the safety of the vaccine (Sever et al., in press). Should information from VAERS reports raise such concerns, AVEC would inform the National Vaccine Injury Compensation Program, which would convey the information to DoD and the AVIP Agency. AVEC can also provide a public alert through a rapid publication, such as a letter to a journal editor.

REPORTS TO VAERS RELATED TO AVA

As of November 29, 2001, roughly 2.1 million doses of AVA had been administered in the United States since 1990. AVEC has reviewed a total of 1,623 unique VAERS reports about adverse events following receipt of the anthrax vaccine. This section provides summary information about the nature of the events reported to VAERS, the conclusions reached by AVEC as to the likelihood of a causal association between vaccination with AVA and the reported adverse event, allergic reactions reported through VAERS, and the IOM committee's conclusions from its own review of the VAERS reports concerning serious adverse events (i.e., a death, a life-threatening illness, or an illness that results in a permanent disability, hospitalization, or prolongation of a hospital stay).

AVEC Conclusions Regarding Reports to VAERS

Of the 1,623 VAERS reports reviewed by AVEC as of October 2, 2001, 57 involved hospitalization, 161 involved a loss of time from duty of 24 hours or more without hospitalization, and the remainder involved neither hospitalization nor loss of time from duty for 24 hours or more (AVIP, 2001). AVEC found that 10 of the 57 hospitalizations were "very likely/certainly" or "probably" caused by receipt of the anthrax vaccine. All 10 involved allergic inflammation reactions at the injection site. Table 5-1 presents the diagnoses and AVEC classifications of the other 47 hospitalizations reported to VAERS.

Of the 161 VAERS reports that involved a loss of time from duty of 24 hours or more without hospitalization, 89 were classified by AVEC as "certainly" or "probably" caused by anthrax vaccination. The events included in these 89 reports are listed in Table 5-2.

Acute Allergic Reactions Following Vaccination with AVA

DoD reexamined VAERS reports to identify reports of acute allergic (anaphylactic) reactions following vaccination with AVA. These were defined as reactions (1) that had an onset within 2 hours of receipt of AVA (usually within minutes) and (2) that involved either airway and cardiovascular collapse (anaphylactic shock) or less severe anaphylactic symptoms such as generalized itching, symptoms of chest tightness with or without evidence of hives, and reactions for which epinephrine or antihistamines

TABLE 5-1 AVEC Classification of Hospitalizations Reported to VAERS (as of October 2, 2001) Following Anthrax Vaccination and Not Classified as "Very Likely/Certainly" or "Probably" Caused by Anthrax Vaccine Adsorbed

Diagnosis	Number of VAERS Reports			
	Unclassifiable	Unrelated	Unlikely	Possible
Abdominal pain	1			
Acute encephalitis		1		
Angioedema		1		
Aplastic anemia	1			
Atrial fibrillation	1		1	
B-cell lymphoma involving central nervous system		1		
Bipolar psychiatric disorder	1	1		
Blackout episode		1		
Cardiac arrest		1		
Cardiomyopathy with atrial fibrillation		1	1	
Diabetes mellitus, insulin requiring	1			
Diabetes mellitus, non-insulin requiring		1		
Dysesthesias (T1 and below)	1			
Dyspnea	2			
Endocarditis with perirectal abscess		1		
Fatigue and injection-site inflammation				1
Febrile illness		1		
Guillain-Barré syndrome	3	2		
Idiopathic thrombocytopenic purpura	1			
Inflammation over olecranon process		1		
Intestinal surgery (appendectomy)		1		
Liver abscess with *Escherichia coli* septicemia		1		
Meningitis, aseptic		1		
Meningitis, viral	1			
Meningitis, unspecified		1		
Multiple sclerosis			1	
Neurological symptoms (facial weakness, slurred speech)			1	
Neutropenia, fever	2			
Pemphigus vulgaris			1	
Progressive paralytic neurological disease			1	
Rash				1
Scleritis, bilateral		1		
Seizure		1		
Syncope		1		
Systemic lupus erythematosus			1	
Toxic epidermal necrolysis syndrome		1		
Viral-like syndrome		2		
Total	15	23	7	2

SOURCE: AVIP (2001).

TABLE 5-2 Adverse Events Reported to VAERS (as of October 2, 2001) Involving Loss of Time from Duty of 24 Hours or More and Considered by AVEC as Certainly or Probably Caused by Anthrax Vaccine Adsorbed

Reported Adverse Event	Number of Events
Injection-site reactions	52
Various rashes	9
Acute allergic reactions	9
Virus-like symptoms	9
Itching	2
Gastroenteritis	2
Muscle aches	2
Bronchiolitis obliterans	1
Tingling sensation	1
Photophobia	1
Swollen lymph nodes	1
Total	89

SOURCE: AVIP (2001).

were given. As of October 2, 2001, no cases of anaphylactic shock had been reported to VAERS. There were 16 cases (7.6 per 1 million doses) of less severe anaphylactic reactions, all of which resolved without sequelae (Grabenstein, 2001a).

IOM Review of Serious VAERS Reports

The IOM committee reviewed the extent, nature, and quality of the information available in VAERS to inform its analysis of VAERS and AVEC. A subcommittee of the IOM committee reviewed all VAERS reports related to AVA that were defined as serious under VAERS criteria and that had been submitted through October 30, 2001—a total of 120 reports. The subcommittee also discussed with AVEC its process for causality assessment. The IOM subcommittee was satisfied with the approach described by AVEC and did not replicate the causality assessments for the cases that the subcommittee reviewed.

The subcommittee undertook a qualitative review and discussion of the collection of cases reported to VAERS in a search for patterns or suggestions of similar clinical pictures or possibly related underlying pathophysiology. For all events or symptoms that appeared in two or more reports of serious events, the subcommittee checked the rates of these (or related) diagnoses among those who had and those who had not been immunized with AVA in the DoD analyses of DMSS data that had previously been presented to the entire committee (see Chapter 6 and Appendix G). No confirmatory increases in the rates of these events in the immunized population were found.

Finding: The committee has reviewed the case materials and the methods applied by VAERS and AVEC to evaluate those materials and concurs with their conclusions that those materials present no signals of previously undescribed serious adverse reactions associated with exposure to AVA.

REFERENCES

AVIP (Anthrax Vaccine Immunization Program). 2001. *Section J: Reports involving anthrax vaccine submitted to the FDA/CDC Vaccine Adverse Event Reporting System (VAERS) and Evaluated by the Anthrax Vaccine Expert Committee. Detailed Safety Review of Anthrax Vaccine Adsorbed.* [Online.] Available: http://www.anthrax.osd.mil/Sit_Files/articles/INDEXclinical/safety_reviews.htm [accessed January 18, 2001].

Bailey S. 1999. Policy for reporting adverse events associated with the anthrax vaccine. Memorandum to Surgeon General of the Army, Surgeon General of the Navy, and Surgeon General of the Air Force. Department of Defense, Washington, D.C.

Buck J. 2001. Written statement. Presentation to the Joint Meeting of the Institute of Medicine Committee to Assess the Safety and Efficacy of the Anthrax Vaccine and the Institute of Medicine Committee to Review the CDC Anthrax Vaccine Safety and Efficacy Research Program, Meeting III, Washington, D.C.

Carlton PK Jr. 2000. Vaccine Adverse Events Reporting System (VAERS). Memorandum for See Distribution. Department of the Air Force, Washington, D.C.

Caserta V. 2000. Anthrax Vaccine Expert Committee (who, what, when, where, and how). Presentation to the Institute of Medicine Committee to Assess the Safety and Efficacy of the Anthrax Vaccine, Meeting I, Washington, D.C.

Chen RT. 2000. Special methodological issues in pharmacoepidemiology studies of vaccine safety. In: BL Strom, ed. *Pharmacoepidemiology.* 3rd ed. West Sussex, England: John Wiley & Sons, Ltd. Pp. 707–732.

Chen RT, Rastogi SC, Mullen JR, Hayes SW, Cochi SL, Donlon JA, Wassilak SG. 1994. The Vaccine Adverse Event Reporting System (VAERS). *Vaccine* 12(6):542–550.

Clinton JJ. 2000. Reactions of the anthrax vaccine. Memorandum to Surgeon General of the Army, Surgeon General of the Navy, and Surgeon General of the Air Force. Department of Defense, Washington, D.C.

Collet JP, MacDonald N, Cashman N, Pless R. 2000. Monitoring signals for vaccine safety: the assessment of individual adverse event reports by an expert advisory committee. Advisory Committee on Causality Assessment. *Bulletin of the World Health Organization* 78(2):178–185.

Department of the Air Force. 1995. Immunizations & Chemoprophylaxis—Air Force Joint Instruction 48-110 (U.S. Army Regulation 40-562; Navy Bureau of Medicine & Surgery Instruction 6230.15; Coast Guard Commandant Instruction M6230.4E). Department of the Air Force, Washington, D.C. *Aerospace Medicine.* [Online.] Available: http://afpubs.hq.af.mil/pubfiles/af/48/afji48-110/afji48-110.pdf [accessed February 20, 2002].

Ellenberg SS, Chen RT. 1997. The complicated task of monitoring vaccine safety. *Public Health Reports* 112(1):10–20.

FDA (Food and Drug Administration). 2001. *Vaccine Adverse Event Reporting System (VAERS) Frequently Asked Questions.* [Online]. Available: http://www.fda.gov/cber/vaers/faq.htm [accessed May 24, 2001].

GAO (General Accounting Office). 2000. *Anthrax Vaccine: Preliminary Results of GAO's Survey of Guard/Reserve Pilots and Aircrew Members.* GAO-01-92T. Washington, D.C.: GAO.

Grabenstein JD. 2001a. Technical review comments. Excerpted draft sections for DoD/AVIP technical review. Anthrax Vaccine Immunization Program Agency, Falls Church, Va., December 7.

Grabenstein JD. 2001b. Vaccine Adverse Events Reporting System. E-mail to Joellenbeck L, Institute of Medicine, Washington, D.C., August 3.

Grabenstein JD. 2001c. Acute allergic reactions after anthrax vaccination. Information paper. Anthrax Vaccine Immunization Program Agency, Falls Church, Va.

IOM (Institute of Medicine). 1994a. Stratton KR, Howe CJ, Johnston RB Jr, eds. *Adverse Events Associated with Childhood Vaccines: Evidence Bearing on Causality.* Washington, D.C.: National Academy Press.

IOM. 1994b. Stratton KR, Howe CJ, Johnston RB Jr, eds. *Research Strategies for Assessing Adverse Events Associated with Vaccines: A Workshop Summary.* Washington, D.C.: National Academy Press.

Irelan, J. 2000. *Anthrax Vaccine Immunization Progam—What Have We Learned?* Statement at the October 3, 2000, hearing of the Committee on Government Reform, U.S. House of Representatives, Washington, D.C.

Iskander J. 2001a. Detection of duplicate VAERS reports. E-mail to Joellenbeck L, Institute of Medicine, Washington, D.C., August 3.

Iskander J. 2001b. Technical review. E-mail to Joellenbeck L, Institute of Medicine, Washington, D.C., June 1.

Iskander J. 2002. Number of VAERS reports filed for all vaccines. E-mail to Joellenbeck L, Institute of Medicine, Washington, D.C., February 8.

Kerrison JB, Lounsbury D, Thirkill CE, Lane RG, Schatz MP, Engler RM. 2002. Optic neuritis after anthrax vaccination. *Ophthalmology* 109(1):99–104.

Mootrey G. 2000. The Vaccine Adverse Event Reporting System (VAERS) and anthrax vaccine. Presentation to the Institute of Medicine Committee to Assess the Safety and Efficacy of the Anthrax Vaccine, Meeting I, Washington, D.C.

Nietupski J. 2001. Statement and documents submitted for the Joint Meeting of the Institute of Medicine Committee to Assess the Safety and Efficacy of the Anthrax Vaccine and the Institute of Medicine Committee to Review the CDC Anthrax Vaccine Safety and Efficacy Research Program, Meeting III, Washington, D.C.

Peake JB. 2000. Reactions to Vaccines. Memorandum to Commanders of the North Atlantic, Southeast, Great Plains, Western, European, and Pacific Regional Medical Commands. Department of the Army, Washington, D.C.

Rosenthal S, Chen R. 1995. The reporting sensitivities of two passive surveillance systems for vaccine adverse events. *American Journal of Public Health* 85(12):1706–1709.

Sever JL, Brenner AI, Gale AD, Lyle JM, Moulton LH, West DJ. In press. Safety of anthrax vaccine: a review by the Anthrax Vaccine Expert Committee (AVEC) of adverse events reported to the Vaccine Adverse Event Reporting System (VAERS). *Pharmacoepidemiology and Drug Safety.*

Singleton JA, Lloyd JC, Mootrey GT, Salive ME, Chen RT. 1999. An overview of the Vaccine Adverse Event Reporting System (VAERS) as a surveillance system. VAERS Working Group. *Vaccine* 17(22):2908–2917.

Surgeon General of the Navy. 2000. Handling persons with reactions to anthrax vaccine. Memorandum. Department of the Navy, Washington, D.C.

Swanson-Biearman B, Krenzelok EP. 2001. Delayed life-threatening reaction to anthrax vaccine. *Journal of Toxicology. Clinical Toxicology* 39(1):81–84.

Tanner J. 2001. Survey results of the 9th Airlift Squadron. Presentation to the Joint Meeting of the Institute of Medicine Committee to Assess the Safety and Efficacy of the Anthrax Vaccine and the Institute of Medicine Committee to Review the CDC Anthrax Vaccine Safety and Efficacy Research Program, Meeting III, Washington, D.C.

Tilson H. 1992. Pharmacosurveillance: public health monitoring of medication. In: Halperin W, Baker EL, Monson RR (consulting ed.), eds. *Public Health Surveillance*. New York, N.Y.: Van Nostrand Reinhold. Pp. 206–229.

U.S. Congress, House of Representatives, Committee on Government Reform. 2000. *The Department of Defense Anthrax Vaccine Immunization Program: Unproven Force Protection*. House Report 106-556. Washington, D.C.: U.S. House of Representatives.

VAERS (Vaccine Adverse Event Reporting System). 2001. A federal program for surveillance of vaccine safety. Brochure. Vaccine Adverse Event Reporting System, Rockville, Md.

Weibel R. 2001. Charge or mission statement for AVEC. E-mail to Joellenbeck L, Institute of Medicine, Washington, D.C., May 16.

6

Safety: Epidemiologic Studies

A small body of published reports as well as results from newer studies by Department of Defense (DoD) researchers provided data regarding adverse events following administration of Anthrax Vaccine Adsorbed (AVA). The studies examined a variety of outcomes, including local and systemic reactions occurring soon after vaccination, hospitalizations and outpatient visits, long-term health status, and reproductive outcomes. Since many of the studies are as yet unpublished, this report discusses them in detail. They are described in this chapter in three general categories: (1) ad hoc studies about immediate-onset adverse events, (2) ad hoc studies about later-onset adverse events, and (3) record-linkage studies. Studies within each of these three categories are described in the following order: (a) randomized controlled trials, (b) other controlled studies, and (c) uncontrolled studies. A few additional studies were known to the committee but were not reviewed. The committee could not obtain sufficient documentation for those studies, despite efforts to do so, to conduct an appropriate scientific review.

The synthesis of studies of local and systemic adverse events following receipt of AVA is hindered by several factors. First, the studies report on different types of adverse events and use different definitions of the events and of the severity of those events. For example, some studies include pruritis (itching), whereas others do not, and some studies count erythema (redness of the skin) only if it exceeds a certain size. Some studies use standardized quantitative definitions for an adverse event following inoculation with AVA, whereas others rely on the recipient's self-reported perception of a reaction. Second, adverse events are monitored or reported for various periods following inoculation, with some study reports not indicating the lengths of such periods. Thus, some adverse event rates apply to the first 24 to 48 hours postimmunization, whereas others may apply to the period from days to weeks following vaccination. Third, studies differ in their methods of ascertaining the presence of adverse events. Some studies used active surveillance to identify local and systemic reactions, with all recipients monitored on a regular basis at specified intervals. Other studies relied on passive surveillance, with vaccine recipients deciding whether an adverse event had occurred and whether to report that event. Fourth, the anthrax vaccine formulation was not constant across studies, and in some studies the anthrax vaccine was administered in combination with other vaccines. In addition, studies differed in the number of anthrax vaccine doses given. Finally, the adverse event rates reported were sometimes based on the number of doses administered and were sometimes based on the number of persons vaccinated. It should be noted that the same considerations affect the evaluation of safety for other vaccines as well.[1] The summary of findings presented below and in Tables 6-1 to 6-4 (referred to as the adverse events tables) should be read with the foregoing considerations in mind.

AD HOC STUDIES

Studies of Health Effects with Immediate Onset

Randomized Controlled Trials

Brachman Study Brachman and colleagues (1962) conducted the only randomized, placebo-controlled trial of the efficacy of a protective antigen anthrax vaccine. Information on events of immediate onset following immunization is presented here; information on the efficacy of the vaccine is reported in Chapter 3. The vaccine studied was not AVA but was an earlier formulation produced from the R1-NP strain of anthrax (see Chapter 7 for more details). The study was carried out from January 1955 through March 1959 in four mills in the eastern United States that processed raw imported goat hair, which was commonly contaminated with anthrax spores.

The worker population eligible for the study included 1,249 men and women with no history of prior anthrax infection. The numbers of study

---

[1]An international effort is under way to standardize case definitions of many of the adverse events that can follow vaccination. The Brighton Collaboration was launched in the autumn of 2000 and has now developed several definitions in draft form (http://brighton collaboration.org/index.cfm).

TABLE 6-1 Ad Hoc Studies of Immediate-Onset Adverse Events Following Anthrax Vaccination: Local Events

Study	Study Population and Observation Period	Data Collection Method(s)	Number of Subjects or Doses	Rates of Overall
Randomized Controlled Trials				
Field study (Brachman et al., 1962)[b]	U.S. goat hair mill workers (4 mills), 1955–1959	Examination at 24 and 48 hours (2 mills)	1,249 persons (4 mills)	35%
Placebo				
Route of administration pilot study (Pittman, 2001b; Pittman et al., 2002)[c]	Military and civilian study volunteers, 1998	Active surveillance	173 persons; 117 with all doses	
Intramuscular			118 doses	
Subcutaneous			203 doses	
Subcutaneous	Men		132 doses	
Subcutaneous	Women		71 doses	
Other Controlled Studies				
Double dose (Gunzenhauser et al., 2001)	ROTC cadets, Ft. Lewis, summer 2000	Self-report; postvaccination survey	73 cadets	
Doubled first dose[e]			25	92%, 72%
Standard doses[e]			48	92%, 67%

Local Events[a]							
Mild	Moderate	Severe	Redness	Induration	Knot, Lump, or Nodule	Edema or Swelling	Other
			+	+	+	2.8%	Itching, pain, warmth, tenderness
3 persons							
			6%	2%	0		Tenderness, 56%; warmth, 5%
			36%	15%	38%		Tenderness, 70%; warmth, 16%
			22.0%	3.0%	24.2%	2.3%	Tenderness, 63%; itching, 6%
			63.4%[d]	38%[d]	63.4%[d]	9.9%[d]	Tenderness, 63%[d]; itching, 30%[d]
			0, 39%		88%, 44%	84%, 50%	Sore arm, 92%, 67%
			0, 19%		42%, 29%	42%, 19%	Sore arm, 83%, 67%

Continued

TABLE 6-1 Continued

Study	Study Population and Observation Period	Data Collection Method(s)	Number of Subjects or Doses	Rates of Overall
Uncontrolled Studies				
Investigational new drug reports (CDC, 1967–1971)[f]	Textile, laboratory workers; 1966–1971		~7,000 persons ~16,000 doses	
Special Immunizations Program (Pittman et al., 2001a,b)[g]	Ft. Detrick laboratory workers, 1973–1999	Passive self-report; reported adverse events assessed and recorded by occupational health clinic medical personnel	1,583 persons 10,722 doses	3.6%
Men[g]			1,249 men 8,797 doses	
Women[g]			334 women 1,925 doses	

Local Events[a]							
Mild	Moderate	Severe	Redness	Induration	Knot, Lump, or Nodule	Edema or Swelling	Other
8.4%	0.9%	0.2%					
1.6%	1.4%	0.2%	2.5%	2.8%	+	0.1%	Tenderness, 1.7%; itching, 0.8%; lymph node enlargement, 0.1%
1.2%	0.9%	0.1%	1.7%	2.0%	+	<0.1%	Tenderness, 1.3%; itching, 0.4%; lymph node enlargement, 0.1%; arm motion limitation, 0.1%
3.5%[d]	3.5%[d]	0.5%[d]	6.3%[d]	6.4%[d]	+	0.3%[d]	Tenderness, 3.6%[d]; itching, 2.4%[d]; lymph node enlargement, 0.4%[d]; arm motion limitation, 0.2%

Continued

TABLE 6-1 Continued

Study	Study Population and Observation Period	Data Collection Method(s)	Number of Subjects or Doses	Rates of Overall
Ft. Bragg Booster Study (Pittman et al., 2002)	Army personnel; Desert Shield/ Desert Storm AVA vaccinees given booster doses of AVA alone or with PBT, 1992, 1994	Active surveillance	495 men	
Recipients of AVA only[g]			43	
AVA arm for recipients of AVA and PBT[g]			452	
U.S. Forces Korea (CDC, 2000; Hoffman et al., submitted for publication)[c]	Personnel covered by Camp Casey Troop Medical Clinic, Aug. 1998–July 1999	Retrospective self-report through questionnaire	2,824	
Men[h]			2,214	31.5– 39.7%[i]
Women[h]			610	59.9– 67.9%[d,i]
Tripler Army Medical Center (Wasserman, 2001)	Military health care workers, 1998–2000	Self-report through questionnaire; medical record review	601	
Men			416	

Local Events[a]							
Mild	Moderate	Severe	Redness	Induration	Knot, Lump, or Nodule	Edema or Swelling	Other
27.9%	4.7%	0					
16.0%	9.3%	0.7%					
7.2–7.7%	3.9–4.8%	0.4–1.1%			21.4–28.9%	2.5–3.4%	Pain, 9.6–10.2%; itching, 5.5–7.5%
11.7–13.5%[d]	10.7–13.3%[d]	2.0–4.1%[d]			49.8–62.4%[d]	3.9–9.4%[d]	Pain, 15–18.8%[d]; itching, 20.4–37%[d]
			15–23%[j]		56–65%	7–10%	Itching, 24–31%; pain limiting motion, 5–10%; muscle soreness, 50–66%

Continued

TABLE 6-1 Continued

Study	Study Population and Observation Period	Data Collection Method(s)	Number of Subjects or Doses	Rates of Overall
Women			185	
Adjusted odds ratios for women versus men (95% CI)				2.44 (2.04–2.93)
Dover Air Force Base (Tanner, 2001)	9th Airlift Squadron, surveyed Jan. 2000	Self-report through questionnaire	252 eligible; 139 responses	Reports on systemic events only

NOTES: AVA, Anthrax Vaccine Adsorbed; PBT, pentavalent botulinum toxoid; +, reaction reported as present.

[a]The rates are per dose.
[b]Study subjects received only the Merck vaccine and not AVA.
[c]Data are for doses 1 to 3.
[d]Significant difference between men and women ($p < .05$).
[e]Data are for doses 1 and 2, respectively.
[f]Reaction rates are for doses of AVA and were calculated by the committee from data in the CDC reports. Mild reactions are defined as areas of erythema (redness) only

Local Events[a]							
Mild	Moderate	Severe	Redness	Induration	Knot, Lump, or Nodule	Edema or Swelling	Other
			37–43%[j]		81–93%	8–15%	Itching, 56–68%; pain limiting motion, 8–17%; muscle soreness, 56–80%
			3.02 (2.52–3.62)[k]		4.48 (3.55–5.65)	1.41 (1.08–1.84)	Itching, 4.45 (3.74–5.31); pain limiting motion, 1.62 (1.23–2.12); muscle soreness, 1.54 (1.29–1.84); muscle ache, 1.44 (1.20–1.72)

or of measurable edema or induration of ≤3 cm in diameter. Moderate reactions are defined as areas of edema or induration of >3 cm to <12 cm in diameter. Severe reactions are defined as any reaction measuring >12 cm in diameter or accompanied by marked limitation of arm motion or axiliary node tenderness.

[g]Mild reactions are areas of erythema (redness) and/or induration (E/I) of < 5 cm in diameter, moderate reactions are areas of E/I of 5 to 12 cm, and severe reactions are areas of E/I of >12 cm.

[h]Data on mild, moderate, and severe events are for areas of redness of <5, 5 to 12, and >12 cm in diameter, respectively.

[i]Local or systemic effects.

[j]Data are for areas of redness of >5 cm in diameter.

[k]The outcome measure is the ratio of reports of areas of redness of >5 cm in diameter to reports of areas of <5 cm in diameter.

TABLE 6-2 Ad Hoc Studies of Immediate-Onset Adverse Events Following Anthrax Vaccination: Systemic Events

Study	Overall	Muscle Aches	Rates of Fever
Randomized Controlled Trials			
Field study (Brachman et al., 1962)[b]	0.2%		
Route of administration pilot study (Pittman 2001b; Pittman et al., 2002)[c]			
Intramuscular		4%	1%
Subcutaneous		4%	2%
Subcutaneous (Men)		3.0%	3.0%
Subcutaneous (Women)		7.0%	1.4%
Other Controlled Studies			
Doubled dose (Gunzenhauser et al., 2001)			
Doubled first dose[d]			12%, 0%
Standard dose[d]			8%, 7%

Systemic Events[a]			Functional Impact or Health Care Use
Headache	Malaise	Other	
	2 persons		Work loss: 6 days
11%	5%	Anorexia, 5%; nausea, 4%; itching, 0	
10%	9%	Anorexia, 1%; nausea, 2%; itching, 2%	
9.1%	9.8%	Anorexia, 2.3%; nausea, 2.3%; itching, 2.3%	
11.3%	8.5%	Anorexia, 0; nausea, 2.8%; itching, 2.8%	
0, 11%		Tiredness, 0, 22%	Decreased performance reported: 17% after second dose Sought medical care: 1 cadet after first dose No hospitalizations or missed training
0, 5%		Tiredness, 0, 7%	Decreased performance reported: 7% after second dose Sought medical care: none No hospitalizations or missed training

Continued

TABLE 6-2 Continued

Study	Overall	Muscle Aches	Rates of Fever
Uncontrolled Studies			
Investigational New Drug reports (CDC, 1967–1971)	4 persons	+	+
Special Immunizations Program (Pittman, 2001a; Pittman et al., 2001a,b)	1%	0.3%	0.1%
Men		0.2%	<0.1%
Women		0.4%	0.2%[e]
Ft. Bragg Booster Study (Pittman et al., 2002)			
Recipients of AVA only		23.3%	2.5%
Recipients of AVA and PBT		31%	2.7%
U.S. Forces Korea (CDC, 2000; Hoffman et al., submitted for publication)			
Men			0.7–1.0%
Women			2.1–4.0%[e]

Systemic Events[a]			Functional Impact or Health Care Use
Headache	Malaise	Other	
+	+	Chills, nausea	
0.4%	0.4%	Nausea, 0.1%; chills, 0.1%; dizziness, 0.1%	
0.3%	0.3%	Nausea, 0.1%; chills, 0.1%; dizziness, <0.1%; hives, 0%	
0.7%[e]	0.6%	Nausea, 0.2%; chills, 0.1%; dizziness, 0.3%[e]; hives, 0.2%[e]	
9.3%	7.0%	Joint pain, 7%; rash, 0; anorexia, 0; nausea, 0; breathing difficulty, 0	
16.6%	16.8%	Joint pain, 13.1%; rash, 17.3%; anorexia, 3.8%; nausea, 3.5%; breathing difficulty, 0.2%	
	3.6–6.5%	Chills, 1.2–2.4%; other, 0.8–4.4%	Among those reporting any local or systemic event:[c] Less active: 2.8–5.7% Work limitation: 0.0–0.4% Work loss: 0.4–0.7% Sought health care: 0.4–1.7% Used medications: 0–0.2%
	8.4–15.4%[e]	Chills, 3–5.5%[e]; other, 2.7–5.2%[e]	Among those reporting any local or systemic effect:[c] Less active: 3.1–6.7% Work limitation: 0.4–1.9%[e] Work loss: 0.0–1.1% Sought health care: 0.8–2.2% Used medications: 0–0.8%

Continued

TABLE 6-2 Continued

Study	Overall	Rates of Muscle Aches	Fever
Tripler Army Medical Center (GAO, 1999; CDC, 2000; Wasserman, 2001)		+	
Men		41%	4%
Women		45%	9%
Dover Air Force Base (Tanner, 2001)[f]	64%	41.7%[g]	7.9[h]

NOTES: AVA, Anthrax Vaccine Adsorbed; PBT, pentavalent botulinum toxoid; +, reaction reported as present.

[a]The rates are per dose unless noted otherwise.
[b]Study subjects received only the Merck vaccine.
[c]Data are for doses 1 to 3.

Systemic Events[a]			Functional Impact or Health Care Use
Headache	Malaise	Other	
+		Joint aches, fatigue	Sought care or time off: 3–8% (doses 1 to 4)
			No significant differences in rates of outpatient care or hospitalization for vaccinated and unvaccinated
17%		Joint ache, 16%; fatigue, 22%	Work limitation: 2–6% (doses 1 to 6) Sought health care: 2–5% (doses 1 to 3)
32%		Joint ache, 22%; fatigue, 36%	Work limitation: 4–12% (doses 1 to 6) Sought health care: 4–14% (doses 1 to 3)
18.7		Itching, 15.1%; loss of energy, 41.7%; sleep problems, 17.3%; nausea/abdominal pain, 6.5%; short-term memory loss, 25.9%; reduced concentration, 27.3%	Sought treatment: 29.5% Missed >1 day of duty: 17.3% Not returned to full duty: 7.2%

[d]Data are for doses 1 and 2, respectively.
[e]Significant difference between men and women ($p < .05$).
[f]Data are the percentage of respondents not rate per dose.
[g]Data are for joint or muscle pain.
[h]Data are for fever or chills.

TABLE 6-3 Ad Hoc Studies of Later-Onset Adverse Events Following Anthrax Vaccination

Study	Study Population and Observation Period	Data Collection Method(s)
Any Health Outcome		
Multiple vaccines cohort (Peeler et al., 1958)[a]	Ft. Detrick workers receiving multiple doses of multiple vaccines, 1944–1956	Medical history, physical exam, retrospective review of medical records
Multiple vaccines cohort (Peeler et al., 1965)[a]	Ft. Detrick workers receiving multiple doses of multiple vaccines, 1944–1962	Medical history, physical exam, retrospective review of medical records
Multiple vaccines cohort (White et al., 1974)[a]	Ft. Detrick workers receiving multiple doses of multiple vaccines, 1944–1971	Medical history, physical exam, retrospective review of medical records
Reproductive Outcomes		
Pregnancy, births, and birth outcomes (Wiesen, 2001a; Wiesen and Littell, 2001)	Ft. Stewart, women on active service, aged 17–44; Jan. 1999–March 2000	Local medical records, DEERS records to identify births among women transferred from Ft. Stewart

[a]Study subjects received the Merck vaccine alone or in combination with AVA.

Number of Subjects	Reported Health Outcomes
99 men	No evidence of illness attributable to immunization
76 men	Laboratory abnormalities of uncertain origin; no evidence of illness attributable to immunization
77 men (alive); 11 deceased cohort members; 26 age- and gender-matched unvaccinated controls	Inconsistent laboratory abnormalities; no evidence of illness attributable to immunization
4,092 women	Vaccinated versus unvaccinated women odds ratio (95% CI): Pregnancy: 0.9 (0.7–1.1) Birth: 0.8 (0.7–1.4) Premature birth or low birth weight: 2.1 (0.6–7.4) Any adverse birth outcome (age adjusted): 1.2 (0.5–2.9)

TABLE 6-4 Record-Linkage Studies of Adverse Events Following Anthrax Vaccination

Study	Study Population and Observation Period	Data Collection Method(s)
Single-Service Databases		
Air Combat Command Study (Rehme, 2001; Rehme et al., 2002)	Air Force personnel with medical visit during 1998 deployment in SWA, 1998–1999	Air Force and DoD databases on vaccination and postdeployment health care visits
Men		
Women		
Army Aviation Epidemiology Register (Mason et al., submitted for publication)	Army aircrew personnel; Jan. 1998–Nov. 2000	Records from aviation physical examinations conducted within 24 months before and after vaccination
DoD Databases		
Naval Health Research Center analysis (Sato, 2001a,b; Sato et al., 2001)	All personnel on active duty; Jan. 1, 1998– March 31, 2000	DoD records on hospitalization in military or civilian facilities linked to DoD records on vaccination and personnel data

Number of Subjects	Findings

5,177 persons	No significant increase in risk for use of ambulatory care or for any specific diagnosis
	
	Selected results as relative risk (vaccinated versus unvaccinated; 95% CI)
	    Any postdeployment outpatient visit: 0.96 (0.90–1.02)
	    Muscle aches: 0.75 (0.41–1.35)
	    Migraine: 0.93 (0.38–2.32)
	    Hearing loss: 0.28 (0.08–0.97)
	    Diabetes: 1.68 (0.20–13.9)
	    Sleep disorders: 2.80 (0.36–21.9)
	    Tinnitus: 0.42 (0.07–2.51)

4,352	Any postdeployment outpatient visit: 0.95 (0.88–1.02)
825	Any postdeployment outpatient visit: 0.99 (0.88–1.12)

3,356 matched pairs of vaccinated and unvaccinated aircrew personnel	No significant increase in risk for any outcome
	Selected results as odds ratio (vaccinated versus unvaccinated; 95% CI)
	    Weight change (>19 lbs [8.6 kg]): 0.61 (0.45–0.83)
	    Intraocular pressure >20 mm Hg: 0.40 (0.13–1.28)
	    Hearing loss >15 dB: 0.94 (0.82–1.08)
	    Diabetes or fasting blood sugar >115 mg/dL: 1.25 (0.34–4.66)

Vaccinated:
  2,651 hospitalizations
  120,870 person-years
 	
Unvaccinated:
  151,609 hospitalizations
  2.3 million person-years
	Risk for hospitalization within 42 days of vaccination for any of 14 summary ICD-9-CM diagnostic categories is significantly lower for vaccinated men and women
	
	Range for adjusted relative risk (vaccinated versus unvaccinated; 95% CI)
	    Men: 0.30 (0.27–0.33) to 0.75 (0.68–0.84)
	    Women: 0.17 (0.11–0.26) to 0.67 (0.47–0.94)

Continued

TABLE 6-4 Continued

Study	Study Population and Observation Period	Data Collection Method(s)
Army Medical Surveillance Activity DMSS analyses (AMSA, 2001a,b,c)		DMSS records on inpatient and outpatient visits and on vaccination history
Screening analyses	All personnel on active duty; Jan. 1, 1998– Dec. 31, 2000	
Hypothesis testing analyses	All personnel on active duty; Jan. 1, 1998– Dec. 31, 2000	
Post- versus prevaccination hospitalization	Vaccinated personnel only, Jan. 1, 1998–Dec. 31, 2000	
Post- versus prevaccination hospitalization; at 0–45 days and >45 days postvaccination	Vaccinated personnel only, Jan. 1, 1998–Dec. 31, 2000	

Number of Subjects	Findings
	See Appendix G for a complete listing of all significantly elevated adjusted rate ratios (RR) from these analyses
Vaccinated: 757,540 person-years Unvaccinated: 3.4 million person-years	No significant elevation of risk among vaccinated personnel for inpatient, outpatient, or incident visits for any of 14 summary ICD-9-CM diagnostic categories
Vaccinated: 515,389 person-years Unvaccinated: 2.8 million person-years	No significant elevation of risk among vaccinated personnel for any of 12 inpatient and 14 outpatient diagnoses

Postvaccination: 738,382 person-years
Prevaccination: 478,093 person-years
	Of 843 diagnoses, adjusted RR significantly lowered for 12 diagnoses and significantly elevated for 15 (see Appendix G, Table G-1). Diagnoses with significantly elevated adjusted RR (95% CI) include
	    Inguinial hernia (ICD-9-CM 550): 1.31 (1.01–1.65)
	    Diabetes mellitus (ICD-9-CM 250): 3.46 (1.51–7.90)
	    Carcinoma in situ of breast and genitourinary system (ICD-9-CM 233): 5.14 (1.81–14.57)

Postvaccination:
  0–45 days: 165,682 person-years
  >45 days: 572,700 person-years
Prevaccination: 478,093 person-years
	For 0–45 days postvaccination: of 843 diagnoses, adjusted RR significantly lowered for 7 diagnoses and significantly elevated for 13 (see Appendix G, Table G-2). Diagnoses with significantly elevated adjusted RR (95% CI) include
	    Diabetes mellitus (ICD-9-CM 250): 3.49 (1.39–8.79)
	    Other disorders of the intestine (ICD-9-CM 569): 4.16 (1.51–11.49)
	
	For >45 days postvaccination: of 843 diagnoses, adjusted RR were significantly lowered for 10 diagnoses and significantly elevated for 20 (see Appendix G, Table G-2). Diagnoses with significantly elevated adjusted RR (95% CI) include
	    Diabetes mellitus (ICD-9-CM 250): 3.44 (1.47–8.06)
	    Other disorders of the intestine (ICD-9-CM 569): 2.61 (1.06–6.44)

Continued

TABLE 6-4 Continued

Study	Study Population and Observation Period	Data Collection Method(s)
Post- versus prevaccination hospitalizations 1–3 doses and 4+ doses	Vaccinated personnel only; Jan. 1, 1998–Dec. 31, 2000	
Prevaccination versus nonvaccinated	All personnel on active duty; Jan. 1, 1998–Dec. 31, 2000	
Post- versus prevaccination, men	Men on active duty; Jan. 1, 1998–Dec. 31, 2000	
Post- versus prevaccination, women	Women on active duty; Jan. 1, 1998–Dec. 31, 2000	

NOTES: ICD-9-CM, *International Classification of Diseases, Ninth Revision, Sixth Edition, Clinical Modification,* 2001, Reston, Va.: St. Anthony's Publishing; SWA, Southwest Asia.

Number of Subjects	Findings

Postvaccination:
  1–3 doses: 184,273 person-years
  4+ doses: 554,109 person-years
Prevaccination:
  478,093 person-years
	For 1–3 doses: of 843 diagnoses, adjusted RR significantly lowered for postvaccination period for 5 diagnoses and significantly elevated for 23 (see Appendix G, Table G-3). Diagnoses with significantly elevated adjusted RR (95% CI) include
	  Diabetes mellitus (ICD-9-CM 250): 4.98 (2.02–12.25)
	  Asthma (ICD-9-CM 493): 2.18 (1.37–3.47)
	  Regional enteritis (ICD-9-CM 555): 4.90 (1.55–15.44)
	
	For 4+ doses: of 843 diagnoses, adjusted RR significantly lowered for 10 diagnoses and significantly elevated for 13 (see Appendix G, Table G-3). Diagnoses with significantly elevated adjusted RR (95% CI) include
	  Malignant neoplasms of the thyroid gland (ICD-9-CM 193): 2.35 (1.01–5.48)
	  Diabetes mellitus (ICD-9-CM 250): 3.05 (1.31–7.09)
	  Other disorders of the intestine (ICD-9-CM 569): 3.24 (1.33–7.89)

Prevaccination:
  478,093 person-years
Never vaccinated:
  2.9 million person-years
	Overall, vaccinated personnel were healthier (had fewer hospitalizations) prior to vaccination than never-vaccinated personnel
	Of 843 diagnoses, adjusted RR significantly elevated for 5 diagnoses (malaria; erythematous conditions; superficial injury of elbow, forearm, and wrist; toxic effect of carbon monoxide; effects of air pressure; see Appendix G, Table G-4)

Postvaccination:
  664,434 person-years
Prevaccination:
  2.9 million person-years
	Of 12 specific diagnoses, none with significantly elevated adjusted RR (see Appendix G, Table G-5).

Postvaccination:
  73,947 person-years
Prevaccination:
  509,265 person-years
	Of 12 specific diagnoses, adjusted RR (95% CI) significantly elevated for multiple sclerosis (see Appendix G, Table G-5):
	  All hospitalizations for MS: 2.14 (1.14–4.01)
	  Incident (first) hospitalizations for MS 1.26 (0.50–3.14)

participants were not reported by sex. Study participants received subcutaneous inoculations of 0.5 milliliters (ml) of either vaccine or placebo (0.1 percent alum). The first three doses were given at 2-week intervals, followed by three additional doses given at 6-month intervals and annual boosters thereafter.

Employees at two mills were examined at 24 and 48 hours after inoculation for evidence of local and systemic reactions. Two measures of local adverse reactions were used: (1) an "erythema value," based on the size of the area of erythema at the injection site, and (2) a "reaction index," based on all objective findings of erythema, induration (hardness), and edema (swelling from accumulation of serous fluid). The reaction index ranged from 0 (no reaction) to 4 (marked reaction). Significant (3 to 4+) reactions were observed in about 2 to 15 percent of immunized persons after the first through the fourth inoculations, in approximately 40 percent of immunized persons after the fifth inoculation, and in 15 percent of immunized persons after the seventh inoculation. The most common local reactions—erythema, pruritis, and a small area of induration—were mild and disappeared within 24 to 48 hours. Overall, local reactions of any type, from mild to severe, were observed following 35 percent of inoculations.

Local reactions of greater severity included edema, an area of erythema of 25 square centimeters (cm^2) or more, local tenderness and pruritis, and small painless nodules that persisted for several weeks. Severe, edema-producing reactions occurred following 2.8 percent of vaccinations, with those reactions peaking at the sixth inoculation and none occurring following the first inoculation. In three inoculees, extensive edema extended from the deltoid to the midforearm or wrist and resolved in 3 to 5 days. Systemic reactions were observed in two of the vaccine recipients who experienced edema. The systemic reactions consisted of "some malaise of 24 hours' duration." Overall, 6 working days were lost as a result of the reactions of edema. In all, three placebo recipients experienced mild reactions, which were not further described. No information about sex differences in adverse effects was reported, nor was there any long-term follow-up of study participants.

The study by Brachman and colleagues (1962) has several strengths in estimating the frequency of reactions following receipt of anthrax vaccine. First, there was a placebo group against which the rates of reported reactions could be compared. Second, the characteristics of the vaccinated and placebo groups were likely to be comparable initially because of the randomized assignment of study participants. Third, recipients were directly monitored for the occurrence of adverse events following vaccination, reducing the possibility of reporting biases. Fourth, the criteria for determination of the presence and magnitudes of the reactions were explicitly defined. Unfortunately, events following vaccination were monitored in only two of the four mills and were monitored only for the first 48 hours following inoculation. The largest disadvantage of the study is its limited size.

Dose Reduction and Route Change Study A pilot study at the U.S. Army Medical Research Institute of Infectious Diseases (USAMRIID) on immune responses to alternative AVA dosing schedules and alternative routes of administration included active surveillance for adverse reactions (Pittman, 2001b; Pittman et al., 2002). In that study, 173 U.S. military and civilian volunteers (109 men and 64 women) were randomized to one of seven groups, defined on the basis of dosing schedule and route of administration. Three experimental dosing schedules were tested: a single injection on day 0, injections on days 0 and 14, and injections on days 0 and 28. For each experimental dosing schedule, two groups were established; one group was inoculated subcutaneously and the other group was inoculated intramuscularly. A control group was administered AVA by the licensed six-dose schedule and subcutaneous administration.

Study participants were evaluated clinically for local and systemic reactions at 30 minutes, 1, 2, and 3 days, 1 week, and 1 month after each vaccination. Local reactions at the injection site were common, with significant differences related to route of AVA administration and to sex. With subcutaneous vaccine administration, tenderness at the injection site was observed following the administration of 70 percent of the doses, erythema was observed following the administration of 36 percent of the doses, and induration was observed following the administration of 15 percent of the doses. With intramuscular administration, those effects were observed following the administration of 56, 6, and 2 percent of the doses, respectively. Subcutaneous nodules, observed following the administration of 38 percent of the subcutaneous doses, were not noted with intramuscular administration. With subcutaneous administration of one to three doses of AVA, some local reactions were significantly more common in women than in men. For example, erythema was observed in 63.4 percent of women and 22 percent of men, a subcutaneous nodule was observed in 63.4 percent of women and 24.2 percent of men, and local tenderness was observed in 84.5 percent of women and 62.9 percent of men.

The incidence of systemic reactions did not vary by route of vaccine administration or sex. For subcutaneous administration, the most common systemic reactions that occurred following administration of the first three doses were headache (9.9 percent of doses), malaise (9.4 percent), and myalgia (4.4 percent). No serious reaction attributable to the vaccine was observed with either subcutaneous or intramuscular administration.

The USAMRIID pilot study has the advantage of being a prospective randomized controlled trial, although it did not have a comparison group that received no active agent. In addition, the critical component of sex was included in the analysis. The study confirms a sex difference in local reactions that cannot be wholly attributable to a bias in reporting. However, it does not find a sex-related difference in systemic reaction rates that has been reported in other studies. The results of the study suggest that the approved subcutaneous route of vaccine administration may produce more local reactions than intramuscular administration. Given the significance of the route of administration, the number of participants in the study was relatively small, and larger studies should be instituted in the future. The Centers for Disease Control and Prevention (CDC) is planning a more extensive study to test the route of administration and the number of doses needed for protection.

Other Controlled Studies

ROTC Cadets Inadvertent administration of higher than recommended doses of anthrax vaccine to Reserve Officer Training Corps (ROTC) cadets provided an opportunity to compare their reports of acute effects with reports from cadets who received the recommended doses (Gunzenhauser et al., 2001). During the summer of 2000, 73 ROTC cadets were scheduled to begin the AVA series before deployment to Korea. Twenty-five cadets received 1.0 ml of vaccine as the initial dose, twice the recommended amount. The other 48 cadets received the standard dose of 0.5 ml. All the cadets received the standard dose of the vaccine for the second immunization.

Information on symptoms experienced by the cadets following vaccination was collected through a voluntary survey administered a few days after receipt of each of the two doses. The recipients of the double dose had been advised of the dosing error, and most of them completed the voluntary surveys after the receipt of both doses (25 and 18 responses, respectively). Of those who received only standard doses, 12 cadets completed the survey administered after the first dose, and 42 cadets completed the survey after the second dose.

Among the cadets who received the double dose, 92 percent reported a sore arm after the first injection, 88 percent reported a lump at the injection site, and 84 percent reported swelling. For cadets who received the standard dose, the reports for these symptoms after the first injection were 83, 42, and 42 percent, respectively. Fever was the only systemic effect reported after administration of the first dose, reported by 12 percent of those who received the double dose and 8 percent of those who received the standard dose. Decreased performance was reported by 28 percent of the cadets who received the double dose and 8 percent of those who received the standard dose. Following administration of the second vaccine dose, 44 percent of cadets who had received a double first dose reported three or more local symptoms, whereas 26 percent of those who received a standard first dose reported three or more local symptoms. In the group that received the double dose, 22 percent reported tiredness and 11 percent reported headache, whereas 7 and 5 percent of those in the standard-dose group reported these symptoms, respectively. Reports of fever (7 percent) and nausea (5 percent) came only from the standard-dose group.

This opportunistic study provides information on adverse events following the receipt of a double vaccine dose and standard vaccine doses. The increased dose produced local and systemic effects similar to those experienced after receipt of the standard dose, but a greater proportion of the recipients experienced the effects. In both groups, there were fewer reports of systemic effects (e.g., fever, tiredness, and headache) than local effects. No severe adverse events or hospitalizations occurred among either group of cadets after the administration of either dose. The number of subjects in the two study groups is small, however; and all ascertainment of health effects was through self-reports.

Uncontrolled Studies

Investigational New Drug Data The committee reviewed five annual reports submitted from 1967 through 1971 by CDC to the Division of Biologics Standards of the National Institutes of Health in support of the Investigational New Drug (IND) application required for licensure of AVA (CDC, 1967–1971). The committee received the information as the result of a Freedom of Information Act request made by an earlier Institute of Medicine (IOM) committee. The committee also received copies of unredacted progress reports from the files of the current vaccine manufacturer, BioPort.

Two vaccine formulations were administered under the IND application. The formulation originally developed at Fort Detrick, Maryland, by Wright and colleagues (1954) and manufactured by Merck, Sharp and Dohme was distributed only during the first reporting year. The other formulation was AVA, which was manufactured by the Michigan Department of Public Health by the methods described by Puziss and colleagues (1963). AVA was administered over the entire course of the study. Because distribution of the older Merck vaccine was discontinued, some study participants received both formulations over the course of their vaccinations.

The annual reports submitted in support of the IND application reflect experience from the administration of almost 16,000 doses of AVA to about 7,000 people in an observational study with no control subjects. The study was designed as an open-label, multicenter study that provided investigational vaccine to individuals at risk of exposure to anthrax at nine U.S. sites and one foreign site. Most of the study participants were textile workers with potential contact with contaminated goat hair or wool; a minority were laboratory personnel engaged in research or diagnostic procedures involving anthrax. Adverse events following vaccination were reported by the investigators administering the vaccines, who were required to record any reaction observed 48 hours after administration of the vaccine and to notify the National Communicable Disease Center (NCDC) of any severe reactions. A reporting form for each vaccinee was returned to NCDC following administration of the initial series of three doses or after the administration of a booster dose. It is not clear whether investigators examined or at least contacted vaccine recipients to ascertain reactions (active surveillance) or whether they relied on reports from recipients (passive surveillance).

Local reactions were classified as mild, moderate, or severe. A mild reaction was defined as an area of erythema (redness) only or of measurable edema or induration of ≤3 cm in diameter. A moderate reaction was defined as an area of edema or induration of >3 cm to <12 cm in diameter. A severe reaction was defined as any reaction measuring >12 cm in diameter or accompanied by marked limitation of arm motion or axiliary node tenderness. Mild reactions were reported following the administration of 8.4 percent of the AVA doses, moderate reactions following the administration of 0.9 percent of the AVA doses, and severe reactions following the administration of 0.2 percent of the AVA doses. Systemic reactions, including chills, fever, aches, and malaise, were reported for four vaccine recipients. All reactions were self-limited. Adverse event rates were not reported by sex, and no surveillance for later-onset effects was conducted.

This study suggests that AVA has a reaction profile comparable to that of other toxin-based vaccines such as tetanus toxoid. No investigations were reported of the mechanisms of the few systemic reactions that were noted. The reactogenicity of the vaccine appeared to vary by lot. The use of one lot manufactured by Merck was discontinued because it was more reactogenic than another available lot. Conclusions from the study are limited by its observational design. Furthermore, reports of adverse events are not available by sex or age, and in the early part of the study more than one vaccine formulation was administered.

Special Immunizations Program Safety Study Additional information on the immediate-onset reactions following administration of AVA is available from observations of inoculations given between 1973 and 1999 through the Special Immunizations Program at USAMRIID at Fort Detrick, Maryland (Pittman, 2001a; Pittman et al., 2001a,b). The study participants were those laboratory and maintenance workers who required access to the biocontainment facilities where *Bacillus anthracis* was studied.

The study population included 1,583 at-risk individuals, of whom 79 percent were men, 81 percent were aged 18 to 40, and 86 percent were of European origin. Over the reporting period, these individuals received 10,722 AVA doses, administered in accordance with the licensed schedule. The median number of doses received was six. A total of 273 (17.2 percent) study participants received 10 or more doses, and 46 (2.9 percent) participants received 20 or more doses. Most participants also received several other vaccines during the study period.

Surveillance for the occurrence of local and systemic adverse events was passive: the vaccine recipients self-reported adverse events if they sought treatment or if they believed the adverse event should be recorded in their health records. When participants came into the clinic to report adverse events, study staff evaluated and recorded the adverse events, classifying them as local or systemic.

Local reactions of some type were reported for 3.6 percent of the 10,722 doses of vaccine administered. Erythema and/or induration (E/I), the most common local reaction, was reported for 3.2 percent of the doses administered. Of the 1925 doses administered to women, E/I was reported following 7.3 percent. Men received 8,797 doses, of which 2.2 percent resulted in reports of E/I. Doses given to individuals ages 18 to 40 were followed by significantly more reports of reactions at the injection site than were doses given to those over age 40, but this result was not adjusted for sex. After adjustment for age and sex, reports of erythema, induration, and injection-site warmth were significantly higher for doses given to participants of European ancestry than for those given to African Americans.

Of the 32 vaccine lots used during the study, 50 or more doses were administered from only 19 lots. There was significant variation by lot in the incidence of injection-site reactions, ranging from 0 to 22.1 percent. Receipt of vaccine from the one lot that was found to have traces of squalene contamination did not produce an elevated rate of local reactions (5.3 percent of doses administered, which was the fifth highest rate of local reactions among the 19 lots). (See Chapter 4 for information on laboratory analysis for the presence of squalene in AVA.)

After controlling for vaccine lot and sex, reporting of E/I after the administration of one dose was found to be associated with an increased likelihood of reporting of E/I after the administration of the next dose (odds ratio [OR] = 13; 95 percent confidence interval [CI] = 8.7 to 21). The relative risks of a second reaction were 6.9 (95 percent CI = 4.3 to 10.9) for women and 14.3 (95 percent CI = 8.8 to 23) for men. However, a reaction to one dose was not a satisfactory predictor of a subsequent reaction for either women or men because most reactions occurred in persons who had received a previous dose with no resulting reaction.

Systemic reactions of any sort were reported following the administration of 101 of the 10,722 doses (1 percent) and were more frequent for doses administered to women than for doses administered to men. Overall, the most commonly reported reactions were headache (0.4 percent of doses), malaise (0.4 percent), myalgia (0.3 percent), nausea (0.1 percent), and dizziness (0.1 percent). For both women and men, those who reported a systemic reaction following the administration of one dose were more likely to report a systemic reaction following the administration of a subsequent dose. However, the majority of systemic reactions occurred after the administration of a dose to individuals who had already received vaccine doses with no systemic reaction. No sustained adverse events were noted, but long-term follow-up was not conducted.

Since the adverse events were self-reported and were not uniformly recorded for all who were vaccinated, this study may be most useful for the establishment of trends in subgroups. Absolute estimates of local or systemic reactions cannot be given. However, the study suggests that females and younger individuals more commonly report local reactions. The rates did vary by vaccine lot, but this may be confounded by secular trends in reporting reactions. The study also confirms that a prior reaction is predictive of a future reaction. However, the study cannot distinguish between elevated rates of reporting of adverse events versus an actual increase in the reaction rates.

Fort Bragg Booster Study Pittman and colleagues (1997, in press; Pittman, 2001c) conducted a study to assess the persistence of antibodies to *B. anthracis* 18 to 24 months after initial vaccination during Operations Desert Shield and Desert Storm and to assess the safety and immunogenicity of a vaccine booster dose. Study participants were recruited from active-duty personnel at Fort Bragg, North Carolina, in 1992 and 1994. All participants were volunteers and signed an informed-consent form to participate in the study.

The study population consisted of 495 male Operations Desert Shield and Desert Storm veterans who received one to three primary doses of AVA in 1990 or 1991. Only 5.5 percent received a single AVA dose; 70.5 percent received two doses, and 24.0 percent received three doses. Of the total, 91.3 percent received both AVA and pentavalent botulinum toxoid (PBT) in separate arms, and 8.7 percent received AVA only. For the booster study, participants who had originally received both vaccines also received (in separate arms) booster doses of both vaccines. Most participants (62 percent) were aged 30 to 39, and 92 percent were non-Hispanic Caucasians.

Adverse reactions to the booster vaccination were monitored through active surveillance. All study participants were assessed at 30 minutes after receiving the booster dose and subsequently on days 1, 2, 3, and 7 following vaccination. In addition, 86 percent of the participants returned after 24 to 36 days for an additional evaluation. Any individuals with reactions that were present at 24 to 36 days were monitored until the reactions resolved.

Because of the field setting of the study and the use of active surveillance, local reactions were common for both vaccines. Among the subjects who received only an AVA booster, an E/I reaction of <5 cm in diameter was observed in 27.9 percent, and an E/I reaction of 5 to 12 cm was observed in 4.7 percent. None of the study participants who received only an AVA booster had an E/I reaction of >12 cm in diameter. Among those who received both AVA and PBT, E/I reactions of these sizes were observed in 16.0, 9.3, and 0.7 percent of participants, respectively. Local reactions commonly occurred within 4 days of receipt of the booster dose.

Systemic reactions were also frequent following receipt of the vaccine booster dose, but the investigators noted that the study participants were also engaged daily in strenuous physical exercise, which could produce systemic reactions as well. The most common systemic reactions reported by those who received only an AVA booster dose were muscle ache (23.3 percent), headache (9.3 percent), malaise (7 percent), joint pain (7.0 percent), and fever (2.5 percent). In the much larger group of individuals who received both the AVA and the PBT booster doses, systemic reactions were reported by a greater percentage of study participants: muscle ache, 31 percent; rash, 17.3 percent; malaise, 16.8 percent; headache, 16.6 percent; joint pain, 13.1 percent; and fever, 2.7 percent. Anorexia (3.8 percent), nausea (3.5 percent), and breathing problems (0.2 percent) were reported only by study participants who received both booster doses simultaneously.

This study prospectively recorded the occurrence of local and systemic reactions following administration of an AVA booster to men previously primed with AVA vaccine. Because most vaccinees also received PBT, the results are difficult to interpret in terms of the effects specifically related to AVA. Those who received both vaccines simultaneously had more systemic reactions. Although fewer local reactions were noted in those who received both vaccines than in those who received AVA only, these reactions may have been recorded less often when systemic reactions were noted. The results do suggest that local and systemic reactions commonly occur within 4 days of vaccination but that these reactions are transient.

U.S. Forces in Korea Hoffman and colleagues (Hoffman et al., submitted for publication; CDC, 2000) analyzed information on adverse events following vaccination of U.S. forces in Korea with AVA between August 1998 and July 1999. The study was conducted at a single military clinic where a structured medical note was used as a survey instrument. In the study, 2,036 men and 495 women reporting to the clinic for vaccination with AVA completed a short questionnaire that requested information on sex, health status, vaccination history, and the occurrence of local or systemic reactions following the previous vaccination.

For both men and women, local reactions were common and were generally minor and did not lead to impairment of work performance. Women and anyone who had a reaction following receipt of a prior dose of AVA or who was taking medications were significantly more likely than their counterparts to report adverse events. Nodules and erythema were statistically more common in women. For example, reported rates of occurrence of nodules following receipt of one of the first three vaccine doses ranged from 49.8 to 62.4 percent for women, whereas the rates were 21.4 to 28.9 percent for men. Women also reported higher rates of localized itching, ranging from 20.4 to 37.0 percent, whereas the rates were 5.5 to 7.5 percent for men. Among those reporting a single reaction, men more consistently reported high rates of pain (12.4 to 16.9 percent) than women (2.9 to 5.0 percent). Decreased activity without a loss of time from work was the most common consequence of adverse events, reported by 6.7 percent of women and 5.7 percent of men following receipt of the third vaccine dose.

These data indicate that minor adverse events following the receipt of AVA are common and that rates are generally higher among women than among men. Since the service personnel reported adverse events at the next vaccine administration, however, there may have been some underreporting of adverse events and some selection bias in the reporting of those events. However, the results confirm those of other studies that women report more adverse events following vaccination with AVA but that they also report less pain than men.

Tripler Army Medical Center Survey The nature and frequency of adverse events following vaccination with AVA were assessed in a group of 601 military health care workers at Tripler Army Medical Center in Hawaii who began receiving vaccinations in September 1998 (AVIP, 2001; CDC, 2000; GAO, 1999; Wasserman, 2001). The study population included 416 men and 185 women, and the overall median age was 28 years. Enlisted personnel accounted for 71 percent of the group. Self-administered questionnaires were used to collect data on adverse events following each dose. Data on localized reactions were collected retrospectively for the first three doses and prospectively for subsequent doses. All data on systemic reactions were collected prospectively.

Local reactions were common and were generally highest following receipt of the first dose. The reactions included an area of redness, a lump or a knot at the injection site, and localized itching. Reports of local reactions were significantly higher for women than men, with an adjusted OR for any local reaction of 2.44 (95 percent CI = 2.04 to 2.93). Redness with a diameter of >5 cm was reported by 37 to 43 percent of women, whereas it was reported by 15 to 23 percent of men. Similarly, a lump or knot at the injection site was reported by 81 to 93 percent of women and 56 to 65 percent of men. Edema involving the lower arm was reported by 8 to 14 percent of women and 7 to 10 percent of men.

Muscle ache was the most commonly reported systemic reaction, reported following 45 percent of doses administered to women and 41 percent of doses administered to men. The study participants also reported whether their ability to perform their duties was affected and whether they had medical visits related to vaccination. For both indicators, reports were higher for women than for men. Four to 12 percent of women and 2 to 6 percent of men reported limitations in their ability to perform their duties. Four to 14 percent of women and 2 to 5 percent of men reported that they made an outpatient medical visit following vaccination with AVA.

This study monitored a group of subjects over the full series of six inoculations, but by the sixth dose about 50 percent of the original participants had been lost due to reassignment, separation from the military, or medical and other exemptions from vaccination. No control group was included, and it is uncertain how reports from medical personnel would compare with those from other military personnel.

9th Airlift Squadron Survey A survey of the members of the 9th Airlift Squadron at Dover Air Force Base in Delaware collected information on the systemic symptoms that they experienced following vaccination with AVA (Tanner, 2001). Vaccination of this squadron with AVA began in the autumn of 1998. In January 2000 a questionnaire was distributed by mail to all members of the squadron except administrative workers, a group that had not yet been vaccinated. Respondents were asked to provide information that included the number of vaccine doses they had received, whether they had experienced any of 16 specified systemic symptoms at any time since receiving their first vaccine dose, and whether they had sought treatment from the flight surgeon's clinic for symptoms or had lost time from duty. Respondents were also asked to describe their symptoms and any formal diagnosis that they had received.

Of 265 questionnaires mailed, 139 (52 percent) were completed and returned by vaccinated squadron members. Two other respondents had not been vaccinated, and so their responses were not included in the tabulations; 11 questionnaires were undeliverable. Responses were received from nine women, but the survey results were not reported separately for men and women. Joint or muscle pain was the most common symptom, reported by 42 percent of the 139 respondents. Other common symptoms included loss of energy or tiredness (31 percent), reduced concentration (27 percent), and short-term memory loss (26 percent). Reports of some systemic symptoms noted in other studies included itchy skin (21 percent), headaches (19 percent), and chills or fever immediately following vaccination (11 percent). Overall, 89 respondents (64 percent) reported one or more symptoms. Of these, 41 reported that they had sought treatment for one or more symptoms. The author noted that an unspecified number of untreated respondents added comments indicating that they had refrained from seeking treatment because of concerns about the quality of care available or the potential loss of flight status. In addition, 24 of the respondents with symptoms reported that they had missed more than 1 day of work; 10 had not returned to full duty.

This survey provides both quantitative and qualitative information on the self-reported systemic symptoms experienced by members of a single Air Force squadron who responded to the survey. An unofficial survey may elicit reports of symptoms from persons who would be reluctant to report those symptoms as part of an official DoD study or disease surveillance program. On the other hand, if persons with symptoms are more likely to respond to the survey, the rates of occurrence of symptoms after vaccination with AVA will be overestimated. In addition, no information is provided about the timing of these self-reported symptoms in relation to the time of receipt of AVA. It is difficult to interpret the results of a survey that asks for the occurrence of events "at any time" since receiving AVA. The author acknowledges that the low response rate and the lack of a control group are important limitations of the study.

Studies of Health Effects with Later Onset

Any Health Outcomes: Uncontrolled Studies

Multiple Vaccines Studies Three published studies (Peeler et al., 1958, 1965; White et al., 1974) provide longitudinal information on a population of skilled laborers and laboratory workers at Fort Detrick, Maryland. The members of this study population received multiple doses of many different vaccines, including an anthrax vaccine, because of the potential for occupational exposure to virulent microorganisms. The 99 white male workers in the initial cohort (Peeler et al., 1958) were selected for the study because they had the longest and most intensive vaccination histories among the 700 employees receiving a continuing schedule of multiple immunizations. The workers began receiving vaccinations in 1944 and were evaluated for these studies in 1956, 1962, and 1971, respectively. Both acute and more persistent changes in health status following vaccination were ascertained through complete medical histories, physical examinations, laboratory tests, and reviews of outpatient and immunization records.

An earlier IOM report (IOM, 2000) described the three studies in some detail. The well-studied cohort showed no evidence of illnesses attributable to intensive immunization over a 25-year period or any serious, unexplained illnesses. Reaction rates for immediate-onset events, whether local or systemic, were not reported for any individual vaccine. The concerns over the high incidence of abnormal liver function test results, lymphocytosis, and abnormalities observed by electrophoresis of serum raised in the two earlier studies (Peeler et al., 1958, 1965) were increasingly dispelled by the third report (White et al., 1974). The laboratory changes were often reversible, as shown in the second study (Peeler et al., 1965), and in the third study (White et al., 1974), conducted 10 months after the termination of the immunization program, laboratory values had normalized. The serum abnormalities seen earlier are probably explainable by an increased level of fast mobility gamma globulins. The overall mortality rate for the cohort was within the expected range.

In general, data from these studies do not suggest that repeated exposure to AVA along with other vaccines is associated with later-onset health effects, but the studies are of limited value for evaluating the safety of AVA. Because the cohort was exposed to many vaccines in addition to an anthrax vaccine, indications of any deleterious effects could have been due to any of the vaccines received. In addition, during the time frame covered by these studies, workers received both earlier anthrax vaccine products and the currently licensed AVA product. Although the number of anthrax vaccine recipients increased over the study period from 28 to at least 76, without apparent coincident changes in the health status of the group, the small size of the cohort provides little statistical power to detect increased risk of illness.

Reproductive Outcomes: Controlled Study

Pregnancy, Births, and Birth Outcomes Wiesen and colleagues (Wiesen, 2001a,b; Wiesen and Littell, 2001) compared the reproductive experiences of vaccinated and unvaccinated women on active duty in the U.S. Army. The study population consisted of 4,092 women, ages 17 to 44 years, who had been assigned to Fort Stewart or Hunter Army Airfield in Georgia between January 1999 and March 2000. Of this group, 3,135 received at least one dose of AVA; 962 were unvaccinated. The vaccinated and unvaccinated women were similar in age and marital status. A similar percentage of women in each group was African American, but a smaller percentage of the vaccinated group was white (28.8 versus 36.4 percent) and a larger percentage was of another race (19.7 versus 12.9 percent).

The analysis compared the two groups in terms of pregnancy rates, the proportion of pregnancies resulting in live births, and the incidence of adverse birth outcomes. The size of the study population provided an 80 percent power to detect a 20 percent decline in the pregnancy rate. Pregnancies, births, and birth outcomes were determined from a review of medical records at Fort Stewart. For 54 of 85 women who left Fort Stewart during their pregnancies, records from the Defense Enrollment Eligibility Reporting System (DEERS) could be used to determine if a birth occurred. Vaccination against anthrax had no effect on pregnancy rates (OR = 0.9, 95 percent CI = 0.7 to 1.1), with or without adjustment for marital status, race, and age. There also was no significant difference between vaccinated and unvaccinated women in terms of the proportion of pregnancies that resulted in a live birth (adjusted OR = 0.8, 95 percent CI = 0.7 to 1.0). In addition, the adjusted ORs for low birth weight (OR = 1.3, 95 percent CI = 0.2 to 6.4) and structural abnormalities of cosmetic or surgical significance (OR = 0.7, 95 percent CI = 0.2 to 2.3) showed that there was no statistically significant elevation of risk for the infants of vaccinated women.

The strengths of this study include the size of the study population and the resulting statistical power to detect changes in pregnancy rates. Also, the retrospective ascertainment of outcomes from a source independent of exposure reduces potential observer and follow-up biases. However, information on certain outcomes was obtained from two sources: medical records and DEERS. It may have been better to use only information from DEERS to ascertain the outcome and then verify agreement with the medical record, where available. The study may be interpreted as providing some assurance that vaccination with AVA has no major adverse effect on reproductive potential or reproductive outcomes. However, because specific birth defects occur at low rates and different birth defects can have different causes, failure to detect an excess overall rate of birth defects does not necessarily rule out an elevation of risk for a specific, although rare, birth defect. In addition, the power of the study to detect meaningful decreases in birth rates or birth weights associated with maternal AVA exposure is unknown. The study does not directly address the risks of vaccination during pregnancy. Women known to be pregnant were exempted from vaccination, but some women with early unconfirmed pregnancies may have been vaccinated. Thus, more definitive conclusions regarding pregnancy outcomes will depend on additional study.

Observations Regarding Ad Hoc Studies

The studies reviewed thus far describe a consistent pattern of relatively frequent, mild to moderate local reactions of immediate onset following receipt of AVA. Severe local reactions and systemic reactions are much less common. These studies are relatively small, however, and none of them provides adequate information concerning the occurrence of later-onset events. In addition, most of these studies do not include adequate comparison groups of unimmunized individuals against which rates of adverse events among vaccinated groups can be compared. The record-linkage studies discussed in the next section are therefore especially valuable because they address many of these limitations. Analyses based on data from record-linkage systems generally involve larger study populations and cover a longer period of experience with AVA than other studies do. More importantly, they provide the opportunity to examine associations of AVA with disease conditions of later onset, and they provide appropriate comparison groups that consist of persons who have not been exposed to AVA. Furthermore, evaluation of the outcome is unrelated to assessment of vaccine exposure.

RECORD-LINKAGE STUDIES

Surveillance and analysis of adverse events following vaccination of military personnel are aided by the availability of databases that permit linkage of personnel and demographic information with information on military experience, immunizations, and medical events for active-duty personnel. The individual branches of the armed services maintain such databases, but even more useful are various DoD-wide databases, particularly the system of databases of health-related information (reported by each of the armed services) called the Defense Medical Surveillance System (DMSS; see http://amsa.army.mil/AMSA/AMSA_DMSS.htm). DMSS is coordinated by the Army Medical Surveillance Activity (AMSA).

The DMSS databases permit linkage of the records for all active-duty personnel. These databases include some historical data, but they have various starting dates. For example, records on inpatient care in military medical facilities date from 1990, whereas those for ambulatory care begin in 1996. Medical data are derived from Standard Inpatient Data Records and the Standard Ambulatory Data Records for all inpatient and outpatient encounters at military facilities. For each hospitalization, up to eight discharge diagnoses are coded using the *International Classification of Diseases, Ninth Revision, Clinical Modification* (ICD-9-CM). Other DMSS databases have records on immunizations and reportable health events. At present, the records on immunizations with AVA are more complete than those for immunizations with other vaccines. Records on reportable health events cover a set of diseases and health conditions named in the list of Tri-Service Reportable Events (AMSA, 1998; Mazzuchi, 1998). This list includes any adverse event following vaccination that results in admission to a health care facility or the loss of time from duty for more than 1 day.

Because DMSS and other DoD-wide databases can produce data on the entire population of active-duty military personnel and on the subpopulation vaccinated under the Anthrax Vaccine Immunization Program, they have denominator data that are unavailable from the Vaccine Adverse Event Reporting System (VAERS), making it possible to assess vaccine-associated adverse event rates (number of adverse events/number of vaccine administrations) for some types of health events following vaccination. Adverse event rates can also be compared between populations that did and that did not receive the vaccine. The DMSS databases also make it possible to monitor postvaccination medical histories over the length of active service. Even though this period is limited (typical Army enlistment is 2 to 6 years [Grabenstein, 2001]), it is a longer period of observation than that available for most vaccine safety studies.

Although DMSS is a substantially richer analytic resource than VAERS, it still has certain limitations. Whereas VAERS has the potential to receive reports on any type of adverse event following vaccination, including mild events, DMSS will capture only events that require inpatient or ambulatory medical care or result in the loss of time from duty. DMSS data may also be affected by administrative and operational differences among the armed services. Many of the data contained in DMSS are originally collected in data systems operated by the individual services and are periodically transmitted to AMSA for incorporation into DMSS databases. Delays in the transfer of data can mean that DMSS records are not up to date. Differences in data collection practices by the individual services may also mean that DMSS records differ in terms of their completeness.

During the course of its work, the committee reviewed record-linkage analyses carried out with data from databases maintained by individual branches of the armed services, as well as the results of analyses conducted by the Naval Health Research Center and AMSA with data available from DMSS or other DoD-wide databases. Discussions of the studies conducted with data from the databases of the individual service branches are followed by discussions of the analyses conducted with data from DoD-wide databases.

Studies Conducted with Data from Single-Service Databases

Air Combat Command Study

Rehme and colleagues (Rehme, 2001; Rehme et al., 2002) performed an opportunistic retrospective cohort study in which they compared the postdeployment use of Air Force ambulatory health care services by AVA-vaccinated and unvaccinated Air Force personnel following their return from Southwest Asia (SWA). The study population was identified by linking Air Force records on visits to a medical treatment facility in SWA between January 1, 1998, and September 10, 1998, with DoD records on vaccination against anthrax. Of the personnel with records of a visit to a medical treatment facility in SWA, 4,045 persons had a record of the receipt of at least one dose of AVA and 1,133 persons had no record of the receipt of any doses of AVA. Men accounted for 84 percent of the vaccinated group and 85 percent of the unvaccinated group.

No difference in the rate of postdeployment use of Air Force ambulatory health care services within the 6 months following vaccination with AVA was found between the vaccinated and the unvaccinated personnel. Women were more likely than men to have had a postdeployment ambulatory health care visit (relative risk 1.38, 95 percent CI = 1.30 to 1.46), but there was no difference between vaccinated and unvaccinated men (relative risk = 0.95, 95 percent CI = 0.88 to 1.02) or between vaccinated and unvaccinated women (relative risk = 0.99, 95 percent CI = 0.88 to 1.12). The analysis also examined ambulatory health care visits in terms of 17 broad ICD-9-CM diagnostic categories as well as 16 specific diagnoses, including diabetes, thyroid disorders, anemia, and headache. For vaccinated personnel, the risks of any of these diagnoses were comparable to or lower than those for unvaccinated personnel.

The uniformly negative results support the general conclusion that AVA does not lead to increased use of health care services by DoD personnel, and the inclusion of only deployed personnel in the study attempts to control for a possible "healthy soldier" effect. This is analogous to the "healthy worker" effect observed in studies of occupational groups compared with the general population.

Nevertheless, the study has important limitations. First, all personnel entered into this study must have visited an ambulatory health care setting at least once during their deployment, and according to the investigators, this eliminated more than 50 percent of the deployed personnel. This eligibility criterion might have the effect of masking an adverse effect of AVA if those not vaccinated experienced other health conditions that made them more likely to have used health care services. The uniformity of the findings, however, argues against (although does not rule out) this potential bias.

Second, there is no control for whether Air Force personnel sought ambulatory care in SWA or in the United States from sources other than Air Force treatment facilities. If personnel were more likely to receive AVA if they were to be deployed for longer periods in SWA and if medical care was less available in SWA, the results may mask a real effect of vaccination with AVA. Again, the uniformity of the results argues against (but does not rule out) this potential bias.

Third, if personnel who received AVA had medical problems that resulted in an early discharge from the military, they would not have been included in the analysis. The investigators clearly note this possibility but suggest that the time required to process a medical discharge would limit its effect. The available data offer no basis for evaluation of this possibility.

Finally, it is not known how service personnel were selected to receive AVA (perhaps it was random, but the committee does not know this).

U.S. Army Aviation Epidemiology Data Register

A study of U.S. Army aircrew members was conducted to assess clinical outcomes reflecting vaccine-associated adverse events among those who had been vaccinated with AVA (Mason et al., 2001, submitted for publication). The study used record linkage to assess those who were vaccinated with AVA and those who were not and to identify clinical outcomes. A total of 3,356 AVA-vaccinated aircrew personnel were matched to an equal number of unvaccinated personnel by age, sex, race, class of flying duties (aviator, flight traffic controller, flight surgeon), and type of service (active, reserve). Changes in medical condition were determined by comparison of information from medical examinations conducted before and after the vaccination date for the AVA-exposed individual in the pair. The clinical outcomes evaluated included weight change, an increase in blood pressure, anemia, increased intraocular pressure, stereopsis, hearing loss, vision loss, proteinuria or glycosuria, and increased fasting blood sugar levels. No outcome showed any positive association with receipt of the AVA vaccine. In fact, those vaccinated with AVA actually showed less weight loss and vision loss than those not vaccinated.

The apparent reduction in risk may be attributable to a healthy soldier effect. Those vaccinated may have been healthier than those not vaccinated, thus producing an apparent but spurious negative association with administration of AVA. In addition, the average time between examinations may have been different for the personnel vaccinated with AVA and those not vaccinated with AVA. Nonetheless, the results do not show any elevation in adverse outcomes due to AVA vaccination.

Analyses of Data from DoD-Wide Databases

Naval Health Research Center DoD-Wide Surveillance of Hospitalizations

Sato and colleagues (2001a,b; Sato et al., 2001) used data from DoD databases on hospitalizations of active-duty military personnel to determine whether those who had received AVA had an excess of hospitalizations within 42 days of AVA vaccination compared with those who had not received AVA. The study included all U.S. military service personnel on active duty during the analysis period, which extended from January 1,

1998, through March 31, 2000. Hospitalizations in both military and nonmilitary facilities were ascertained. Hospitalization data were linked with the vaccination, demographic, and personnel data in DoD records. All personnel received other standard vaccinations.

The analysis was based on 2,651 hospitalizations and 120,870 person-years of observation in the group vaccinated with AVA (the vaccinated group) and 151,609 hospitalizations and more than 2.3 million person-years in the group not vaccinated with AVA (the unvaccinated group). For the vaccinated group, the risk interval was counted from the date of AVA vaccination until either the date of the first hospital admission, the date of receipt of the next dose of AVA, or the end of the analysis period (March 31, 2000). The hospitalization rates for this group were calculated per person-years of observation within 42 days of receipt of any AVA dose. For the unvaccinated group, the risk interval started January 1, 1998, and extended to the date of the first hospital admission, the date of separation from the military, or March 31, 2000. Hospitalizations were assigned to 14 major ICD-9-CM categories of disease on the basis of discharge diagnoses. Subsequent hospitalizations for the same condition were not counted for either group.

Relative risks for the vaccinated group versus the unvaccinated group were adjusted for age (in quartiles), sex, number of hospitalizations in the previous year, marital status, race/ethnicity, pay grade, duty occupation category, branch of service, and number of days deployed (in quartiles). Analyses were done separately for men and women. No adjustments for multiple comparisons were made in the interim analysis presented to the committee.

Vaccinated men and women had significantly lower relative risks than unvaccinated personnel for hospitalizations for each of the 14 broad ICD-9-CM categories examined. Adjusted relative risks for women ranged from a low of 0.18 for diseases of the blood to a high of 0.66 for neoplasms. For men the lowest relative risk was 0.30 for mental conditions, and the highest relative risk was 0.75 for diseases of the digestive system.

In these analyses, receipt of AVA was not associated with a significant increase in the risk of hospitalization within 42 days of vaccination for 14 major groups of disease, and, in fact, vaccinated personnel were hospitalized significantly less than unvaccinated personnel. The relative risks for hospitalization (the group vaccinated with AVA versus the group not vaccinated with AVA) were very low, with the relative risks for most personnel falling between 0.2 and 0.6. Relative risks less than 1.0 would be expected if service personnel who received AVA were also more likely to be deployed and deployment is associated with a healthy soldier effect. The possibility thus cannot be discounted that differences in the risk of hospitalization between personnel who received AVA and personnel who did not reflect differences in deployment status. Although analyses were statistically adjusted for quartiles of number of days deployed, this approach may not have been adequate to fully control for differences between deployed and undeployed military personnel in their underlying health status or in the manner in which health-related issues are addressed for predeployment personnel. Also affecting the interpretation of the current results is the possibility that the disease categories used may be too broad to detect increases in risks of individual diseases in the group vaccinated with AVA.

AMSA Analyses of DMSS Data Regarding Health Outcomes Following Vaccination Against Anthrax

In 2000 and 2001, AMSA prepared several reports that described analyses that were carried out with data available from DMSS to assess whether inpatient or outpatient medical visits are associated with vaccination with AVA. AMSA also carried out analyses in response to specific questions raised by the IOM committee. As a result, several different approaches to the analyses of the data available from DMSS were taken over the course of the committee's work. Each is described separately.

Screening Analyses In 2001, AMSA began a process of regularly using DMSS data for screening purposes. It has since produced two quarterly reports describing screening analyses of data available from DMSS and DoD's electronic immunization tracking system database (AMSA, 2001a,b). The databases were used to compare rates of hospitalization and outpatient visits between military personnel who had and those had not been vaccinated against anthrax on the basis of 14 major disease categories and 824 specific diagnoses (identified on the basis of three-digit ICD-9-CM codes). A third analysis on incident visits (first visits for a diagnosis) to inpatient or outpatient facilities was also conducted. For the April 2001 quarterly report on data for January 1998 to December 2000, a total of 757,540 person-years of observation for the group that had received AVA and 3,430,459 person-years of observation for the group that had not received AVA were included in the analyses.

The analyses found that, for all major diagnostic categories, crude and adjusted rates of hospitalization and of outpatient visits and incident visits (incident visits include inpatient and outpatient visits combined) were lower in the group that received AVA than in the cohort that did not. For specific diagnoses within each database (hospitalization, outpatient, and incident data; a total of 2,472 comparisons), however, the rates of some diagnoses were statistically significantly higher for the group that received AVA than for the group that did not. In many cases, these diagnoses (e.g., malaria, wounds, and trauma) were ones that are expected to occur at higher rates in service members deployed overseas than in those remaining in the United States. Since personnel receiving the anthrax vaccine were those most likely to be deployed to areas where risks of exposure to infectious disease are higher, these statistical associations do not raise questions for further analysis. Statistically significant elevations in rates for outpatient visits were also found for certain malignant neoplasms, portal vein thrombosis, and acute pulmonary heart disease, among others. These statistical associations can raise hypotheses to be tested further in additional analyses, such as those described in the sections that follow to try to account for the healthy soldier effect. AMSA plans to continue these screening analyses as additional data accrue.

Hypothesis Testing Analyses AMSA also presented data to the committee to address specific concerns that had been raised regarding AVA (Lange et al., 2001a). As described above, the analyses compared rates of hospitalization and of outpatient visits for selected conditions among active-duty personnel who received one or more doses of AVA with the rates among those who had not yet been given AVA or who had never received AVA. Rate ratios were adjusted for differences between AVA recipients and AVA nonrecipients in terms of age, sex, rank, deployment, service, ethnicity, previous hospitalizations, calendar year, and occupation. Separate analyses for men and women were also done. Both the group that had received AVA and the group that had not received AVA could have received other types of vaccines.

Rates were calculated for the interval from January 1998 to June 2000 and included 515,389 person-years of observation for the group vaccinated with AVA and 2,873,751 person-years of observation for the group not vaccinated with AVA. The 12 inpatient and the 14 outpatient diagnoses selected for comparison were those for which concern in relation to AVA exposure had been publicly expressed or those that have been investigated in association with other vaccines. Inpatient conditions included arthropathies, asthma, connective tissue diseases, diabetes mellitus, Guillain-Barré syndrome, cardiac dysrhythmias, multiple sclerosis, thyroid disorders, and lymphatic cancers. Outpatient conditions included circulatory problems; endocrine or immunological conditions; genitourinary problems; connective tissue diseases; ill-defined conditions; and respiratory, skin, and nervous system diseases.

For each of the diagnostic categories examined, both the unadjusted and the adjusted rate ratios for hospitalization or outpatient visit rates for the group that received AVA compared with those for the group that did not receive AVA did not differ significantly from 1.0 (the ratio observed when the rates are equal). The rate ratios were less than 1.0 for nearly all of the diagnoses examined (ranges, 0.67 to 1.11 for hospitalizations and 0.68

to 0.84 for outpatient conditions), indicating lower hospitalization and outpatient visit rates in the group that received AVA than in the group that did not receive AVA. Lower rates in the group that received AVA were observed for all personnel combined and for the separate analyses among male and female soldiers.

These data indicate that there was no excess risk of selected adverse health events that required either hospitalization or an outpatient visit among active-duty military personnel receiving AVA over a 2.5-year period. In fact, the group that received AVA tended to have fewer hospitalizations or outpatient visits than the group that did not receive AVA.

Inferences about the safety of AVA based on these hypothesis-testing data are limited for several reasons. First, only selected diagnoses were examined, and thus the analyses do not address all possible risks. In addition, many of the diagnostic categories subsumed multiple medical conditions. Thus, risks associated with specific conditions within these categories might have been missed. Although deployment status was included as a covariate in the adjusted rate ratio analyses, this approach may not have been sufficient to account for the many differences in health status and reporting biases for those who are eligible for deployment and those who are not eligible for deployment.

Subsequent Analyses to Address the Healthy Soldier Effect To address concerns about inherent health-related differences in personnel who did and did not receive AVA because of deployment and to examine a wider range of diagnoses, in response to the committee's request, a second set of analyses were performed with the DMSS data (AMSA, 2001c). Again, several approaches were used, and in most of these analyses, service members served as their own controls. Tables are found in Appendix G.

Postimmunization Versus Preimmunization Analyses: Overall Analyses In the first analysis, the hospitalization rates in the time period after the receipt of one or more doses of AVA were compared with the rates in the period before the receipt of AVA for the population of service members who had received at least one dose of AVA. The analyses included the active-duty personnel who had received one or more doses of AVA between January 1, 1998, and December 31, 2000. Pre- and postimmunization cohorts were established on the basis of each individual's daily immunization status during that time frame. Therefore each individual could contribute a different amount of preimmunization time depending upon his or her time in the military prior to receiving AVA. Rate ratios (the rate after vaccination with AVA versus the rate before vaccination with AVA) were calculated for hospitalizations for 843 specific diagnoses (identified on the basis of three-digit ICD-9-CM codes) and were adjusted by Poisson regression methods for up to 11 covariates. Ratios were calculated only for diagnoses with at least five hospitalizations in each comparison group.

The results of these analyses were based on 11,436 hospitalizations during 478,093 person-years of observation in the preimmunization time period (crude rate, 23.92 per 1,000 person-years) and 21,436 hospitalizations during 738,382 years of observation in the postimmunization time period (crude rate, 29.03 per 1,000 person-years). The unadjusted overall rate ratio (the rate after vaccination with AVA versus the rate before vaccination with AVA) for hospitalization was 1.21. Hospitalization rates in the period after vaccination with AVA were higher than those in the period before vaccination for about one-half (414 of 843) of the diagnoses and were lower than those in the period before vaccination for the others. Of the conditions with rate ratios significantly different from 1.0, hospitalization rates in the period after vaccination were statistically significantly elevated for 15 conditions (see Appendix G, Table G-1) and were statistically significantly reduced for 12 conditions. One would have expected rates for about 42 diagnoses to be significantly different in the intervals before and after vaccination with AVA just by chance, given the large number of conditions examined. The significantly elevated rate ratios ranged from 1.31 (95 percent CI = 1.04 to 1.65) for inguinal hernia (ICD-9-CM code 550) to 5.14 (95 percent CI = 1.81 to 14.57) for carcinoma in situ of the breast and genitourinary system (ICD-9-CM code 233). The rate of hospitalization for diabetes mellitus was increased 3.46-fold (95 percent CI = 1.51 to 7.90) in the interval after vaccination with AVA.

Comparison of rates of hospitalization in the same individual before and after the receipt of AVA removes many of the biases inherent in comparing groups vaccinated with AVA and groups not vaccinated with AVA. However, one limitation of comparisons based on a single individual is that for very serious medical conditions (e.g., aplastic anemia or multiple sclerosis) the interval before vaccination with AVA will by definition have few or no events, since if such events had occurred, the soldier would likely never have been eligible to receive AVA.

Similarly, for a diagnosis generally made on an outpatient basis, such as diabetes, it is possible for the rate before vaccination with AVA to be artificially and differentially lower since those who had the disease and who had been hospitalized for it would be less likely to be deployed and therefore less likely to be vaccinated. A normal rate of hospitalization for the disease after vaccination would then appear to be an increase over the rate before vaccination, thus explaining the higher rate after vaccination with AVA without indicating that the vaccine caused the problem (particularly in the instance when that rate after vaccination with AVA remains below the expected rate for the population). In other words, the frequency of diabetes after receipt of AVA may appear to be elevated only because the rate in the time period before vaccination is especially low due to the healthy soldier effect. Whether this phenomenon explains the apparent higher risk after vaccination with AVA can be determined by comparing the rate before vaccination with AVA with the rate in those who never received AVA. If the rate before vaccination with AVA is significantly lower than that in those who were never vaccinated (as it is in the case of diabetes), it supports the conclusion that there is no increased risk attributable to AVA.

Postimmunization Versus Preimmunization Analyses by Time Window A second, similar analysis compared hospitalization rates for the same individuals for the period before immunization with AVA and two time periods after immunization: 0 to 45 days and more than 45 days. This analysis was intended to determine whether any excess risks following exposure to AVA might have been obscured in the previous analysis, which used a longer, open-ended postvaccination time frame. The approach to the analysis was the same as that described above, except that the period after immunization was divided into two time intervals. The unadjusted overall hospitalization rate ratio for the first time interval (0 to 45 days postvaccination versus prevaccination) was 1.08 (25.81 versus 23.92 per 1,000 person-years) and that for the second time interval was 1.25 (29.96 versus 23.92 per 1,000 person-years). Compared with the hospitalization rates before receipt of AVA, rates of hospitalization within 45 days of being given AVA were significantly greater than 1.0 for 13 of the 843 diagnoses examined (Appendix G, Table G-2) and significantly less than 1.0 for 7 diagnoses. Diagnoses for which adjusted rate ratios were statistically significantly greater than 1.0 included diabetes mellitus (adjusted rate ratio = 3.49, 95 percent CI = 1.39 to 8.79) and other disorders of the intestine (ICD-9-CM code 569; adjusted rate ratio = 4.16, 95 percent CI = 1.51 to 11.49). Most of the significantly elevated rate ratios in the first time period were associated with nonspecific diagnostic categories, such as other and unspecified disorders of the back (ICD-9-CM code 724). Given the number of diagnoses examined, significantly elevated rate ratios would have been expected for approximately 42 diagnostic categories just by chance.

In the second time interval (>45 days after vaccination with AVA), adjusted rate ratios for hospitalization were significantly greater than 1.0 for 20 of the diagnoses examined (Appendix G, Table G-2), including ratios of 3.44 (95 percent CI = 1.47 to 8.06) for diabetes mellitus and 2.61 (95 percent CI = 1.06 to 6.44) for other disorders of the intestine (ICD-9-CM code 569). Adjusted rate ratios significantly less than 1.0 were observed for 10 of the 843 diagnoses examined. No consistent pattern was observed when rate ratios for the first interval (0 to 45 days postimmunization) were compared with those for the second interval (>45 days postimmunization). That is, ratios were not uniformly either larger or smaller in the first interval than they were in the second interval. This suggests that any excess risks following vaccination with AVA did not aggregate in the immediate period after vaccination, nor were excess risks specifically identified for conditions that may take some time to develop and be recognized, resulting in hospitalization in the later interval after vaccination.

Postimmunization Versus Preimmunization Analyses by Dose A third analysis among persons ultimately vaccinated with AVA compared rates of hospitalization before receipt of AVA and after receipt of either one to three doses or four or more doses of vaccine. This analysis was designed to determine whether there is a dose-response effect between the amount of exposure to AVA and the risk of hospitalization for specific diseases. Results were based on 11,436 hospitalizations during 478,093 person-years of observation in the preimmunization time period (crude rate, 23.92 per 1,000 person-years), 5,832 hospitalizations during 184,273 years of observation in the cohort that received one to three doses of AVA (crude rate, 31.65 per 1,000 person-years), and 15,604 hospitalizations during 554,109 person-years of observation (crude rate, 28.16 per 1,000 person-years) in the cohort that received four or more doses of AVA. The ratios of crude overall hospitalization rates in the postimmunization time period compared with the hospitalization rates in the preimmunization time period were 1.32 for the cohort that received one to three doses and 1.18 for the cohort that received four or more doses.

In the cohort that received one to three doses, hospitalization rates for 23 diagnoses were significantly higher than the rates before vaccination with AVA (Appendix G, Table G-3), and those for 5 diagnoses were significantly lower than the rates before vaccination with AVA. Conditions with significantly elevated adjusted rate ratios included diabetes mellitus (rate ratio = 4.98, 95 percent CI = 2.02 to 12.25), asthma (rate ratio = 2.18, 95 percent CI = 1.37 to 3.47), and regional enteritis (rate ratio = 4.90, 95 percent CI = 1.55 to 15.44). In those who received four or more doses, the hospitalization rates were significantly elevated for 13 diagnoses (Appendix G, Table G-4) and were significantly reduced for 10 diagnoses compared with the rates in the prevaccination time period. Significantly elevated adjusted rate ratios in the cohort that received four or more doses included malignant neoplasms of the thyroid gland (rate ratio = 2.35, 95 percent CI = 1.01 to 5.48), diabetes mellitus (rate ratio = 3.05, 95 percent CI = 1.31 to 7.09), other disorders of the intestine (ICD-9-CM code 569; rate ratio = 3.24, 95 percent CI = 1.33 to 7.89), and osteochondropathies (ICD-9-CM code 732; rate ratio = 2.17, 95 percent CI = 1.09 to 4.32).

Rate ratios were not calculated for multiple sclerosis since there was only one case in the preimmunization time period (hospitalization rate, 0.21/100,000 population). The rates of hospitalization for multiple sclerosis were 7.60 and 3.25 per 100,000 population in the cohort that received one to three doses and the cohort that received four or more doses, respectively. The corresponding rate for those who never received AVA was 3.5/100,000 population. Thus, the rates of hospitalization for multiple sclerosis were similar in those receiving the greater number of AVA doses and in persons who had never been immunized with AVA.

It is also noteworthy, as mentioned earlier, that the prevaccination disease history of service members who received AVA because they were going to be deployed will, by definition, not include any severe, chronic conditions that would have disqualified them from deployment. For nearly all diagnostic groups, hospitalization rate ratios were smaller rather than larger for the higher-dose cohort. Thus, no dose-response effects of AVA and the risk of hospitalization were observed. A dose-response effect may not be observed, however, if persons with significant health conditions that required hospitalization, whether or not these conditions occurred in conjunction with exposure to AVA, did not receive additional doses of the vaccine. If this were the case, even in the presence of a true association, higher risk ratios would be expected for the cohort that received one to three doses.

Preimmunization Versus Nonimmunization Analyses The fourth analysis was somewhat different from the first three in that hospitalization rates in the time period before vaccination with AVA for those ultimately vaccinated were compared with the rates for those who were never vaccinated with AVA. This comparison would allow assessment of inherent differences in disease risk among those who received AVA at some time and those who never did. The results of these analyses were based on 11,436 hospitalizations during 478,093 person-years of observation in the cohort evaluated before immunization (crude rate, 23.92 per 1,000 person-years) and 109,893 hospitalizations during 2,890,037 person-years of observation in the cohort that was never immunized (crude rate, 38.02 per 1,000 person-years). The unadjusted overall rate ratio for hospitalization (preimmunization versus never immunized) was 0.63. The rate ratios for all major categories but one (diseases of the skin; adjusted rate ratio = 1.01) were less than 1.0, as would be expected if those who would receive AVA were healthier than those who never received AVA. These rate ratios ranged from 0.29 to 0.91, indicating for many conditions a substantial healthy soldier effect. Hospitalization rates for specific diagnoses of diabetes mellitus, regional enteritis, other disorders of the intestine, and multiple sclerosis were also significantly lower in the preimmunization cohort (rates provided in the interpretation section below). For five diagnoses (malaria; erythematous conditions; superficial injury of elbow, forearm, and wrist; toxic effect of carbon monoxide; and effects of air pressure), hospitalization rates were statistically significantly higher for the preimmunization cohort than in those never immunized (Appendix G, Table G-4). Overall, the results of these analyses confirm that those who ultimately received AVA were healthier as a group, even before receipt of the vaccine, than those who never received AVA.

Postimmunization Versus Preimmunization Analyses, Including Those Unvaccinated The final analyses, done separately for men and women, compared the rates of hospitalization for specific diagnoses during the period before receipt of AVA with the rates after receipt of the first dose of AVA. The population included all personnel on active duty between January 1, 1998, and December 31, 2000. In this comparison, the rates for the preimmunization cohort were based on those for all active-duty personnel, including those who never received AVA, whereas the postimmunization time period covered the interval after receipt of the first dose of AVA among those who were vaccinated. Twelve specific diagnoses were investigated: arthropathies and related disorders; asthma; diffuse disease of connective tissue; diabetes mellitus; disease of the ear and mastoid process; inflammatory and toxic neuropathy; cardiac dysrhythmias; lymphosarcoma and reticulosarcoma; multiple sclerosis; acute myocardial infarction; disorders of the thyroid gland; and diseases of the esophagus, stomach, and duodenum (Appendix G, Table G-5).

Among the women, there were 1,847 hospitalizations and 509,265 person-years of observation in the preimmunization cohort and 268 hospitalizations and 73,947 years of observation in the postimmunization cohort. Among the men, there were 11,684 hospitalizations and 2,858,865 person-years of observation in the preimmunization cohort and 2,361 hospitalizations and 664,434 years of observation in the postimmunization cohort. Among the men, none of the adjusted rate ratios (rates before vaccination with AVA versus the rates after vaccination with AVA) were significantly greater than 1.0, and the rate ratios ranged from 0.65 to 1.02. Among the women, however, the rate of hospitalization for multiple sclerosis was significantly increased for the postimmunization cohort compared with that for the preimmunization cohort (rate ratio = 2.14, 95 percent CI = 1.14 to 4.01). When analyses were restricted to incident cases so that multiple hospitalizations of the same woman would not be counted, the adjusted rate ratio for multiple sclerosis in the postimmunization interval versus that in the preimmunization interval was no longer significantly elevated (rate ratio = 1.26; 95 percent CI = 0.50 to 3.14).

The major limitation of this sex-specific analysis is that postimmunization rates (which are, by definition, based only on those for persons who received AVA) were compared with the preimmunization rates among all active-duty personnel. The latter group includes both those who would go on to receive AVA and those who were never immunized with AVA. Use of this comparison group would likely reduce the magnitude of any AVA-associated hospitalizations. On the other hand, it provides a somewhat "fairer" comparison for rates of hospitalization for severe conditions, such as aplastic anemia, that would have precluded ever receiving AVA.

Interpretation of Analyses of Data from DMSS Databases The committee emphasizes that the statistically significant associations observed above are not necessarily causal associations and, indeed, most likely are not causal associations. The interpretation of data such as these requires careful attention to several important but often subtle matters. For example, upon initial review of the postexposure versus the preexposure data (i.e., the initial analyses performed to evaluate risks while controlling for the healthy soldier effect), the results appeared to suggest an elevated risk of hospitalization for diabetes mellitus after receipt of AVA. At first blush, this could be evidence that AVA uncovers cases of diabetes that otherwise might not have been detected, as has been postulated for viral infections (Robles and Eisenbarth, 2001).

However, upon closer examination, a causal link appears to be unlikely. One possibility for observing a significant increase in rates of hospitalization for diabetes would simply be chance. In fact, 27 different conditions were found to be statistically significantly associated with AVA (15 conditions with rate ratios greater than 1.0 and 12 conditions with rate ratios less than 1.0), but 42 diagnoses would be expected to be significantly different in the periods before and after vaccination with AVA purely by chance because of the large number of conditions examined. By use of a conventional p value standard of .05, one would expect 1 in 20 findings to be statistically significant just by chance. However, in this situation that explanation appears to be unlikely. In examining the results stratified by sex, they are completely consistent. Yet there is only a 1 in 400 probability (0.05×0.05) that the results could be significant for both men and women independently purely by chance.

Instead, other patterns in the data make it clear that this association is unlikely to be causal. First, the elevated risk is present to the same degree in the time period >45 days after vaccination as in the time period 0 to 45 days after vaccination. This seems unlikely, although not impossible, if the mechanism was causal.

Diabetes is a common disease that is normally treated on an outpatient basis. Data on outpatient care, however, do not appear in the detailed DMSS analyses available to the committee at the time the report was written. A selection bias may affect data on hospitalizations for diabetes. If soldiers with known diabetes who were treated as outpatients were less likely to be deployed, they would be less likely to receive AVA. The result would be a lower than normal rate of hospitalization for diabetes before vaccination among those who would ultimately receive AVA. Comparison of a normal rate of hospitalization for diabetes after vaccination with this lower rate before vaccination would produce the false appearance of a positive association, and this false signal would persist, regardless of whether one were examining the time period right after the vaccination (0 to 45 days) or the time period thereafter (>45 days).

How can one be confident that the true explanation is this selection bias rather than a causal connection? A separate analysis compared the rates of hospitalization for any of 843 diagnoses in the prevaccination period with the rates for those who were never vaccinated. In general, the rates of hospitalization prevaccination were lower than the rates in the group that was never vaccinated, confirming the healthy soldier effect. The adjusted rate ratios varied, but most often they were about 0.7 or 0.8. However, for diabetes the comparable adjusted rate ratio was 0.12 (95 percent CI = 0.06 to 0.24). Thus, those who received AVA were dramatically less likely to be hospitalized for diabetes than those who were never vaccinated. The normal rate of spontaneous development of diabetes after vaccination would therefore falsely appear as an increased risk. The same was true when the prevaccination rates were compared with the rates in those who never received AVA for some of the other apparent signals, such as regional enteritis (rate ratio = 0.14, 95 percent CI = 0.06 to 0.35) and other disorders of the intestine (rate ratio = 0.28, 95 percent CI = 0.12 to 0.64). For multiple sclerosis a selection bias seems even more likely, with a hospitalization rate ratio of about 0.06 for the preimmunization cohort versus those never vaccinated with AVA (based on only one preimmunization case of multiple sclerosis).

Overall, the analyses of data from DMSS were very reassuring. They indicate that exposure to AVA is not associated with a significantly increased risk for any condition of later onset that cannot be otherwise explained by biases inherent in this type of analysis. Several possible "signals" were observed, however. Signals are the earliest indication of a *possible* causal relationship between an exposure and a health event. These conditions include diabetes, regional enteritis, and multiple sclerosis. The committee's judgment is that these signals are probably not causally linked to exposure to AVA but most likely are due to random error or biases. However, a causal link cannot be completely excluded. Thus, these signals deserve continued surveillance; in addition, ad hoc studies are required to further explore the possible links of these signals with exposure to AVA. Such studies could involve additional analyses with data from DMSS, as well as examination of medical records to validate the diagnosis and the timing of the onset of symptoms in relation to the vaccine exposure.

The committee was impressed by the creativity and rigor of the military professional staff working with the data in the DMSS databases and their productivity. However, the committee also counsels great caution in the use of approaches that use such data collected through automated systems for signal generation. As expected by chance alone, the rates of several diseases and conditions will predictably appear to be elevated in one group or another. Although random error and bias are likely explanations for these increases, other conclusions might also be drawn. In other words, these preliminary findings should lead to further examination of the data. The current DoD approach and organization focus on screening DMSS data for hypotheses. DoD should, however, devote more attention and resources to the evaluation of these hypotheses, as was begun in response to the committee's inquiries. As has been articulated in a set of good epidemiology practices developed for use with similar administrative and clinical data sets in civilian practice (Andrews et al., 1996), analysis of such data requires the exercise of great caution and a commitment to devote the necessary resources to explore the possible associations that might surface from such exercises. Chapter 8 discusses recommended improvements for use of DMSS data.

Thus, finding an increased rate of occurrence of one or more adverse events must be considered a signal until proper review provides an alternative explanation. Criteria for determination of which signals should be further evaluated need to be developed and routinely applied. At a minimum, a system for retrieval and review of primary medical records is required to be able to rule out coding and classification errors, to search for subtle but possibly explanatory variables that may confound an association, or to differentiate a true signal from a statistical chance event.

Finding: DMSS data are screened quarterly to identify statistically significant elevations in hospitalization and outpatient visit rate ratios associated with receipt of AVA. In this way, DMSS promises to be very useful as a tool for hypothesis generation.

Finding: The elevated rates of specific diagnoses in the various analyses of DMSS data are not unexpected per se; that is, they appear to be explicable by chance alone. The bias of selection of healthy individuals for receipt of AVA is also a likely explanation for some observed associations. Thus these elevated rates should not be automatically viewed as an indication of a causal association with the receipt of AVA. However, additional follow-up is needed.

Recommendation: AMSA staff should follow up the currently unexplained elevations in hospitalization rate ratios for certain diagnostic categories among the cohorts of AVA recipients. Studies might include additional analyses with the database or examination of medical records to validate and better understand the exposures and outcomes in question. A protocol should be developed to ensure that such follow-up regularly and reliably occurs after a potential signal is generated.

Finding: Examination of data from the DMSS database to investigate potential signals suggested by VAERS reports related to vaccination with AVA has not detected elevated risks for any of these signals for the vaccinated population, although continued monitoring is warranted.

PRELIMINARY INFORMATION ON ANALYSIS OF DATA ON BIRTH DEFECTS

As it was completing its work, the committee received information about a record-linkage study at the DoD Center for Deployment Health Research by Ryan and colleagues (Ryan, 2002) of the risk of birth defects among children born to women in the military who were vaccinated with AVA. Although the analysis was not complete as of February 2002, preliminary results suggesting a possible increase in risk were noted in the January 2002 revision of the product insert for AVA and in informed-consent documents provided in December 2001 to individuals who were offered vaccination with AVA as supplemental prophylaxis following possible exposure to anthrax spores in the autumn 2001.

The analysis compares the prevalence of birth defects among children born to women in the military who received AVA during the first trimester of pregnancy with the prevalence of birth defects among children of military women who received AVA at any other times, according to records in the DoD Birth Defects Registry and the DoD database that stores information on AVA immunizations given to military personnel. Established in 1998, the DoD Birth Defects Registry contains information on infants with birth defects (ICD-9-CM codes 740.0–760.71) diagnosed within the first year of life (Ryan et al., 2001). The registry data are captured from databases on DoD-financed hospitalizations and ambulatory care in military and civilian facilities.

For the period 1998-1999, approximately 3,000 infants were born to military women with a record of having received at least one dose of AVA. Comparisons were adjusted for maternal age, race, marital status, service branch, rank, and occupational group. No quantitative results from this study were available to the committee, but they were reported to indicate a small but statistically significant association between anthrax vaccine exposure in the first trimester of pregnancy and the frequency of birth defects diagnoses.

The authors acknowledge several of the limitations of their preliminary analysis. The timing of exposure to AVA (i.e., whether or not it occurred in the first trimester) was not precisely known for each infant but rather was estimated based on traditional gestational age cut points for term, preterm, and very preterm infants. Thus, time of exposure was subject to mis-classification because of the manner in which exposure periods were estimated. Inexact vaccination dates could also contribute to misclassification of time of exposure. In addition, it appears that all "major" birth defects were combined, which may not be biologically appropriate. The accuracy of identification of birth defects is uncertain, and analyses were not adjusted for differences between groups in other factors that might influence risk of birth defects such as maternal alcohol use, exposure to medications, or use of folic acid supplements. The number of infants exposed during the first trimester is relatively small, making estimates of risk derived from such analyses highly uncertain. These limitations again emphasize the need to distinguish possible "signals" generated by exploration of large databases, which require further and more definitive studies, from findings of causal associations.

These study results remain preliminary and therefore may change with further analysis. Because of the importance of this issue, the study investigators are working rapidly to validate both exposures and outcomes using primary data sources, which is highly appropriate. In the meantime, the standing DoD policy to avoid immunization of women during pregnancy has been reiterated, which is also appropriate. Further conclusions about the safety of AVA during pregnancy must await the results of this and other studies.

CONCLUSIONS REGARDING AVA VACCINATION AND ADVERSE EVENTS

The committee has reviewed information from a variety of sources, including VAERS and DMSS, on the association between vaccination with AVA and adverse events. For AVA, as with any vaccine, it is essential in assessing questions regarding the safety of the vaccine to distinguish between immediate-onset health events that are observable within hours or days following vaccination and later-onset events that would be observable only months or years following vaccination.

On the question of immediate-onset health events, substantial amounts of data are now available from VAERS, DMSS, and epidemiologic studies. The committee concluded that vaccination with AVA is associated with certain acute local and systemic effects. Epidemiologic studies have consistently found, using either active surveillance (Brachman et al., 1962; Pittman, 2001b,c; Pittman et al., 1997, 2002, in press) or passive surveillance (Hoffman et al., submitted for publication; Pittman, 2001a; Pittman et al., 2001a,b; Wasserman, 2001), that some AVA vaccinees experience local reactions at the injection site that include redness, induration, edema, itching, or tenderness. Systemic events, such as fever, malaise, and myalgia, are also associated with vaccination with AVA, but these reactions are generally less common than reactions at the injection site. The types of local and systemic reactions associated with AVA and the rates at which they were observed are comparable to those observed with other vaccines regularly administered to adults, such as diphtheria and tetanus toxoids and influenza vaccines (Treanor, 2001). The available data also indicate that although these immediate-onset health effects can be serious enough in some individuals to result in brief limitation of activities or the loss of time from work (Hoffman et al., submitted for publication; Wasserman, 2001), the effects are self-limited and result in no serious, permanent health impairments (AMSA, 2001a,b,c; Grabenstein, 2000; Lange et al., 2001a,b; Mason et al., 2001, submitted for publication; Rehme, 2001; Rehme et al., 2002; Sato, 2001a,b; Sato et al., 2001).

Questions have been raised about differences between men and women in their reactions following vaccination with AVA. The committee concluded that the available data from studies that have used both active and passive surveillance indicate that there are sex differences in local reactions at the injection site following vaccination with AVA. Women are more likely than men to experience and report erythema, local tenderness, subcutaneous nodules, itching, and edema (Hoffman et al., submitted for publication; Pittman, 2001a,b; Pittman et al., 2001a,b, 2002; Wasserman, 2001). In addition, some systemic effects, including fever, headache, malaise, and chills, were sometimes reported more often by women than by men (Hoffman et al., submitted for publication; Pittman, 2001a; Pittman et al., 2001a,b), but, unlike local reactions, the rates of systemic reactions did not differ substantially between men and women when the outcomes were evaluated clinically (Pittman, 2001b; Pittman et al., 2002). For female service members, reactions following vaccination with AVA may be more likely to have an adverse effect on their ability to perform their duties (Hoffman et al., submitted for publication; Wasserman, 2001). Studies of other vaccines have generally found higher rates of local reactions among women but similar rates of systemic reactions between men and women (Treanor, 2001). The factors that account for these sex differences are not known, but they could be a function of differences in muscle mass, the dose per unit of body mass, physiologic factors, or care-seeking behavior. Because of the reported sex differences in reactions following vaccination with AVA, it will be important that future studies of vaccination with AVA continue to analyze data separately for men and women.

Some of the data reviewed by the committee provided evidence of lot-to-lot differences in the reactogenicity of AVA (Pittman, 2001a; Pittman et al., 2001a,b; CDC, 1967–1971). The information presented to the committee on the recertification of the AVA manufacturing process suggests that AVA lots released for use in the future may show less variation in reactogenicity because of greater consistency in production, but there is no a priori basis for prediction of the level of reactogenicity. This and other concerns related to the future use of AVA are discussed further in Chapter 7.

AVA is unusual compared with other vaccines in that it is licensed for subcutaneous rather than intramuscular administration. The limited evidence available from a small study that tested changes in the dosing schedule and route of administration of the vaccine (Pittman, 2001b; Pittman et al., 2002) points to subcutaneous administration as a contributing factor in the local reactions associated with AVA. The route of administration did not appear to affect rates of systemic reactions. A few studies of other vaccines (Treanor, 2001) have also shown that subcutaneous administration is associated with higher rates of local erythema or induration, reactions commonly reported following administration of AVA. The committee concluded that further investigations should be conducted to confirm whether a change from subcutaneous to intramuscular administration of AVA could reduce the rates of local reactions without impairing the efficacy of the vaccine.

Service members and others have also expressed concerns about potential later-onset and chronic health effects resulting from receipt of AVA. The committee examined the available information regarding later-onset health effects, but the data are limited, as they are for all vaccines. DMSS, which provides the best source of data for studying later-onset health effects, currently has data on service personnel who have documented histories of vaccination with AVA and other vaccines and who have been observed for up to a maximum of 3 years. Although AVA has been administered to military personnel for more than 3 years, unreliable documentation of vaccinations before 1998 limits the use of DMSS data for observation of potential vaccine-related health effects over longer periods. The evidence available to date from analyses of DMSS data (AMSA, 2001a,b,c; Grabenstein, 2000; Lange et al., 2001a,b; Mason et al., 2001, submitted for publication; Rehme, 2001; Rehme et al., submitted for publication; Sato, 2001a,b; Sato et al., 2001) provides no convincing evidence at this time of elevated risks of later-onset health events among personnel who have received AVA. Repeated examination of a small population of heavily vaccinated laboratory workers provides no indication that vaccination with AVA is associated with an obvious increase in the risk of illness with later onset (Peeler et al., 1958, 1965; White et al., 1974).

The committee notes that the studies reviewed did not examine the use of AVA in children, elderly individuals, or persons with chronic illnesses. In addition, information regarding outcomes of pregnancy following use of the vaccine is limited. These limitations would have to be taken into account if AVA were being considered for use in the general population.

FINDINGS AND RECOMMENDATIONS

Immediate-Onset Health Events

Finding: The data available from VAERS, DMSS, and epidemiologic studies indicate the following regarding immediate-onset health events following receipt of AVA:

- Local events, especially redness, swelling, or nodules at the injection site, are associated with receipt of AVA, are similar to the events observed following receipt of other vaccines currently in use by adults, and are fairly common.
- Systemic events, such as fever, malaise, and myalgia, are associated with receipt of AVA, are similar to the events observed following receipt of other vaccines currently in use by adults, but are much less common than local events.
- Immediate-onset health effects can be severe enough in some individuals to result in brief functional impairment, but these effects are self-limited and result in no permanent health impairments.
- There is no evidence that life-threatening or permanently disabling immediate-onset adverse events occur at higher rates in individuals who have received AVA than in the general population.

Finding: The available data from both active and passive surveillance indicate that there are sex differences in local reactions following vaccination with AVA, as there are following the administration of other vaccines. For female service members, reactions following vaccination with AVA can have a transient adverse impact on their ability to perform their duties. The factors that account for these sex differences are not known.

Recommendation: Future monitoring and study of health events following vaccination(s) with AVA (and other vaccines) should continue to include separate analyses of data for men and women.

Finding: The currently licensed subcutaneous route of administration of AVA and the six-dose vaccination schedule appear to be associated with a higher incidence of immediate-onset, local effects than is intramuscular administration or a vaccination schedule with fewer doses of AVA. The frequencies of immediate-onset, systemic events were low and were not affected by the route of administration.

Recommendation: DoD should continue to support the efforts of CDC to study the reactogenicity and immunogenicity of an alternative route of AVA administration and of a reduced number of vaccine doses.

Later-Onset Health Events

Finding: The available data are limited but show no convincing evidence at this time that personnel who have received AVA have elevated risks of later-onset health events.

Recommendation: DoD should develop systems to enhance the capacity to monitor the occurrence of later-onset health conditions that might be associated with the receipt of any vaccine; the data reviewed by the committee do not suggest the need for special efforts of this sort for AVA.

REFERENCES

AMSA (Army Medical Surveillance Activity). 1998. *Tri-Service Reportable Events: Guidelines and Case Definitions.* Washington, D.C.: Army Medical Surveillance Activity, U.S. Army Center for Health Promotion and Preventive Medicine.

AMSA. 2001a. *Quarterly Report—January 2001. Surveillance of Adverse Effects of Anthrax Vaccine Adsorbed.* Washington, D.C.: Army Medical Surveillance Activity, U.S. Army Center for Health Promotion and Preventive Medicine.

AMSA. 2001b. *Quarterly Report—April 2001. Surveillance of Adverse Effects of Anthrax Vaccine Adsorbed.* Washington, D.C.: Army Medical Surveillance Activity, U.S. Army Center for Health Promotion and Preventive Medicine.

AMSA. 2001c. *Surveillance of Adverse Effects of Anthrax Vaccine Adsorbed: Results of Analyses Requested by the Institute of Medicine Committee to Assess the Safety and Efficacy of the Anthrax Vaccine.* Washington, D.C.: Army Medical Surveillance Activity, U.S. Army Center for Health Promotion and Preventive Medicine.

Andrews EB, Avorn J, Bortnichak EA, Chen R, Dai WS, Dieck GS, Edlavitch S, Freiman J, Mitchell AA, Nelson RC, Neutel CI, Stergachis A, Strom B. L., Walker AM. 1996. Guidelines for good epidemiology practices for drug, device, and vaccine research in the United States. *Pharmacoepidemiology and Drug Safety* 5:333–338.

AVIP (Anthrax Vaccine Immunization Program). 2001. *Section H: TAMC-601 Survey. Detailed safety review of Anthrax Vaccine Adsorbed.* [Online]. Available: http://www.anthrax.osd.mil/Site_Files/articles/INDEXclinical/safety_reviews.htm [accessed January 18, 2001].

Brachman PS, Gold H, Plotkin S, Fekety FR, Werrin M, Ingraham NR. 1962. Field evaluation of a human anthrax vaccine. *American Journal of Public Health* 52:632–645.

CDC (Centers for Disease Control and Prevention). 1967–1971. *Application and Report on Manufacture of Anthrax Protective Antigen, Aluminum Hydroxide Adsorbed (DBS-IND 180). Observational Study.* Atlanta, Ga.: Centers for Disease Control and Prevention.
CDC. 2000. Surveillance for adverse events associated with anthrax vaccination—U.S. Department of Defense, 1998–2000. *MMWR (Morbidity and Mortality Weekly Report)* 49(16):341–345.
GAO (General Accounting Office). 1999. *Medical Readiness: Issues Concerning the Anthrax Vaccine.* GAO/T-NSIAD-99-226. Washington, D.C.: GAO.
Grabenstein JD. 2000. The AVIP: status and future. Presentation to the Institute of Medicine Committee to Assess the Safety and Efficacy of the Anthrax Vaccine, Meeting I, Washington, D.C.
Grabenstein JD. 2001. VAERS information; average length of active duty. E-mail to Joellenbeck L, Institute of Medicine, Washington, D.C., November 13.
Gunzenhauser JD, Cook JE, Parker ME, Wright I. 2001. Acute side effects of anthrax vaccine in ROTC cadets participating in advanced camp, Fort Lewis, 2000. *MSMR (Medical Surveillance Monthly Report)* 7(5):9–14.
Hoffman K, Costello C, Engler RJM, Grabenstein J. Submitted for publication. Using a patient-centered structured medical note for aggregate analysis: determining the side-effect profile of anthrax vaccine at a mass immunization site.
IOM (Institute of Medicine). 2000. Fulco CE, Liverman, CT, Sox HC, eds. *Gulf War and Health.* Washington, D.C.: National Academy Press.
Lange JL, Lesikar SE, Brundage JF, Rubertone MV. 2001a. Screening for adverse events following anthrax immunization using the Defense Medical Surveillance System. Presentation to the Institute of Medicine Committee to Assess the Safety and Efficacy of the Anthrax Vaccine, Meeting II, Washington, D.C.
Lange JL, Lesikar SE, Brundage JF, Rubertone MV. 2001b. Update: surveillance of adverse events of Anthrax Vaccine Adsorbed. Presentation to the Institute of Medicine Committee to Assess the Safety and Efficacy of the Anthrax Vaccine, Meeting IV, Washington, D.C.
Mason KT, Grabenstein JD, McCracken LR. 2001. Hearing loss after anthrax vaccination among US Army aircrew members. Unpublished manuscript.
Mason KT, Grabenstein JD, McCracken LR. Submitted for publication. US Army Aviation Epidemiology Data Register: physical findings after anthrax vaccination among US Army aircrew members, a prospective matched-pair, case-control study.
Mazzuchi JF. 1998. Tri-service reportable events document. Memorandum to Deputy Surgeon General of the Army, Deputy Surgeon General of the Navy, and Deputy Surgeon General of the Air Force. Department of Defense, Washington, D.C.
Peeler RN, Cluff LE, Trever RW. 1958. Hyper-immunization of man. *Bulletin of the Johns Hopkins Hospital* 103:183–198.
Peeler RN, Kadull PJ, Cluff LE. 1965. Intensive immunization of man: evaluation of possible adverse consequences. *Annals of Internal Medicine* 63(1):44–57.
Pittman PR. 2001a. Anthrax vaccine: an analysis of short-term adverse events in an occupational setting—the Special Immunization Program experience over 30 years. Presentation to the Institute of Medicine Committee to Assess the Safety and Efficacy of the Anthrax Vaccine, Meeting II, Washington, D.C.
Pittman PR. 2001b. Anthrax vaccine: dose reduction/route change pilot study. Presentation to the Institute of Medicine Committee to Assess the Safety and Efficacy of the Anthrax Vaccine, Meeting II, Washington, D.C.
Pittman PR. 2001c. Anthrax vaccine: the Fort Bragg Booster Study. Presentation to the Institute of Medicine Committee to Assess the Safety and Efficacy of the Anthrax Vaccine, Meeting II, Washington, D.C.

Pittman PR, Sjogren MH, Hack D, Franz D, Makuch RS, Arthur JS. 1997. *Serologic Response to Anthrax and Botulinum Vaccines.* Protocol No. FY92-5, M109, Log No. A-5747. Final report to the Food and Drug Administration. Fort Detrick, Md.: U.S. Army Medical Research Institute of Infectious Diseases.

Pittman PR, Gibbs PH, Cannon TL, Friedlander AM. 2001a. Anthrax vaccine: short-term safety experience in humans. Manuscript.

Pittman PR, Gibbs PH, Cannon TL, Friedlander AM. 2001b. Anthrax vaccine: short-term safety experience in humans. *Vaccine* 20(5–6):972–978.

Pittman PR, Kim-Ahn G, Pifat DY, Coon K, Gibbs P, Little S, Pace-Templeton J, Myers R, Parker GW, Friedlander AM. 2002. Anthrax vaccine: safety and immunogenicity of a dose-reduction, route comparison study in humans. *Vaccine* 20(9–10):1412–1420.

Pittman PR, Hack D, Mangiafico J, Gibbs P, McKee KT Jr, Friedlander AM, Sjogren MH. In press. Antibody response to a delayed booster dose of anthrax vaccine and botulinum toxoid. *Vaccine.*

Puziss M, Manning LC, Lynch JW, Barclay E, Abelow I, Wright GG. 1963. Large-scale production of protective antigen of *Bacillus anthracis* in anaerobic cultures. *Applied Microbiology* 11(4):330–334.

Rehme P. 2001. Ambulatory medical visits among anthrax-vaccinated and unvaccinated personnel after return from Southwest Asia. Presentation to the Institute of Medicine Committee to Assess the Safety and Efficacy of the Anthrax Vaccine, Meeting IV, Washington, D.C.

Rehme PA, Williams R, Grabenstein JD. 2002. Ambulatory medical visits among anthrax-vaccinated and unvaccinated personnel after return from Southwest Asia. *Military Medicine* 167:205–210.

Robles DT, Eisenbarth GS. 2001. Type 1A diabetes induced by infection and immunization. *Journal of Autoimmunity* 16(3):355–362.

Ryan M. 2002. Assessment of birth defects among infants of women who received anthrax vaccine: information for the Institute of Medicine, Washington, D.C. Microsoft Power Point slides.

Ryan MA, Pershyn-Kisor MA, Honner WK, Smith TC, Reed RJ, Gray GC. 2001. The Department of Defense Birth Defects Registry: overview of a new surveillance system. *Teratology* 64(Suppl 1):S26-S29.

Sato PA. 2001a. DoD-wide surveillance of hospitalizations for long-term adverse events potentially associated with anthrax immunization. Presentation to the Institute of Medicine Committee to Assess the Safety and Efficacy of the Anthrax Vaccine, Meeting IV, Washington, D.C.

Sato PA. 2001b. Questions on updated data. E-mail to Joellenbeck L, Institute of Medicine, Washington, D.C., November 21.

Sato PA, Reed RJ, Smith TC, Wang LZ. 2001. DoD-wide medical surveillance for potential long-term adverse events associated with anthrax immunization: hospitalizations. Provisional report for IOM of data from January 1998 to March 2000. Unpublished manuscript.

Tanner J. 2001. Survey results of the 9th Airlift Squadron. Presentation to the Joint Meeting of the Institute of Medicine Committee to Assess the Safety and Efficacy of the Anthrax Vaccine and the Institute of Medicine Committee to Review the CDC Anthrax Vaccine Safety and Efficacy Research Program, Meeting III, Washington, D.C.

Treanor JJ. 2001. Adverse reactions following vaccination of adults. Commissioned paper. Committee to Assess the Safety and Efficacy of the Anthrax Vaccine, Institute of Medicine, Washington, D.C.

Wasserman GM. 2001. Analysis of adverse events after anthrax vaccination in U.S. Army medical personnel. Presentation to the Institute of Medicine Committee to Assess the Safety and Efficacy of the Anthrax Vaccine, Meeting IV, Washington, D.C.

White CS, Adler WH, McGann VG. 1974. Repeated immunization: possible adverse effects. *Annals of Internal Medicine* 81(5):594–600.

Wiesen AR. 2001a. Lack of effect of anthrax vaccination on pregnancy. Presentation to the Institute of Medicine Committee to Assess the Safety and Efficacy of the Anthrax Vaccine, Meeting IV, Washington, D.C.

Wiesen AR. 2001b. Clarifications of the research presented to the Institute of Medicine Committee to Assess the Safety and Efficacy of the Anthrax Vaccine held July 10–11, 2001. E-mail and attached letter to Joellenbeck L, Institute of Medicine, Washington, D.C., July 16.

Wiesen AR, Littell CT. 2001. Lack of effect of anthrax vaccination on pregnancy, birth, and adverse birth outcome among women in active service with the U.S. Army. Unpublished abstract.

Wright GG, Green TW, Kanode RG Jr. 1954. Studies on immunity in anthrax. V. Immunizing activity of alum-precipitated protective antigen. *Journal of Immunology* 73:387–391.

7

Anthrax Vaccine Manufacture

Anthrax Vaccine Adsorbed (AVA) is licensed for manufacture only by the firm BioPort, which acquired the vaccine production facility from the Michigan Biologic Products Institute (MBPI) in September 1998. Production of the vaccine had been suspended in early 1998 when the facility was closed for renovations. Production resumed in 1999. However, vaccine was not released for routine use until the Food and Drug Administration (FDA) approved the license supplement for the renovations, change in labels and package insert, and change to an outside contractor for filling on January 31, 2002. Therefore during the period that the committee held its meetings and most of its deliberations, the vaccine had not yet been released for use following the renovations.

Among the issues that the committee was charged with addressing is "validation of the manufacturing process focusing on, but not limited to, discrepancies identified by the Food and Drug Administration in February 1998." This chapter provides some background to clarify this portion of the charge, including a description of the role of the FDA in regulating the manufacture and marketing of vaccines, the history of the manufacturing process, and problems particular to the currently licensed anthrax vaccine. The committee's findings regarding the manufacture of the anthrax vaccine are also presented. The committee's first step was to interpret the charge.

COMMITTEE'S INTERPRETATION OF THE CHARGE

"Manufacturing process validation" is the formal and detailed definition of each step in a controlled manufacturing process. The 1987 FDA *Guideline on General Principles of Process Validation* defines process validation as "establishing documented evidence which provides a high degree of assurance that a specific process will consistently produce a product meeting its pre-determined specifications and quality attributes" (FDA, 1987, p. 4). A manufacturer carries out this validation through careful documentation of all aspects of the manufacturing process, and it is overseen and deemed acceptable or unacceptable by FDA. The Institute of Medicine (IOM) committee could not itself validate the manufacturing process, nor was the committee in a position to second-guess FDA's inspection and determination of validity. The committee could, however, review and evaluate the process by which BioPort was working to validate the manufacturing process for AVA.

The committee took the following approach to evaluating BioPort's validation process. The committee requested from BioPort copies of the Form FDA 483s (Form FDA 483 is a list of observations provided by an FDA investigator at the conclusion of an inspection) from FDA inspections conducted since 1998, as well as BioPort's responses to these inspection reports. The committee was specifically interested in the subset of materials focusing on product characterization and process validation.

BioPort provided these documents, as well as copies of the MBPI strategic plan with updates. The documents provide detailed information about the responsiveness of the company to the FDA's findings and the FDA's evaluations of the manufacturer's progress.

REGULATORY OVERSIGHT OF VACCINE MANUFACTURE

All vaccines are regulated by FDA's Center for Biologics Evaluation and Research (CBER). As with other biologics, the development of a new vaccine involves preclinical research (before administration of a vaccine to humans), research in studies with humans in which the product is administered under limited study conditions, an application for licensure, and continued monitoring after licensure and marketing.

The application for licensure must be approved by FDA, which reviews the results of clinical trials and other data and information on safety and efficacy. FDA also reviews detailed information on the manufacturing process and the facility where the product will be produced and tests the products. Previously, sponsors of new biological product applications were required to apply separately for approval of the product and approval of the manufacturing facility (Product License Application and Establishment License Application, respectively), but in 1999 the regulations were modified to combine the two into a single Biologics License Application (BLA) for all products licensed by CBER.

A vaccine product must be produced in compliance with good manufacturing practices (GMPs), as specified in the *Code of Federal Regulations*.[1] To ascertain compliance, FDA conducts periodic GMP surveillance inspections. In the case of vaccines, the inspections are carried out by a team of experts in GMPs and experts in the product in question, an approach adopted in 1999 under the Team Biologics program. The Team Biologics program is a partnership between CBER and FDA's Office of Regulatory Affairs, designed to increase both consistency and focus in FDA's inspections of biologics manufacturers. When a manufacturer makes a change in the facility or the production process that could have a moderate to substantial potential to affect adversely the quality of the product, the manufacturer must submit a supplemental application for FDA approval of the change.

Because vaccines are produced through complex procedures that depend upon living organisms, there are many points in the process where variance could be introduced into the final product. To ensure consistency, each lot of the product must be individually tested and approved before its release for marketing. The vaccine manufacturer must submit a sample of the lot along with a lot release protocol to FDA, which then reviews the lot testing data and, if necessary, performs additional tests.

In the case of AVA, BioPort resumed manufacture of the vaccine in 1999 after a pause for plant renovation. The BLA supplement for the renovations has been approved, and release of lots manufactured after renovation of the facility was approved in January 2002. One of the sources of difficulty in the regulatory history of AVA may be that the standard regulatory expectations for vaccines in general changed between the licensing of AVA in 1970 and 2001. Vaccines may, in some sense, have been victims of their own success: for many vaccines the decline in the disease burden from communicable diseases was so clear and the effectiveness of the vaccine was so great that there was little incentive to modify the production process. However, as part of its continuing quality improvement effort, FDA instituted more explicitly defined process validation requirements for the manufacture of vaccines and other products licensed before these requirements were codified. As a result, manufacturers of vaccines, including AVA, must now ensure that their production processes are validated.

---

[1] Current Good Manufacturing Practice in Manufacturing, Processing, Packing, or Holding of Drugs; General (21 C.F.R. § 210 [2001]) and Current Good Manufacturing Practices for Finished Pharmaceuticals (21 C.F.R. § 211 [2001]).

ANTHRAX VACCINE DEVELOPMENT

Research was conducted at Camp Detrick (later Fort Detrick), Maryland, to develop an anthrax vaccine based on *Bacillus anthracis* cultures grown in synthetic medium without proteins or other macromolecules (Turnbull, 2000). In 1954, Wright and colleagues described a chemically defined medium that could be used to grow the bacteria and provided evidence that protective antigen in culture filtrates could be concentrated, stabilized, and partially purified by precipitation with alum to make a vaccine. Further refinements to simplify large-scale production included microaerophilic incubation (Wright and Puziss, 1957; Wright et al., 1962), use of a different growth medium (Puziss et al., 1963; Wright et al., 1962), and adsorption onto aluminum hydroxide gel (Alhydrogel) instead of precipitation with alum (Puziss and Wright, 1963). Different strains of *B. anthracis* were evaluated for use as the vaccine strain (Auerbach and Wright, 1955; Puziss and Wright, 1963), and ultimately, Vollum strain V770-NP1-R was adopted and used for the licensed anthrax vaccine (see Table 7-1 for a list of significant events in AVA development and manufacture).

Anthrax Vaccine Licensure

It is noteworthy that the landmark study evaluating the efficacy of the anthrax vaccine was carried out not with the vaccine that was ultimately licensed but with the earlier vaccine described above. The previously discussed study by Brachman and colleagues (1962), which evaluated the efficacy of a protective antigen-based anthrax vaccine in wool mill workers, was carried out over a 4-year period between 1955 and 1959. The vaccine they evaluated was made by Merck Sharpe & Dohme (hereafter referred to as the Merck vaccine) using a nonencapsulated, nonpro-teolytic mutant of the Vollum strain of *B. anthracis* called R1-NP that was grown in 599 medium (Puziss and Wright, 1954) to produce protective antigen that was precipitated and concentrated with aluminum potassium sulfate (alum). It differed from the currently licensed vaccine in terms of the *B. anthracis* strain used to generate protective antigen, in the medium in which it was grown, in the mode of growth (aerobic rather than microaerophilic [fermentation]), and in the mode of antigen concentration and purification (alum precipitation rather than adsorption to aluminum hydroxide gel). In addition, the Merck vaccine used 0.01 percent thimerosal as a preservative, whereas the licensed vaccine uses 0.0025 percent benzethonium chloride (see Table 7-2).

The package insert calls for subcutaneous administration of a basic series of six doses of 0.5 ml each. After the initial dose, subsequent doses are administered at 2 weeks, 4 weeks, 6 months, 12 months, and 18 months.

TABLE 7-1 Events in AVA Development and Manufacture

1955–1959	Brachman et al. conduct a field evaluation of the anthrax vaccine manufactured by Merck and publish their results in 1962.
1966	CDC submits an Investigational New Drug (IND) application for Anthrax Vaccine Adsorbed (AVA).
Nov. 10, 1970	Division of Biologics Standards issues a product license to Michigan Department of Public Health (MDPH) to manufacture anthrax vaccine.
1973–1975	FDA convenes an external review of AVA using safety data from CDC trials and efficacy data from the field evaluation of Brachman et al. (1962). The panel finds sufficient evidence that AVA is safe and effective "under the limited circumstances for which the vaccine is employed."
Dec. 13, 1985	Findings from an FDA external review are published in the *Federal Register*.
1993	FDA inspects the MDPH anthrax vaccine manufacturing facilities in January; FDA approves the renovations in July.
1996	MDPH becomes known as MBPI, an entity controlled by the Michigan State government.
Nov. 1996	FDA conducts a surveillance inspection of MBPI (not including the anthrax vaccine manufacturing facilities) in which it finds numerous deviations from regulations.
March 1997	FDA issues MBPI a Notice of Intent to Revoke (NOIR) letter based on the Nov. 1996 inspection.
April 1997	MBPI responds to the NOIR letter with its Strategic Plan for Compliance.
Jan. 1998	MBPI halts production of AVA sublots to begin comprehensive renovation.
Feb. 1998	FDA conducts a comprehensive inspection of the MBPI facility to evaluate MBPI's compliance with its strategic plan.
May 18, 1998	Secretary of Defense William Cohen implements the Anthrax Vaccine Immunization Program for all U.S. armed forces.
Sept. 1998	MBPI transfers ownership to BioPort Corporation.
Oct. 1998	FDA's GMP inspection of BioPort Corporation notes continuing improvement.
Sept. 1999	Submission of BLA supplement for renovation of BioPort's AVA manufacturing facility.
Nov. 1999	Preapproval inspection and complete review letter from FDA.
Oct. 2000	FDA inspects BioPort and observes numerous deviations from regulations, including problems with the filling suite.
April 2001	BioPort responds to FDA with modifications.
2001	BioPort decommissions the filling suite and contracts with Hollister-Stier Laboratories to perform the AVA filling operation.
Dec. 2001	Preapproval inspection of BioPort; FDA approval of the BLA supplement for the facility renovations.
Jan. 2002	Inspection of the Hollister-Stier Laboratories filling operation facility.
Jan. 31, 2002	FDA approval of BLA supplement for the filling operations and labeling change.

TABLE 7-2 Comparison of AVA and Merck Vaccine

Characteristic	Vaccine Product	
	AVA	Merck
Strain	Nonproteolytic, nonencapsulated strain V770-NP1-R	Nonproteolytic, nonencapsulated strain R1-NP
Medium	1095, chemically defined	599, chemically defined
Growth conditions	Microaerophilic (fermentation)	Aerobic (static culture)
Means of removal of bacteria	Filtration (hydrophobic, low protein binding)	Filtration (sintered glass)
Purification and concentration procedure	Adsorption (aluminum hydroxide)	Precipitation (alum and acid)
Recovery	Decantation, centrifugation	Decantation, centrifugation
Concentration factor from culture filtrate	10×	10×
Aqueous vehicle	Normal saline	Normal saline
Adjuvant	Aluminum hydroxide (0.65 mg of aluminum/dose)	Aluminum potassium sulfate (0.52 mg of aluminum/dose)
Preservative	0.0025% Benzethonium chloride	0.01% Thimerosal
Stabilizer	0.01% Formaldehyde	None
Schedule (0.5 ml/dose)	0, 2, 4 weeks; 6, 12, 18 months; annual booster	0, 2, 4 weeks; 6, 12, 18 months; annual booster
Route	Subcutaneous	Subcutaneous
Amount of protein per dose	Approximately 50 µg	Unknown

SOURCES: Giri et al. (2001), Myers et al. (2001).

Annual boosters are required. The evidence to justify this dosing schedule is limited. An alum-precipitated predecessor of AVA was given to 55 volunteers in two 0.5-milliliter (ml) injections given subcutaneously 2 weeks apart and found to be acceptable (Wright et al., 1954). A group of 660 people were then given three subcutaneous injections of this same vaccine at 2-week intervals, followed by a booster dose of 0.25 ml after 6 months. No significant local reactions were reported after the first dose, but 0.6

percent of 650 people receiving the second dose and 2.2 percent of 537 people receiving the third dose reported significant local reactions. Of 445 people receiving a booster dose, 2.6 percent reported significant local reactions. Systemic reactions were reported after 0.7 percent of doses, but information was not provided by dose (Wright et al., 1954). Brachman and colleagues (1962) used the same vaccine with a schedule of three 0.5-ml subcutaneous injections given at 2-week intervals, followed by three 0.5-ml booster doses given at 6-month intervals (see Chapters 3 and 6 for additional discussion of this study). Thereafter booster doses were given at yearly intervals. This schedule was then used for the studies leading to licensure of AVA. As mentioned in Chapters 3 and 6, a pilot study has been conducted to evaluate changes in both the route of administration and the dosing schedule (Pittman, 2001; Pittman et al., 2002). A clinical trial will soon begin to further evaluate these modifications.

The Centers for Disease Control and Prevention (CDC) submitted an Investigational New Drug (IND) application for anthrax vaccine to the Division of Biologics Standards (DBS) of the National Institutes of Health on April 14, 1966 (Elengold, 2000). Although Merck Sharp & Dohme had produced one of the vaccine lots evaluated early in the study, the Michigan Department of Public Health (MDPH) made the remainder of the lots evaluated. In 1968, MDPH was awarded a 3-year contract to produce the vaccine. The manufacturing process was that described by Puziss and colleagues in 1963. The process was also described in the materials provided with the progress reports to DBS under the IND application (CDC, 1967–1971). (Safety and efficacy data from the five annual progress reports submitted as part of the IND application are presented elsewhere in this report.) Additional data indicating that the vaccine protected guinea pigs from challenge were also submitted (Pittman, 1969). An ad hoc committee involved with review of the vaccine expressed the desire for additional efficacy data as well as for comparisons of sera from human recipients of the Merck vaccine with sera from recipients of the MDPH vaccine but recommended that licensure be granted (Feeley et al., 1969; Pittman, 1969). On the basis of the information submitted, DBS issued a product license to MDPH to manufacture AVA on November 10, 1970 (Elengold, 2000).

Rereview of Anthrax Vaccine

In 1972, DBS was moved from NIH to become part of FDA, where it was called the Bureau of Biologics (Parkman and Hardegree, 1999). FDA began a process of reexamining the vaccines that had already been licensed to evaluate their safety and efficacy. FDA assigned initial review of each category of biological products to a separate independent advisory panel that was charged with preparing a report for the FDA commissioner to

1. Evaluate the safety and effectiveness of the biological products,
2. Review labeling of the biological products, and
3. Identify the biological products under review that are safe, effective, and not misbranded (FDA, 1985, p. 51002).

The advisory report includes recommendations classifying products into one of three categories:

- Category I designates those biological products determined by the panel to be safe, effective, and not misbranded;
- Category II designates those biological products determined by the panel to be unsafe, ineffective, or misbranded; and
- Category III designates those biological products determined by the panel not to fall within either Category I or II on the basis of the panel's conclusion that the available data are insufficient to classify such biological products and for which further testing is therefore required (p. 51002).

The panel appointed to review data on bacterial vaccines, toxoids, related antitoxins, and immune globulins evaluated AVA. The panel met numerous times from 1973 to 1975. Its final report on all the products that it reviewed was published in the *Federal Register* in 1985. In that report the panel recommended that AVA be placed in Category I, the category of products determined to be safe, effective, and not misbranded "because there is substantial evidence of safety and effectiveness for this product" (p. 51058). The panel found the vaccine to be "fairly well tolerated with the majority of reactions consisting of local erythema and edema. Severe local reactions and systemic reactions are relatively rare" (p. 51058). The panel found that the safety of the product was "not a major concern, especially considering its very limited distribution and the benefit-to-risk aspects of occupational exposure in those individuals for whom it is indicated" (p. 51058). The panel noted that the product was intended solely for use for immunization of high-risk individuals such as industrial populations working with animal hides and other products and laboratory workers handling the organism. In considering efficacy, it found protection against cutaneous anthrax in fully immunized subjects to be adequately established by the study by Brachman and colleagues (1962), who used "the very similar Merck . . . vaccine" (p. 51058). The panel reported that "no meaningful assessment of its value against inhalation anthrax is possible due to its low incidence" (p. 51058).

Anthrax Vaccine Manufacturing Process and Vaccine Constituents

Briefly, the process for manufacturing the licensed vaccine is as follows

(Giri et al., 2001; CDC, 1967–1971; Puziss et al., 1963): an inoculum of nonencapsulated, nonproteolytic, avirulent B. *anthracis* strain V770-NP1-R is placed into sterile growth medium 1095. This chemically defined growth medium, described by Wright and colleagues in 1962, contains amino acids, minerals, glucose, and other specified ingredients found to be optimal for growth of B. *anthracis*. Bacterial growth takes place through fermentation under microaerophilic (limited oxygen) conditions. The inoculated medium is slowly agitated and held at 37 ± 0.5°C for 23 ± 1 hours in each of two fermentors (volumes of 10 and 100 liters, respectively) while pH and glucose levels are monitored (Puziss et al., 1963; Myers, 2001).

After incubation, the mixture is filtered by use of hydrophobic, low-protein binding filters. On completion of filtration, sterile aluminum hydroxide gel is added and the mixture is stirred for 17 ± 1 hours. The supernatant (fluid) is removed after a period of settling (73 ± 1 hours) and again after a centrifugation step. The aluminum hydroxide-adsorbed antigen is resuspended in a physiological saline solution that contains formaldehyde (final concentration: 0.01 percent) as a stabilizer and benzethonium chloride (final concentration: 0.0025 percent) as a preservative. Tests for stability, purity, and potency are carried out, and the vaccine is filled in 10-dose vials, stoppered, and sealed before it is labeled and packaged for use.

The time required to manufacture a lot of AVA is approximately 22 weeks from the initiation of sublot production to release for distribution by FDA. The approximate timeline is shown in Table 7-3, but actual times for any given lot may be longer or shorter.

Vaccines are licensed with defined dating periods, but the regulations[2] provide that FDA may grant an extension of the expiration dates if the lot in question passes potency and sterility tests. AVA was previously licensed for up to 36 months from the date of manufacture when stored at 2 to 8°C, including both time in manufacturer's storage and time in distribution (Elengold, 2001).

One example of the evolution in vaccine standards that has taken place over the last 30 years lies in the characterization of vaccine constituents. In contrast to the development of AVA and other vaccines of an earlier era, consider the analytical data assembled for recombinant hepatitis B vaccines for adults, which were licensed in the late 1980s. In the prelicensing phase of research, physicochemical, immunological, and molecular biological test methods were all used to provide evidence of the identity, purity, and genetic stability of the protein product (Parkman and Hardegree, 1999). Protein characterization techniques included sodium dodecyl sulfate-polyacrylamide gel electrophoresis (SDS-PAGE), peptide mapping, amino acid

---

[2]Date of Manufacture. 21 C.F.R. § 610.50 (2001).

TABLE 7-3 Timeline for Production of AVA

Activity	Week
Initiate sublot production	1
Formulate bulk lot	7
Fill into vials	9
Complete testing	15
Submit release protocol to FDA	17
Release for distribution by FDA	22

SOURCE: Myers (2002b).

composition analysis, amino-terminal sequencing, and high-performance size-exclusion chromatography. Immunological techniques included Western blotting for hepatitis B surface antigen and contaminating yeast proteins, radioimmunoassay, enzyme-linked immunosorbent assay (ELISA), and immunogenicity in mice.

Few protein characterization and immunological techniques were available, however, to describe or specify the constituents of the anthrax vaccine when it was developed and refined in the 1950s and 1960s. Evaluations of the product relied heavily on comparison of relative potency in animals. For example, the relative success of various vaccine formulations was assessed on the basis of the production of effective immunity in rabbits, guinea pigs, and monkeys. Puziss and Wright's assay of protective antigen (1954) consisted of estimating "protective antigen activity" by immunization and challenge of guinea pigs. In their study described in a 1962 paper, Wright and colleagues also used complement fixation titrations (McGann et al., 1961) to estimate levels of protective antigen.

Detailed characterization of vaccine constituents was not routine in the 1960s. The anthrax vaccine was licensed in 1970, and the specifications of vaccine constituents consisted only of the amounts of stabilizer, preservative, and adjuvant added. No required amount of protective antigen was originally specified in the vaccine license, nor are the maximum (or minimum) amounts of other components that might be of interest or concern, such as edema factor (EF) or lethal factor (LF). The criteria for lot release were simply that the vaccine pass the necessary potency, safety, and purity tests.

Today, with detailed characterization of vaccine constituents clearly feasible, BioPort has undertaken analyses to characterize AVA in support of ongoing process validation studies (Winberry et al., 2001). One challenge is the development of an easy and reliable desorption procedure for the separation of vaccine constituents from Alhydrogel. Because of the difficulty of conducting desorption from Alhydrogel, BioPort investigators analyzed aliquots of the fermentation filtrate before adsorption. By use of the Bradford (1976) method to determine protein concentration, SDS-PAGE separation, Western blotting, and ELISA, a typical fermentation filtrate was determined to contain 10 micrograms (µg) of Bradford protein per milliliter; over 40 percent protective antigen, based on SDS-PAGE and Western blotting; and 2 to 4 µg of protective antigen per milliliter, based on ELISA. No detectable EF was found by Western blotting, but LF was determined by ELISA to be present in the range of 10 to 30 nanograms per milliliter of filtrate (Winberry et al., 2001).

To explore the biological activity of the LF in the vaccine, the mouse macrophage cytotoxicity assay was performed on 11 vaccine lots. Initial results indicated that the small-molecular-weight additives Phemerol (benzethonium chloride) and formaldehyde have minor toxic effects on macrophage cells. After their removal by dialysis, no toxic effect on the cells was evident. BioPort investigators concluded that the small amount of LF present in the vaccine is inactive and noted that further studies on characterization of the filtrate and the final formulated vaccine were ongoing (Winberry et al., 2001).

In agreement with FDA, BioPort has changed several manufacturing parameters for the production of AVA to provide greater assurance of product consistency. As depicted in Figure 7-1, these changes apply to aspects of production from temperature and time of fermentation to characteristics of the final product. Manufactured lots of vaccine must contain between 5 and 20 µg of total protein per milliliter, with no less than 35 percent of this protein consisting of the 83-kilodalton (kDa) protective antigen (precursor), to be acceptable (Giri et al., 2001). Data from 36 sublots combined as groups of 12 to obtain three consistent lots of filtrate found the Bradford protein to be present at a mean concentration of 7.7 µg/ml, with a concentration range of 5.1 to 15.8 µg/ml. The mean percentage of protective antigen, based on densitometric scans of the 83-kDa band on SDS-polyacrylamide gels, was 65.6 percent (range, 48.2 to 84.6 percent) for the 36 sublots (Myers, 2002a).

REGULATORY ACTIONS CONCERNING AVA MANUFACTURE

MDPH, a state-owned and -run facility, received the license to manufacture AVA in 1970 and produced vaccine until the facility was transferred to MBPI in 1995. In September 1998 the facility was sold to the private company BioPort, but the existing MBPI management team was retained (see Table 7-1).

FDA conducted an inspection of the MDPH anthrax vaccine manufacturing facility in January 1993, which was followed in July 1993 by FDA approval of amendments to the license application for new equipment and

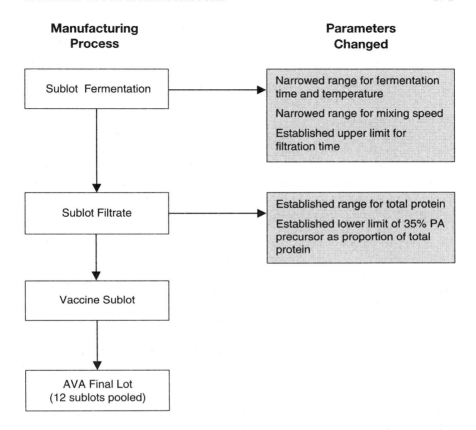

FIGURE 7-1 Changes to parameters of the Anthrax Vaccine Adsorbed manufacturing process.
SOURCES: Giri et al. (2001), Myers (2002a,b).

facilities (Donlon, 1993; FDA, 1993). Meanwhile, FDA inspections of MDPH product lines other than AVA in 1993 and 1995 resulted in findings of significant deviations from GMP and an official warning letter.

During a follow-up inspection of MBPI conducted in November 1996 that did not include the facilities for manufacture of AVA, FDA documented many deviations from the Food, Drug, and Cosmetic Act, FDA regulations, and current GMPs for the manufacture of blood-derived products and bacterial vaccines other than AVA (Elengold, 2000, 2001; Zoon, 1997). FDA issued a Notice of Intent to Revoke (NOIR) letter to MBPI in March 1997, stating that if MBPI's corrective actions proved to be inadequate, FDA might revoke its licenses. The letter did not mandate closure of the facility or involve seizure of finished product (Zoon, 1997). MBPI's response to the NOIR letter was a Strategic Plan for Compliance, provided to FDA in April 1997. Periodic updates to the strategic plan that reported on MBPI's progress were also provided to FDA (Michigan Biologic Products Institute, 1997–1998). In January 1998, after completion of renovation planning, MBPI shut down the anthrax vaccine production facility for planned renovations.

In February 1998, FDA conducted a comprehensive inspection covering all product lines of the facility to evaluate MBPI's compliance with the strategic plan. The inspection, which covered the manufacture and testing of all lots of AVA as well as other products, found that MBPI had made progress in achieving its compliance goals but that there were "significant deviations from FDA's regulations" (Elengold, 2000, p. 2; FDA, 1998a). The FDA inspection report noted that the manufacturing process for anthrax vaccine was not validated and included detailed lists of equipment or processes that had not been adequately described, specified, or documented. It reported a lack of written procedures or specifications for examination, rejection, and disposition of sublots of vaccine and problems with sample selection for potency testing, assignment of expiration dates, and documentation of justification for redating of expired lots. Many problems were also identified in the stability program (FDA, 1999a). As a result of this inspection, MBPI voluntarily quarantined several lots of vaccine after consultation with FDA (FDA, 1999a, p. 14). The facilities were transferred to BioPort in September 1998.

Another FDA inspection of the facility (now BioPort's facility) took place in October 1998. The inspection covered AVA and other product lines. Regarding AVA, the inspection found problems in the program for monitoring the stability of the vaccine (FDA, 1998b), but it also noted progress in many of the areas of observations made in the February 1998 Form FDA 483 (FDA, 1999a, pp. 20–23).

In September 1999, BioPort submitted a supplement to its BLA to FDA covering the renovations to the manufacturing facility. As part of its review of that application, FDA carried out a preapproval inspection of the BioPort plant in November 1999. The Establishment Inspection Report from that inspection identified observations and possible deviations in the areas of "validation, failure to investigate, manufacturing deviations, deviation reporting, aseptic processing, filling operations, standard operating procedures, stability testing, and environmental monitoring" (Elengold, 2000, p. 3; FDA, 1999b). The next inspection was in October 2000. Again, the inspection noted several items in need of attention, including the filling suite, which was among the categories listed as needing attention in the 1999 inspection (FDA, 2000). In April 2001, BioPort submitted a response detailing the company's modifications and improvements. In regard to the filling suite, BioPort decided to decommission the area and, subject to CBER approval, outsource the filling operation, at least temporarily.

The most recent inspection of the BioPort anthrax vaccine production facilities took place from December 12 to 19, 2001. The inspection report (FDA, 2001a) noted seven observations that needed attention, many of which BioPort successfully addressed during the inspection (FDA, 2001b). FDA approved the supplement to BLA on December 27, 2001, with acknowledgment that BioPort has made three commitments for additional postapproval work (Masiello, 2001).[3] Before lots of new AVA could be released and become available for shipment, however, FDA also had to approve a supplemental BLA for Hollister-Stier Laboratories, which is performing the filling operation under contract to BioPort. A preapproval inspection of that facility took place in January 2002, and FDA approved the supplement to the BLA for the contract filler on January 31, 2002, with the specification that additional stability data be collected (Maseillo, 2002). Under the approval, lots of AVA filled at Hollister-Stier will have an expiration date 18 months from the date of manufacture when the vaccine is stored at 2 to 8 degrees C, but as before the dating period may be extended with submission of supporting data to FDA.

For purposes of clarity, the committee has categorized the AVA product according to whether it was produced before or after the plant renovation. The available remaining vaccine was produced before January 1998, when MBPI halted production to carry out a comprehensive renovation. The committee heard testimony that FDA believes that the previously manufactured and CBER-released lots of AVA, not presently quarantined by BioPort, are safe and effective for the labeled indications (Elengold, 2000). While FDA has now released postrenovation lots for use, they had not been shipped as of late February 2002. Therefore, all AVA currently or previously used is prerenovation product, regardless of when the particular lot in question may have been released, and any vaccine subsequently manufactured by BioPort will be referred to as "postrenovation vaccine."[4]

---

[3]According to the approval letter from FDA, BioPort committed to (1) submit three successful consecutive media fill simulation studies evaluating the pooling of 12 sublots into the bulk formulation tank, (2) complete the validation of a protein nitrogen assay, and (3) develop an in vitro method for the assay of residual LF protein in AVA.

[4]Postrenovation vaccine was offered under an IND application to postal workers and congressional staff who were probably exposed to anthrax spores in the autumn of 2001. This vaccine was offered under an IND application because the lots had not yet been approved for release by FDA and because AVA was offered at a dosing schedule different from that for which it was licensed.

The General Accounting Office recently reported on changes to the manufacturing facilities not separately reported to FDA (GAO, 2001). In 1990 the manufacturer (then MDPH) changed its filter type from ceramic to nylon and thereafter used several different nylon filters (Elengold, 2001). In 1997 it changed filter types to match the industry standard, a polyvinylidene (nonshedding) filter. According to BioPort, these changes were within the specifications for filters in the original approved license. FDA learned of the changes and contacted BioPort in February 2001. The agency requested data and then accepted the changes in July 2001. On the basis of the data regarding the filter changes that BioPort submitted to FDA, which the company also provided to the IOM committee, all the lots of vaccine used by the Department of Defense not only as part of the Anthrax Vaccine Immunization Program but also, importantly, for safety studies were manufactured after the change from ceramic to nylon filters. Thus, several examinations of the safety of the product produced since the change to nylon filters have, in effect, been conducted. (The safety studies were discussed in Chapter 6.)

FINDINGS AND RECOMMENDATIONS

The committee assembled and reviewed the evidence it received in the course of its study. This evidence includes numerous Form FDA 483s and responses to those reports between FDA and BioPort, as well as statements and explanations to the IOM committee from officials of both FDA and BioPort on July 11, 2001. Furthermore, the committee took into consideration the recent and increasing BioPort and Department of Defense investments in facility renovations and process improvements, including the major action of shutting down the inadequate filling operations and transferal of those operations, with CBER approval, to a contractor meeting GMP standards. Finally, the committee noted the evident availability of technical support and assistance from CBER and Department of Defense research and development resources and the results that have been achieved in the form of progress in correcting the deficiencies noted in the Form FDA 483, as reported by BioPort and confirmed by FDA at the committee's meeting of July 10 and 11, 2001. As noted at the start of the chapter, FDA has now approved BioPort's BLA supplements for facility renovation, the changed package insert and label, and the contract filler (Goldenthal, 2002; Masiello, 2001, 2002).

The committee deliberated about the historical evidence concerning regulatory practice with regard to biologics and the special case of the AVA manufacturing facility. The committee took special note of the changes, modernizations, and improvements that FDA has undertaken, including normalization of inspections and creation of the Team Biologics program (the partnership between CBER and FDA's Office of Regulatory Affairs). In addition, the committee took special note of the continuing effort at constructive criticism and response between the agency and the manufacturer. The committee also considered the history of the AVA manufacturer, in particular, the switch from a state-owned to a privately owned and operated interstate commercial venture and the coincident changes in FDA oversight and validation requirements. Finally, the committee was most mindful of the changes in scientific and technical knowledge in the process of vaccine manufacture and characterization that have occurred since the original licensure of the AVA product.

Finding: FDA's process of plant inspection and FDA's validation of the vaccine manufacturing process have changed and have become more stringent with time.

Finding: With high-priority efforts by the manufacturer and FDA, the manufacturing process for AVA has been validated so that vaccine manufactured postrenovation has been approved for release and distribution.

The manufacturing facility licensed to produce AVA has been the subject of numerous specific citations regarding the manufacturing process and equipment on FDA inspection reports. The manufacturer also responded, however, and worked toward full compliance with FDA requirements and lot release. As a result of the regulatory changes mentioned in the finding above and changes in the myriad important details of materials and equipment and in scientific knowledge, the committee believes that greater consistency will be assured in the postrenovation AVA product.

Finding: AVA will now be produced by a newly validated manufacturing process under strict controls, according to current FDA requirements. As a result the postrenovation product has greater assurance of consistency than that produced at the time of original licensure.

REFERENCES

Auerbach BA, Wright GG. 1955. Studies on immunity in anthrax. VI. Immunizing activity of protective antigen against various strains of *Bacillus anthracis*. *Journal of Immunology* 75:129–133.

Brachman PS, Gold H, Plotkin S, Fekety FR, Werrin M, Ingraham NR. 1962. Field evaluation of a human anthrax vaccine. *American Journal of Public Health* 52:632–645.

Bradford MM. 1976. A rapid and sensitive method for the quantitation of microgram quantities of protein utilizing the principle of protein-dye binding. *Analytical Biochemistry* 72:248–254.

CDC (Centers for Disease Control and Prevention). 1967–1971. *Application and Report on Manufacture of Anthrax Protective Antigen, Aluminum Hydroxide Adsorbed (DBS-IND 180). Observational Study.* Atlanta, Ga.: Centers for Disease Control and Prevention.

Donlon JA. 1993. FDA approval of Michigan Department of Public Health ammendment to establishment license application. Letter to Myers RC, Michigan Department of Public Health, Lansing, Mich.

Elengold, M, Deputy Director, Operations, Center for Biologics Evaluation and Research, FDA. 2000. *Anthrax Vaccine Immunization Program—What Have We Learned?* Statement at the October 3, 2000, hearing of the Committee on Government Reform, U.S. House of Representatives, Washington, D.C.

Elengold M. 2001. Technical review. E-mail to Joellenbeck L, Institute of Medicine, Washington, D.C., December 12.

FDA (Food and Drug Administration). 1985. Biological products: bacterial vaccines and toxoids: implementation of efficacy review. Proposed rule. *Federal Register* 50(240): 51002–51117.

FDA. 1987. *Guideline on General Principles of Process Validation.* Rockville, Md.: Food and Drug Administration.

FDA. 1993. Form FDA 483 issued to Michigan Department of Public Health. Period of inspection: January 14–15, 1993. Letter to Myers R, Michigan Department of Public Health, Lansing, Mich.

FDA. 1998a. Form FDA 483 issued to Michigan Biologic Products Institute. Period of inspection: February 4–20, 1998. Letter to Myers RC, Michigan Biologic Products Institute, Lansing, Mich.

FDA. 1998b. Form FDA 483 issued to BioPort Corporation. Period of inspection: October 19–23, 1998. Letter to El-Hibri F, BioPort Corporation, Lansing, Mich.

FDA. 1999a. *Establishment Inspection Report of BioPort Corporation, October 19–23, 1998.* Rockville, Md.: FDA.

FDA. 1999b. Form FDA 483 issued to BioPort Corporation. Period of inspection: November 15–23, 1999. Letter to El-Hibri F, BioPort Corporation, Lansing, Mich.

FDA. 2000. Form FDA 483 issued to BioPort Corporation. Period of inspection: October 10–26, 2000. Letter to Kramer RG, BioPort Corporation, Lansing, Mich.

FDA. 2001a. Form FDA 483 issued to BioPort Corporation. Period of inspection: December 12–19, 2000. Letter to Kramer RG, BioPort Corporation, Lansing, Mich.

FDA. 2001b (December 19). Press Release: Pre-approval Inspection of the BioPort Facility. Rockville, Md.: FDA.

Feeley JC, Manclark CR, O'Malley JP, Kolb RW. 1969. Michigan Department of Public Health anthrax vaccine, evaluation of clinical data submitted under IND-180 on January 22, 1969. Memorandum to Pittman M, U.S. Department of Health, Education, and Welfare, Washington, D.C.

GAO (General Accounting Office). 2001. *Anthrax Vaccine: Changes to the Manufacturing Process.* GAO-02-181T. Washington, DC: GAO.

Goldenthal K. 2002. The labeling supplement to your license application for Anthrax Vaccine Adsorbed has been approved. Letter to Giri L, BioPort Corporation, Lansing, Mich.

Giri L, Kramer R, Myers R, Brennan-Root K, Waytes T, Winberry L. 2001. BioPort response to committee questions. Presentation to the Institute of Medicine Committee to Assess the Safety and Efficacy of the Anthrax Vaccine, Meeting IV, Washington, D.C.

Masiello SA. 2001. FDA approval of a BioPort Corporation biologics license application supplement. Letter to Giri L, BioPort Corporation, Lansing, Mich.

Masiello SA. 2002. Your request to supplement your BLA to include Hollister-Stier Laboratories LLC, Spokane, Washington, as a contract manufacturer has been approved. Letter to Giri L, BioPort Corporation, Lansing, Mich.
McGann VG, Stearman RL, Wright GG. 1961. Studies on immunity in anthrax. VIII. Relationship of complement-fixing activity to protective activity of culture filtrates. *Journal of Immunology* 86:458–464.
Michigan Biologic Products Institute. 1997–1998. *Strategic Plans and Updates.* Lansing, Mich.: BioPort Corporation.
Myers R. 2001. Technical review. E-mail to Joellenbeck L, Institute of Medicine, Washington, D.C., December 15.
Myers R. 2002a. Follow-up questions. E-mail to Joellenbeck L, Institute of Medicine, Washington, D.C., January 9.
Myers R. 2002b. Timeline for vaccine manufacture. E-mail to Joellenbeck L, Institute of Medicine, Washington, D.C., February 19.
Myers R, Winberry L, Park S. 2001. Components of the Anthrax Vaccine Adsorbed and contrast with Merck vaccine. Presentation to the Institute of Medicine Committee to Assess the Safety and Efficacy of the Anthrax Vaccine, Meeting II, Washington, D.C.
Parkman PD, Hardegree MC. 1999. Regulation and testing of vaccines. In: Plotkin SA, Orenstein WA, eds. *Vaccines*, 3rd ed. Philadelphia, Pa.: W.B. Saunders Company. Pp. 1131–1143.
Pittman M. 1969. Michigan Department of Health: application for license for anthrax vaccine. Memorandum to Gibson ST, Department of Health, Education, and Welfare, Washington, D.C.
Pittman PR. 2001. Anthrax vaccine: dose reduction/route change pilot study. Presentation to the Institute of Medicine Committee to Assess the Safety and Efficacy of the Anthrax Vaccine, Meeting II, Washington, D.C.
Pittman PR, Kim-Ahn G, Pifat DY, Coon K, Gibbs P, Little S, Pace-Templeton J, Myers R, Parker GW, Friedlander AM. 2002. Anthrax vaccine: safety and immunogenicity of a dose-reduction, route comparison study in humans. *Vaccine* 20(9–10):1412–1420.
Puziss M, Wright GG. 1954. Studies on immunity in anthrax. IV. Factors influencing elaboration of the protective antigen of *Bacillus anthracis* in chemically defined media. *Journal of Bacteriology* 68:474–482.
Puziss M, Wright GG. 1963. Studies on immunity in anthrax. X. Gel adsorbed protective antigen for immunization of man. *Journal of Bacteriology* 85:230–236.
Puziss M, Manning LC, Lynch JW, Barclay E, Abelow I, Wright GG. 1963. Large-scale production of protective antigen of *Bacillus anthracis* in anaerobic cultures. *Applied Microbiology* 11(4):330–334.
Turnbull PCB. 2000. Current status of immunization against anthrax: old vaccines may be here to stay for a while. *Current Opinion in Infectious Diseases* 13(2):113–120.
Winberry LK, Bondoc L, Park S, Simon L, Shih CN, Giri L. 2001. Characterization of the US-licensed anthrax vaccine. In: *Program and Abstracts Book of the Fourth Annual Conference on Anthrax.* Washington, D.C.: American Society for Microbiology.
Wright GG, Puziss M. 1957. Elaboration of protective antigen of *Bacillus anthracis* under anaerobic conditions. *Nature* 179:916–917.
Wright GG, Hedberg MA, Slein JB. 1954. Studies on immunity in anthrax. III. Elaboration of protective antigen in a chemically-defined, non-protein medium. *Journal of Immunology* 72:263–269.
Wright GG, Puziss M, Neely WB. 1962. Studies on immunity in anthrax. IX. Effect of variations in cultural conditions on elaboration of protective antigen by strains of *Bacillus anthracis*. *Journal of Immunology* 83:515–522.
Zoon KC. 1997. Inspections of Michigan Biologic Products Institute, November 18 and 27, 1996. Letter to Myers R, Michigan Biologic Products Institute, Lansing, Mich.

8

Future Needs

As described in detail in preceding chapters, the committee found that the available evidence shows that the currently licensed anthrax vaccine, Anthrax Vaccine Adsorbed (AVA), is reasonably safe and effective, with the caveat that the studies reviewed were carried out in populations of healthy adults only. The committee's research also suggested that the manufacturing process could be validated.

As discussed in Chapter 3, the efficacy of the licensed anthrax vaccine—indeed, of any anthrax vaccine—for the stimulation of protective immunity against inhalational anthrax in humans cannot be demonstrated in clinical trials or field trials, as clinical trials that challenged humans with the anthrax bacillus would be impossible—and intolerable—and humans naturally encounter aerosolized *Bacillus anthracis* spores in few situations. The committee did, however, review evidence from a field trial that showed that a vaccine similar to AVA is effective against *B. anthracis* infection, that AVA itself is effective in stimulating immunity against inhalational challenge in animals, and that AVA and experimental vaccines that contain protective antigen are effective in protecting immunized animals against challenge with *B. anthracis*.

The standard of reasonable safety does not mean that no adverse events are associated with AVA; indeed, local adverse events including tenderness, erythema, nodules, and some swelling are fairly common and seem to be more frequent in women than in men (Pittman et al., 2002). In addition, some vaccinees experienced systemic effects such as fever, but these effects were less common than local reactions and were transient. Some members of the armed services have been concerned that AVA may cause later-onset systemic or multisystem adverse effects. To date there is limited information pertaining to any possible association between vaccination with AVA and later-onset health conditions, as with most vaccines. The available data, however, provide no evidence of a causal connection between receipt of AVA and later-onset or long-term adverse outcomes.

The history of the facility that manufactures AVA has been fraught with difficulties. Over the course of the study, the committee reviewed extensive and detailed exchanges between the manufacturer, BioPort, and the Food and Drug Administration (FDA) regarding the changes to the manufacturing process that were needed. That BioPort has successfully met FDA requirements is welcome news.

Nevertheless, the committee is convinced that relying only on the current anthrax vaccine and the current specifications for its use is far from satisfactory. Not only are many avenues for important research toward the development of a different and better vaccine available, but particular improvements in how the current vaccine is used are also urgently needed. Many of these improvements are feasible, which makes their implementation even more compelling. This chapter suggests some directions for further research and action.

FUTURE USE OF AVA

Finding: Current events in both the military and the civilian arenas highlight and confirm the importance of ensuring both the availability and the quality of the nation's anthrax vaccine.

Less than a month before this report went to press, BioPort received approval for the first release of lots of AVA produced since 1998. Because the supply of AVA has been limited, the Department of Defense's (DoD's) Anthrax Vaccine Immunization Program (AVIP) was proceeding at a reduced rate. Renewed availability of AVA will make possible the resumption of the AVIP schedule. Current events, including the deployment of U.S. troops to Afghanistan and surrounding areas and sabotage of the U.S. mail with items contaminated with *B. anthracis* spores, strongly suggest not only the resumption but also possibly the expansion of vaccination against anthrax. As stated in the new product label (see Appendix D), the licensed product is indicated for "individuals between 18 and 65 years of age who come in contact with animal products such as hides, hair, or bones that come from anthrax endemic areas, and that may be contaminated with *B. anthracis* spores. AVA, now carrying the brand name BioThrax,[1] is also

---

[1]Biothrax is the name under which AVA will be manufactured as of January 31, 2002.

indicated for individuals at high risk of exposure to *B. anthracis* spores such as veterinarians, laboratory workers, and others whose occupation may involve handling potentially infected animals or other contaminated materials." This labeled indication has not changed from the original, which was developed in view of the plausible exposures at the time of licensure of the vaccine and was supported by field and observational studies of animal product processors.

The subsequent weaponization of *B. anthracis*, however, changed for DoD the definition of the groups identified as "high-risk persons" to include not only veterinarians but also members of the armed services who were or who might be deployed to areas near countries where *B. anthracis* had been weaponized. As a result of the recent bioterrorist release of anthrax spores through the U.S. mail system, the definition of "high-risk persons" may be expanded further to include other occupational groups. The population receiving AVA has thus become considerably wider than that anticipated at the time of original licensure.

Meanwhile, the supply of the currently licensed vaccine had been limited by manufacturing difficulties, which have now been overcome. As mentioned above and as discussed in more detail in Chapter 7, the AVA manufacturing facility and the AVA production process have both been the subject of numerous FDA citations and responses. Indeed, the manufacturer undertook a thorough renovation of its manufacturing facility starting in 1998 and modernized several aspects of the production process. These modifications, although certainly intended to improve the overall process of vaccine production, are still changes. Changes in facilities or processes, however, can result in changes in the product, and FDA is responsible for monitoring those changes (see Chapter 7).

Noting the possibility that these changes may affect the final AVA product does not mean that the changes are necessarily bad; in this case they are surely improvements. On the basis of the information provided in presentations and in papers from both BioPort and FDA, the committee notes that modifications were undertaken to incorporate more modern technology into the manufacturing process and to increase assurance of the consistency of the final product (e.g., in the concentration of protective antigen), which still remains a relatively crude vaccine by current standards.

Although greater assurance of product consistency will result from the modifications of the manufacturing facility and the production process that have been undertaken by BioPort and certified by FDA, the levels of immunogenicity, safety, and stability of the postrenovation AVA product must be characterized empirically, as the committee recommends below. The committee emphasizes that the surveillance methods recommended below are the same as those that would be expected for any widely used vaccine and are not unique to AVA.

Finding: The AVA product produced in a renovated facility by a newly validated manufacturing process could differ from the prerenovation product in terms of its reactogenicity, immunogenicity, and stability. The information available to the committee suggests that AVA lots manufactured postrenovation may show less variation in reactogenicity because of greater consistency in the production process, and there is no a priori basis to believe that the postrenovation product will be more reactogenic or less immunogenic than the older vaccine.

Recommendation: As with all vaccines, AVA lots produced postrenovation should continue to be monitored for immunogenicity and stability, and individuals receiving these lots should be monitored for possible acute or chronic events of immediate or later onset.

SURVEILLANCE FOR ADVERSE EVENTS

In addition to issuing statements about appropriate filing of reports to the Vaccine Adverse Event Reporting System (VAERS), DoD has supported the review of each VAERS report associated with AVA by an independent civilian advisory panel called the Anthrax Vaccine Expert Committee (AVEC), described in Chapter 5.

The Future and AVEC

A subgroup of the Institute of Medicine (IOM) committee participated in discussions with members of AVEC to explore their approach to the review of reports and their operating procedures. Although the committee found AVEC's expert scrutiny of the reported cases and vigilance for signals that might require further action to be an important component of surveillance for concerns about the safety of AVA, the important aspects of the review may not be specific to AVA. The IOM committee is also skeptical of the general approach of attribution of causality from reports in surveillance systems. The way in which events are interpreted and used in analyses should take into account the inherent uncertainties of determining "cause" in such a system. There remains considerable potential for misclassification of reported events when considering them as possibly related or unrelated to vaccination. It is important to recognize that reviews of case reports only generate hypotheses. More emphasis should therefore be placed on the use of AVEC-derived hypotheses to trigger formal analyses, such as those that can be performed with data from the Defense Medical Surveillance System (DMSS). Toward that end, AVEC and the Army Medical Surveillance Activity (the office responsible for DMSS) should maintain regular and frequent communication, with signals from the former leading to analyses by the latter. "Signals" are the earliest indication of a possible causal relationship between an exposure and a health event. Such signals can come from the anecdotal experiences of patients with an adverse event after the exposure or from preliminary analyses of data. A signal does not mean that a causal relationship exists, as there may be other explanations for the apparent association. Instead, a signal is merely an indication that further investigation is needed.

Furthermore, AVA appears to be associated with certain adverse events that, although by no means desirable, are self-limited or that, in worst cases, seem to respond to palliative treatment with analgesics or antipyretics. The committee observes that no data to indicate the need for the continuation of special monitoring programs for AVA have emerged, but it recognizes the real concerns of service members ordered to take the vaccine. Vaccine safety in general, and the safety of less commonly used vaccines that members of the U.S. military in particular are required to receive, remains a concern. In the course of reviewing information from monitoring systems, the committee observed several areas in which surveillance for the safety of vaccines in general, including AVA, might be improved.

> **Finding:** Given the concerns raised by some service members about the safety of the anthrax vaccine, the creation of AVEC was an appropriate complement to other resources in FDA, the Centers for Disease Control and Prevention (CDC), and DoD for the monitoring of vaccine safety concerns. The results of the extra monitoring did not indicate the existence of any sentinel events that were not detected in the existing FDA and CDC reviews. The committee finds no scientific reason for the continued operation of AVEC in its present form.

The IOM committee's observation about AVEC reflects no fault with the members of AVEC or its performance as that committee is constituted; rather, the IOM committee observes that AVEC was designed to pay extra attention to concerns regarding the safety of AVA and that the data do not warrant the continuation of such exceptional attention. The resources supporting AVEC activities related to AVA alone could be more wisely invested in improved monitoring of the safety of vaccines in general.

> **Recommendation:** DoD should disband AVEC in its current form and instead assist FDA and CDC in establishing an independent advisory committee charged with overseeing the entire process of evaluating vaccine safety. The proposed advisory committee can also assist on an ad hoc basis in the interpretation of potential signals detected in VAERS or other sources regarding the safety of any vaccine. The newly established FDA Drug Safety and Risk Management Advisory Committee might be an appropriate model.

Because AVEC was designed to review VAERS reports for signals of unexpected adverse events caused by AVA, AVEC had to attempt to discriminate correlation and causality on the basis of the VAERS reports. The VAERS reports, however, are not able to capture data sufficient to support conclusions related to causality. The committee therefore believes that DoD should recommend a shift in focus from making attributions of causality in individual cases to seeking evidence of any patterns or rate thresholds that have been crossed in terms of the serious adverse events reported to VAERS. AVEC's replacement could then develop criteria for signals from VAERS data for any vaccine that warrant additional follow-up and could in general further systematize its processes by developing standard operating procedures and a regular schedule for examination of aggregate VAERS data. Background rates of illnesses as well as the biological plausibility of hypothesized effects must be taken into consideration as part of the method used to identify signals of possible safety concerns regarding AVA. Different roles for the panels that might replace AVEC are described in Table 8-1.

TABLE 8-1 Functions of AVEC and Post-AVEC Panels

Function	AVEC	Redeployed AVEC	Panel Replacing AVEC
Mission	Individual review of VAERS reports to assess causal relationship of AVA and adverse events	Provide ad hoc advice as needed on interpretation of potential signals in VAERS or other sources relevant to vaccine safety	Provide oversight and advice on safety evaluations and advice in specific cases
Scope	All AVA-related VAERS reports	All vaccines administered to service personnel	Entire process of vaccine safety evaluations, plus provision of advice as needed on interpretation of potential signals from VAERS or other sources relevant to the safety of any vaccine
Model	Advisory Committee on Causality Assessment (Canada)	Advisory committee (responding to ad hoc agency requests for advice on specific products)	FDA Drug Safety and Risk Management Advisory Committee (broad mandate and oversight, as well as ad hoc advice)

Recommendation: If DoD chooses to continue AVEC, DoD should consider redefining the panel's role so that it serves as an independent advisory committee that responds on an ad hoc basis to specific requests to assist in the interpretation of potential signals detected by others (e.g., CDC and FDA) and reported to VAERS or other sources regarding the safety of all vaccines administered to service personnel rather than continuing the panel's current role of rereviewing each VAERS report related to AVA.

Although there are serious obstacles and some impassable informational gulfs between VAERS reports and conclusions related to causality for any vaccine, there are some additional difficulties for AVA because, at least to date, the population receiving the vaccine is small. More than 2 million doses of AVA have been distributed since 1990, and about 500,000 members of the armed forces have received the vaccine. By contrast, multiple doses of many other vaccines, such as the diphtheria and tetanus toxoid and acellular pertussis vaccine, the *Haemophilus influenzae* type b vaccine, or inactivated polio vaccine, are administered to some 3 million to 4 million children each year.

Finding: The possibility of detecting a signal in VAERS will be even more limited for AVA than for many other vaccines given the relatively small population (primarily military personnel) exposed to the vaccine and the low rates at which the hypothesized health effects of greatest concern might be expected to occur in that population.

Additional Sources of Data on Adverse Events

Although the IOM committee does not recommend continuation of AVEC as a program that monitors AVA-specific reports in VAERS, the committee does believe that it is essential for DoD to continue to work with CDC and FDA to ensure that VAERS reports are regularly and carefully monitored for any signals that vaccines administered to military service personnel might be associated with adverse health effects. Ensuring the best use and interpretation of VAERS reports, however, requires complementary information from other sources that can be used to help analyze the signals that may be suggested by VAERS reports. One such resource, as discussed earlier, is DMSS. DMSS can be used both to generate and test hypotheses. If VAERS raises a hypothesis, it can be further evaluated in DMSS. DMSS data can also be used to generate hypotheses (as in its quarterly screening reports); these then need to be evaluated in more detail within DMSS, including more detailed data analyses and efforts that might involve review of medical records, for example. Formal testing of these hypotheses would require additional studies, however, in separate datasets.

Finding: VAERS is a critically important source of signals, that is, hypotheses about potential associations between a vaccine and a health event, but these hypotheses must be tested through other means. DMSS gives DoD a unique resource with which to conduct such testing.

A formal mechanism for the direct examination of signals from VAERS using DMSS data should be established. The committee was impressed with information presented on the types of data maintained in DMSS datasets on medical encounters for any reason in the military health care system.

Finding: DMSS is a unique and promising population-based resource for monitoring the emergence of both immediate-onset and later-onset (perhaps up to 5 years) health concerns among military personnel and for testing hypothesized associations between such health concerns and exposures resulting from military service, including vaccines.

Because DMSS is designed to capture records for all medical encounters without depending on the decision of a patient or a physician to report a particular encounter, DMSS data may be cross-checked with the more open-ended but much less complete case reports collected through VAERS. DoD personnel have already conducted some analyses of this sort, and such analyses should continue on a regular basis. But conducting these analyses on a timely basis will require additional analytic resources. The committee believes that DoD must enhance its internal analytic capacity. A proposed collaboration between CDC and the Army Medical Surveillance Activity (Schwartz, 2002) holds promise for increasing the human resources available to apply to hypothesis testing, while AMSA personnel retain their focus on surveillance. In addition, DoD should explore ways to take advantage of the analytic resources of the civilian research community as other federal agencies do. The Centers for Medicare and Medicaid Systems, for example, have developed mechanisms to give researchers access to large databases with information on individual program participants and their medical claims while maintaining appropriate protections for privacy and confidentiality. Similarly, research partnerships with the Canadian province of Saskatchewan may offer another useful model.

Recommendation: DoD should develop a capability for the effective use of DMSS to regularly test hypotheses that emerge from VAERS and other sources regarding vaccine-related adverse events.

Finding: DoD personnel have used DMSS to conduct valuable analyses in response to concerns about health effects that might be associated with vaccination with AVA. Yet DoD personnel working with DMSS data are necessarily limited in time and focus. DMSS data could therefore yield valuable insights in the hands of civilian researchers.

Recommendation: DoD should actively support and advance the development of DMSS data resources and the staffing of units that will allow the continuing rapid and careful analysis of these data, including but not limited to the proposed collaboration between CDC and the Army Medical Surveillance Activity.

Recommendation: DoD should investigate mechanisms that can be used to make DMSS data available to civilian researchers, as is done by civilian agencies, with appropriate controls and protections for privacy.

The main limitations of the DMSS databases with respect to the study of adverse events associated with vaccination are actually related to its main strength. That is, although DMSS collects records of all medical encounters, it cannot capture the adverse events that a vaccine recipient experiences but for which the recipient does not seek medical attention within the military medical system. Because most vaccine-related adverse events are relatively mild and self-limiting, they will not appear in the DMSS database.

Finding: DMSS cannot be used to study mild adverse events, even if they are common.

This limitation can be mitigated with prospective studies and active surveillance of limited populations of vaccinees.

Recommendation: DoD should develop ad hoc prospective cohort studies in one or more military settings to test hypotheses that emerge from VAERS, DMSS, or other sources. However, the committee does not recommend that such studies targeted at AVA be conducted at present since no convincing evidence of new adverse events in AVA recipients sufficient to merit a prospective investigation has been presented. Rather, further studies of the effects of AVA should be performed in the context of studies of the effects of all vaccines administered to members of the military.

Another aspect of the DMSS database that must be taken into consideration for overall monitoring of vaccine safety is that DMSS contains data on medical encounters only for active-duty personnel. Most service members do not become career military personnel, so DoD surveillance systems can monitor their health for only a few years. Later-onset effects of vaccines, if any, would thus not be captured for most service members.

Finding: Because DMSS captures health care data only for military personnel on active duty, it cannot be used to study the later-onset effects of vaccines over periods of time beyond the normal length of active military service.

As discussed in Chapter 6, data on the later-onset adverse effects of vaccines are available for few, if any, vaccines. Although the committee found no data indicating that vaccination with AVA is associated with later-onset adverse events or with any serious or lasting adverse events, some service members have had serious concerns about possible links between AVA and such adverse events. To make it possible to conduct studies of later-onset health concerns, DoD could take steps to improve access to data on the chronic or later-onset effects, if any, of vaccines in general.

Recommendation: DoD should carefully evaluate options for longer-term follow-up of the possible health effects of vaccination against anthrax (and other service-related exposures). The committee recommends consideration of the following specific steps:

- Encourage participation in the Millennium Cohort Study[2] as part of a program to ensure adequate monitoring for any possible later-onset health effects that might be associated with vaccination with AVA or other service-related exposures.
- Collaborate with the Department of Veterans Affairs (VA) to monitor service members who receive medical care through VA facilities after separation from military service. Linking of data from DMSS to data from VA is a possible tool. Even though those who receive their medical care through VA may be an unrepresentative minority of all former military personnel, valid comparisons may be possible between those within that population who received a vaccine or other exposure and those who did not.
- Collaborate with VA to obtain fact-of-death information from the Beneficiary Identification and Records Locator System and with the Social Security Administration to obtain death files. Data on the cause of death should be obtained from the National Death Index as needed.
- Ensure the long-term maintenance of DMSS and other relevant paper and electronic records so that retrospective studies will be feasible if health concerns are identified in the future.

NEW ANTHRAX VACCINE DEVELOPMENT

Although AVA appears to be sufficiently safe and effective for use and its use is certainly preferable to a substantial threat of contracting anthrax,

---

[2]The Millennium Cohort Study is a survey recommended by the U.S. Congress and sponsored by the DoD. The study will monitor a total of 140,000 U.S. military personnel during and after their military service for up to 21 years to evaluate the health risks of military deployment, military occupations, and general military service (see http://www.millenniumcohort.org/about.html).

AVA is far from optimal whether it is considered from the point of view of the potential recipient, the manufacturer, or any involved party.

Finding: The current anthrax vaccine is difficult to standardize, is incompletely characterized, and is relatively reactogenic (probably even more so because it is administered subcutaneously), and the dose schedule is long and challenging. An anthrax vaccine free of these drawbacks is needed, and such improvements are feasible.

The committee urges that improvements in the route of administration and the number of injections of the existing licensed anthrax vaccine, AVA, be made as quickly as possible. As mentioned earlier in this report, the committee believes that the lot-to-lot consistency of AVA will be better assured when the vaccine is produced in the fully renovated facility using the newly certified manufacturing processes and that such an improvement is desirable. The committee also believes that it is likely that the rate of adverse events and the general acceptability of AVA will improve with a change in the route of administration and a reduction in the total number of injections required and that such improvements would be desirable. Research to assess the effects of those changes in the route of administration was under way as this report was being prepared. Any improvements to the way the current vaccine is used that can limit the occurrence of common local and systemic effects will be welcome by all parties involved. But the committee concludes that a new vaccine, developed according to more modern principles of vaccinology, is urgently needed. The committee proposes characteristics, based on experience with other vaccines, that might reasonably be sought in a new vaccine (see Box 8-1).

It was beyond the committee's charge to comment on any particular program to develop a new vaccine against anthrax or to review research related to the development of a new vaccine. The committee does understand that research on new vaccines against anthrax is well under way in several areas in DoD, the National Institutes of Health, and various university laboratories and strongly encourages continued and further support of work on promising new vaccines. The knowledge that has been and that is still being gained from research with AVA on topics such as correlates of immunity in animals, the components necessary to stimulate protective immunity, and the best way to administer the vaccine should be helpful in the development of new and improved vaccine products for protection against anthrax. Research to date shows anthrax to be a complex disease, with complicated protective immune responses. Additional research should speed the urgently needed development of improved means of protection against this disease.

> **BOX 8-1**
> **Goals of Anthrax Vaccine Development**
>
> **Product characteristics**
>
> • Antigen: The vaccine antigen, which must be demonstrated to stimulate protective immunity, should consist of a purified protein, a mixture of defined and purified proteins, or a conjugate of a purified protein and the capsule.
> • Dose requirements: The vaccine should require only two or three injections to elicit high titers of antibodies against the antigen.
> • Immunogenicity: The vaccine should be sufficiently immunogenic to elicit protective antibodies within 30 days so that antibiotics given to exposed individuals could be safely discontinued at 30 days.
> • Stability: The potency of the vaccine should remain stable for a long period of time, allowing it to be stockpiled.
>
> **Product performance**
>
> • Efficacy: The vaccine should be demonstrated to protect monkeys challenged by the aerosol route, with immunity retained for at least a year after the completion of immunization.
> • Local reactions: The vaccine should not cause severe local reactions. This is important not only for better tolerability but also because severe local reactions may create a perception that a vaccine is dangerous, even when the local effects are transient and self-limited.
> • Systemic reactions: The vaccine should not cause severe systemic adverse reactions, as is expected of all vaccines.
>
> **Manufacturing**
>
> • Production process: The production process for the vaccine should be easily scaled up and should ensure maintenance of product consistency.

Recommendation: DoD should continue and further expedite its research efforts pertaining to anthrax disease, the *B. anthracis* organism, and vaccines against anthrax. Research related to anthrax should include, in particular, efforts such as the following:

• DoD should pursue and encourage research to develop an anthrax vaccine product that can be produced more consistently and that is less reactogenic than AVA;
• DoD should pursue and encourage research regarding the *B. anthracis* capsule;
• DoD should pursue and encourage research on the mechanisms of action of the anthrax toxins; such research could lead to the development of small-molecule inhibitors;

- DoD should pursue and encourage research to map the epitopes of the protective antigen that correlate with specific functional activities;
- DoD should pursue and encourage research to test the therapeutic potential of antitoxin proteins or antibodies; and
- DoD should pursue and encourage research into additional potential virulence factors in *B. anthracis* and into other possible vaccine candidates.

REFERENCES

Pittman PR, Kim-Ahn G, Pifat DY, Coonan K, Gibbs P, Little S, Pace-Templeton JG, Myers R, Parker GW, Friedlander AM. 2002. Anthrax vaccine: immunogenicity and safety of a dose-reduction, route-change comparison study in humans. *Vaccine* 20(9-10):1412-1420.

Schwartz B. 2002. Hypothesis testing using the DMSS: outline for a CDC-AMSA collaboration. Presentation to the Institute of Medicine Committee to Review the CDC Anthrax Vaccine Safety and Efficacy Research Program, Meeting V, Washington, D.C.

Appendixes

Appendix A

Statement of Task

The committee will analyze available information, hold workshops, and make specific recommendations on technical aspects regarding the safety and efficacy of the licensed anthrax vaccine. The issues include the types and severity of adverse reactions, including gender (sex) differences; long-term health implications; inhalational efficacy of the vaccine against all known anthrax strains; correlation of animal models to safety and effectiveness in humans; validation of the manufacturing process focusing on, but not limited to, discrepancies identified by the Food and Drug Administration in February 1998; definition of vaccine components in terms of the protective antigen and other bacterial products and constituents; and identification of gaps in existing research.

Appendix B

Biographical Sketches

Brian L. Strom, M.D., M.P.H. (*Chair*), is professor of biostatistics and epidemiology, professor of medicine, professor of pharmacology, director of the Center for Clinical Epidemiology & Biostatistics, and chair of the Graduate Group in Epidemiology & Biostatistics at the University of Pennsylvania School of Medicine. His clinical training and research training are in internal medicine, clinical pharmacology, and epidemiology, with a major research interest in the field of pharmacoepidemiology. He holds editorial positions on numerous journals and has authored more than 300 original papers, as well as one of the first textbooks in the field. Dr. Strom has served as president of the International Society of Pharmacoepidemiology and as a member of the Board of Regents of the American College of Physicians. He is now on the Board of Directors for the American College of Epidemiology. He served on both the Medication Use Task Force of the Joint Commission on the Accreditation of Healthcare Organizations and the Drug Utilization Review Advisory Committee on the United States Pharmacopoeia Convention. He has been elected to the Association of American Physicians, the American Epidemiologic Society, the American Society for Clinical Investigation, and the Institute of Medicine.

William E. Barlow, Ph.D., is a senior scientific investigator at the Center for Health Studies, the research arm of the consumer-governed nonprofit health care organization Group Health Cooperative. He is also research professor of biostatistics at the University of Washington. His scientific research interests are breast cancer screening and the safety and efficacy of childhood immunizations. His statistics interests include practice variation, influence diagnostics, surrogate outcomes, and efficient sampling procedures. Dr. Barlow's work on immunization and vaccines has included work on a comprehensive collection of data on links between medical events and immunization. He directs the Statistical Coordinating Center for the National Breast Cancer Surveillance Consortium, funded by the National Cancer Institute. He is a member of the American Statistical Association, the Biometric Society, and the Society for Clinical Trials.

Dan G. Blazer II, M.D., M.P.H., Ph.D., is the J. P. Gibbons Professor of Psychiatry and Behavioral Sciences, a professor of community and family medicine, and former dean of medical education at the Duke University School of Medicine. He is also adjunct professor in the Department of Epidemiology at the University of North Carolina School of Public Health. Dr. Blazer is the author or editor of more than 20 books and author or coauthor of more than 250 peer-reviewed articles on topics including depression, epidemiology, and liaison psychiatry. He has served on several Institute of Medicine committees and recently chaired the Committee on the Evaluation of the Department of Defense Clinical Evaluation Protocol. He is a fellow of the American College of Psychiatry and the American Psychiatric Association and is a member of the Institute of Medicine.

Linda D. Cowan, Ph.D., is the George Lynn Cross Research Professor in the Department of Biostatistics and Epidemiology at the University of Oklahoma Health Sciences Center. Her interests include cardiovascular disease and the relative importance of different risk factors in men and women, neurological disorders, perinatal epidemiology, and the application of epidemiology in the legal setting. Her recent research includes evaluating risk factors for abnormal fetal growth, identifying cardiovascular disease risk factors in Native American populations, and evaluating multiple approaches to surveillance of hemophilia in Oklahoma. Dr. Cowan is an elected member of the American Epidemiological Society and is the recipient of several teaching awards. She has served on the Institute of Medicine Vaccine Safety Forum and on the Committee to Review the Adverse Consequences of Pertussis and Rubella Vaccines.

Kathryn M. Edwards, M.D., is professor of pediatrics and associate director of the Division of Pediatric Infectious Diseases at Vanderbilt University. Dr. Edwards's work has focused on the evaluation of new vaccines for the prevention of infectious diseases in adults and children. She has conducted large efficacy trials of a live-attenuated intranasal influenza virus vaccine and has coordinated multicenter trials of the safety and immunogenicity of new generations of the *Haemophilus influenzae* type b and *Bordetella per-*

tussis vaccines. Studies of the efficacy of *Streptococcus pneumoniae* vaccines are in progress. Her laboratory efforts have focused on the standardization of serologic markers of vaccine response and correlates of protection against natural disease. Dr. Edwards is a member of the Society for Pediatric Research and is a fellow of the Infectious Diseases Society of America and the American Academy of Pediatrics. She has previously served as a member of the Advisory Committee on Immunization Practices of the Centers for Disease Control and Prevention and the Vaccines and Related Biological Products Advisory Committee of the Food and Drug Administration.

Denise L. Faustman, M.D, Ph.D., is an associate professor of medicine at Harvard Medical School and director of immunobiology at the Massachusetts General Hospital. Her research interests include diabetes, autoimmune diseases, and transplantation. Many of her experimental approaches capture the molecular and genetic bases of preferential autoimmune disease expression in women. She was the inventor of the concept of modifying donor antigens on cells before transplantation, which serves as the platform technology for the use of cloning technology in this clinical arena. Over the past 10 years she discovered two deranged biological pathways in autoimmune lymphocytes that now serve as potential therapeutic sites for the permanent reversal of autoimmunity. In the case of murine autoimmune models, the complete reversal of established diabetic autoimmunity has yielded the first data demonstrating the regeneration in situ of the missing islet tissue. She serves as co-editor-in-chief of the *Journal of Women's Health and Gender-Based Medicine* and since 2000 has served as chairman of the board for the Society for the Advancement of Women's Health Research. She has served on several National Research Council and Institute of Medicine committees, including the Committee on Methods for Producing Monoclonal Antibodies, Committee for Xenograft Transplantation, and the Committee on Gender Differences in Susceptibility to Environmental Factors.

Emil C. Gotschlich, M.D., is vice president for medical sciences at the Rockefeller University, where he is also R. Gwin Follis-Chevron Professor and head of the Laboratory of Bacterial Pathogenesis and Immunology. His early work led to the development of a vaccine for the prevention of group A and C meningococcal meningitis. His research has also been directed at the surface structures responsible for the pathogenicity of group B streptococci and gonococcus. Dr. Gotschlich is a fellow of the American Academy of Microbiology and is a member of both the National Academy of Sciences and the Institute of Medicine.

Dennis L. Kasper, M.D., is executive dean for academic programs, William Ellery Channing Professor of Medicine, and professor of microbiology and molecular genetics at Harvard Medical School. He also serves as director of the Channing Laboratory and as a senior physician at Brigham and Women's Hospital. With his colleagues and students, Dr. Kasper studies the molecular basis of bacterial pathogenesis, applying the resulting knowledge to enhance understanding of the interactions of bacterial surface virulence factors with host defenses. Dr. Kasper's studies focus on the molecular and chemical characterization of important bacterial virulence factors such as capsular polysaccharides, surface proteins, and toxins. The ultimate goal is to develop vaccines and immunomodulatory molecules to prevent bacterial infections and their complications. Dr. Kasper is a fellow of the American Academy of Microbiology and the American Association for the Advancement of Science as well as a member of the Institute of Medicine.

Don P. Metzgar, Ph.D., is a vaccine developer with a career spanning 34 years in research, manufacturing, development, and testing of vaccines. He has developed and licensed or supervised the development and licensing of 16 new or improved vaccines. Dr. Metzgar retired in 1994 from Connaught Laboratories, Ltd., as senior vice president with responsibilities for product development, including manufacturing, quality operations, medical affairs, regulatory affairs, engineering, and maintenance for the United States and Canada. He has served on the National Vaccine Advisory Committee. Dr. Metzgar maintains a relationship with his former employer as a consultant.

Hugh H. Tilson, M.D., Dr.P.H., is clinical professor of epidemiology and health policy and senior adviser to the dean at the University of North Carolina School of Public Health. Dr. Tilson is a practicing epidemiologist and outcomes researcher, with a career in preventive medicine and public health that spans more than 30 years and that includes service as a director of both state and local health departments and as vice president for worldwide epidemiology, surveillance, and policy research at GlaxoWellcome. He is the author of more than 100 papers in the fields of epidemiology, outcomes and policy research, and public health; he is a fellow of the American College of Epidemiology; and he is former vice-chair of the American Board of Preventive Medicine. Dr. Tilson also served as president of the American College of Preventive Medicine from 1995 to 1997 and was founding co-president of the International Society for Pharmacoepidemiology. He serves as an adviser and consultant in health outcomes, drug safety, and evidence-based health policy to regulatory and government agencies as well as pharmaceutical companies.

Appendix C

Information-Gathering Meeting Agendas

Meeting I
October 3, 2000

The Foundry Building
1055 Thomas Jefferson Street, NW
Washington, DC

Agenda

Tuesday, October 3rd

Open Session

8:00 a.m.	Introductory remarks and review of charge *Dr. Brian Strom, Chair, Committee to Assess the Safety and Efficacy of the Anthrax Vaccine*
8:15	Introductions by committee members and meeting attendees
8:30	Sponsor presentation on the study charge *Major General John Parker, Commander, U.S. Army Medical Research and Materiel Command*

APPENDIX C   219

	Congressional comment on the study charge *Mr. Robert Neal, Legislative Assistant, Office of Representative George Nethercutt, Jr.*
9:15	Concerns Regarding the Safety or Efficacy of Anthrax Vaccine *Dr. Meryl Nass* *Dr. George Robertson*
10:00	Break
10:15	Anthrax the Disease, and Anthrax Vaccine Development and History *LTC John D. Grabenstein, Deputy Director for Clinical Operations, Anthrax Vaccine Immunization Program* *LTC Mark G. Kortepeter, Chief, Education and Training, Operational Medicine Division, U.S. Army Medical Research Institute of Infectious Diseases*
11:00	The DoD Anthrax Vaccine Immunization Program (AVIP) Status and Projected Future *LTC John D. Grabenstein, Deputy Director for Clinical Operations, Anthrax Vaccine Immunization Program*
11:45	Working lunch
12:30 p.m.	How Are Safety and Efficacy Determined by FDA? *Dr. Juli Clifford, Division of Vaccines and Related Products Applications, Center for Biologics Evaluation and Research, FDA* *Dr. Karen Midthun, Director, Office of Vaccines Research and Review, Center for Biologics Evaluation and Research, FDA*
1:15	The Vaccine Adverse Events Reporting System (VAERS) *Dr. Gina Mootrey, VAERS Project Officer, National Immunization Program, CDC*
2:00	The Anthrax Vaccine Expert Committee (AVEC) *Dr. Vito Caserta, Health Resources and Services Administration, DHHS*
2:30	Adjourn Open Session

Meeting II
January 29–30, 2001

The Foundry Building
1055 Thomas Jefferson Street, NW
Washington, DC

Meeting Objectives

- Review several completed studies of anthrax vaccine safety and efficacy
- Evaluate knowledge of vaccine components
- Define needs for additional information gathering
- Plan future meetings

Agenda

Monday, January 29, 2001

12:00 p.m. Open Session
A review of some of the studies of the anthrax vaccine

12:00 The CDC Observational Study
Dr. Juli Clifford, Center for Biologics Evaluation and Research, FDA

12:30 Components of the Anthrax Vaccine Absorbed and Contrast with Merck Vaccine
Dr. Robert Myers, BioPort Corporation

1:00 Working lunch

1:30 Field Evaluation of a Human Anthrax Vaccine
Dr. Stanley Plotkin

2:00 Ft. Detrick Multi-Dose, Multi-Vaccine Safety Studies
LTC Phillip Pittman, U.S. Army Medical Research Institute of Infectious Diseases

2:30 Ft. Detrick Special Immunization Program
LTC Phillip Pittman

APPENDIX C 221

3:00	Ft. Bragg Booster Study *LTC Phillip Pittman*
3:30	Break
3:45	Reduced Dose/Route of Administration Pilot *LTC Phillip Pittman*
4:15	Surveillance of Adverse Effects of Anthrax Vaccine Adsorbed *Dr. Jeff Lange, U.S. Army Center for Health Promotion and Disease Prevention*
4:45	Adjourn Open Session

Tuesday, January 30, 2001

Open Session

8:00 a.m.	Breakfast
8:30	U.S Forces in Korea Survey *Dr. Ken Hoffman, Military and Veterans Health Coordinating Board* Vaccine Research Portfolio *LTC John Grabenstein, Anthrax Vaccine Immunization Program Agency*
9:30	Adjourn Open Session

Meeting III
April 17–18, 2001

The Cecil and Ida Green Building
2001 Wisconsin Avenue, NW
Washington, DC

Meeting Objectives

- Review information about anthrax pathology and anthrax vaccine efficacy in animal models
- Review information about variations in anthrax strains and discuss implications for vaccine efficacy
- Gather additional information regarding anthrax vaccine safety and efficacy from public input

Agenda

Tuesday April 17, 2001

Open Session

10:00 a.m.   Anthrax Pathology in Humans
Dr. David Walker, Professor and Chairman, Department of Pathology, University of Texas Medical Branch at Galveston

Discussion

10:45   The Pathology of Experimental Anthrax in Rabbits and Nonhuman Primates
LTC Gary Zaucha, Walter Reed Army Institute of Research

Discussion

11:30   Animal Models for Anthrax Vaccine Efficacy
Dr. Louise Pitt, U.S. Army Medical Research Institute of Infectious Diseases

Discussion

APPENDIX C 223

12:15 p.m. Working lunch

12:45 Group Discussion:
What Outstanding Questions Remain About Animal Models for Vaccine Efficacy?
Moderator, Dr. Dennis Kasper, Member, Committee to Assess the Safety and Efficacy of the Anthrax Vaccine

1:15 Genetic Diversity in *B. anthracis*
Dr. Paul Jackson, Environmental Molecular Biology Group, Los Alamos National Laboratory

Discussion

2:00 Break

2:15 Efficacy of AVA in Different Animal Models Against Challenge by *B. anthracis* Strains of Diverse Geographical Origin
COL Art Friedlander, U.S. Army Medical Research Institute of Infectious Diseases

Discussion

3:00 Group Discussion:
What Outstanding Questions Remain About Vaccine Efficacy Against Varying Anthrax Strains?

3:45 Adjourn Open Session

Joint Meeting of the Institute of Medicine Committee to Assess the Safety and Efficacy of the Anthrax Vaccine and the Institute of Medicine Committee to Review the CDC Anthrax Vaccine Safety and Efficacy Research Program

Wednesday, April 18, 2001

10:30 a.m. Open Session, Oral statements

Master Sergeant (ret) Thomas Starkweather

Mr. Sonnie Bates

Col. (ret) Redmond Handy, National Organization of Americans Battling Unnecessary Servicemember Endangerment (NO ABUSE)

Ms. Nancy Rugo

Capt. John Buck, M.D.

MAJ Jon Irelan

Capt. Jean Tanner

Technical Sergeant Jeffrey Moore

Discussion

12:30 p.m.   Adjourn

Meeting IV
July 10-11, 2001

The Foundry Building
1055 Thomas Jefferson Street, NW
Washington, DC

Meeting Objectives

- Review studies of the safety of the anthrax vaccine
- Gather information regarding manufacturing issues surrounding the anthrax vaccine

APPENDIX C

Agenda

Tuesday, July 10, 2001

10:15 a.m.   Open Session

Welcome and introductory remarks
Dr. Brian Strom, Chair, Committee to Assess the Safety and Efficacy of the Anthrax Vaccine

A review of additional studies of the anthrax vaccine

10:20   Tripler Army Medical Center Survey of AVA Safety
COL Glenn Wasserman, Tripler Army Medical Center

10:50   DoD-Wide Medical Surveillance for Potential Long-Term Adverse Events Associated with Anthrax Immunization
Dr. Paul Sato, Naval Health Research Center

11:20   Surveillance of Adverse Effects of Anthrax Vaccine Adsorbed
Dr. Jeff Lange, U.S. Army Center for Health Promotion and Preventive Medicine

12:30 p.m.   Working lunch

1:00   Lack of Effect of Anthrax Vaccination on Pregnancy, Birth, and Adverse Birth Outcome Among Women in Active Service with the U.S. Army
MAJ Andrew Wiesen, 3rd Infantry Division Surgeon

1:30   Ambulatory Medical Visits Among Anthrax Vaccinated and Unvaccinated Personnel After Return from Southwest Asia
Lt. Col. Paul Rehme, Air National Guard Readiness Center

2:00   Status of the Anthrax Vaccine Research Portfolio
LTC John Grabenstein, Anthrax Vaccine Immunization Program Agency

2:30   Adjourn Open Session

Closed Session

Wednesday, July 11, 2001

Open Session

8:30 a.m.   Welcome and introductory remarks
Dr. Brian Strom, Chair, Committee to Assess the Safety and Efficacy of the Anthrax Vaccine

Dr. Don Metzgar, Member, Committee to Assess the Safety and Efficacy of the Anthrax Vaccine

BioPort presentation responding to questions from IOM committee
Dr. Larry Winberry, Vice President, Operations
Dr. Lallan Giri, Vice President, Quality, Compliance, and Regulatory Affairs

Discussion

10:30   Break

10:45   Commentary from FDA
Mr. Mark Elengold, Deputy Director, Center for Biologics Evaluation and Research

Discussion

12:30 p.m.   Adjourn Open Session

Appendix D

Anthrax Vaccine Adsorbed Package Inserts

50483   Rev. 3/99

ANTHRAX VACCINE ADSORBED

DESCRIPTION

Anthrax Vaccine Adsorbed is a sterile product made from filtrates of microaerophilic cultures of an avirulent, nonencapsulated strain of *Bacillus anthracis* which elaborates the protective antigen during the growth period. The cultures are grown in a synthetic liquid medium and the final product is prepared from sterile filtered culture fluid. The potency of this product is confirmed according to the U.S. Food and Drug regulations (21 CFR 620.23): Additional Standards for Anthrax Vaccine Adsorbed. The final product contains no more than 2.4 mg aluminum hydroxide (equivalent to 0.83 mg aluminum) per 0.5 mL dose. Formaldehyde, in a final concentration not to exceed 0.02%, and benzethonium chloride, 0.0025%, are added as preservatives.

CLINICAL PHARMACOLOGY

Anthrax Vaccine Adsorbed is used in man to promote increased resistance to *Bacillus anthracis* by active immunization (1,2).

INDICATIONS AND USAGE

Immunization with Anthrax Vaccine Adsorbed is recommended for individuals who may come in contact with animal products such as hides, hair, or bones which come from anthrax endemic areas and may be contaminated with *Bacillus anthracis spores;* and for individuals engaged in diagnostic or investigational activities which may bring them into contact with *B. anthracis spores* (1,5). It is also recommended for high risk persons such as veterinarians and others handling potentially infected animals. Since the risk of exposure to anthrax infection in the general population is slight, routine immunization is not recommended.

If a person has not previously been immunized against anthrax, injection of this product following exposure to anthrax bacilli will not protect against infection.

CONTRAINDICATIONS

A history of a severe reaction to a previous dose of anthrax vaccine is a contraindication to immunization with this vaccine.

WARNINGS

1. Any acute respiratory disease or other active infection is generally considered to be adequate reason for deferring an injection.
2. Persons receiving cortico-steroid therapy or other agents which would tend to depress the immune response may not be adequately immunized with the dosage schedule recommended. If the therapy is short termed, immunization should be delayed. If the therapy is long termed, an extra dose of vaccine should be given a month or more after therapy is discontinued.

PRECAUTIONS

1. *General:* Epinephrine solution, 1:1000, should always be available for immediate use in case an anaphylactic reaction should occur, even though such reactions are rare.
2. *Carcinogenesis, Mutagenesis, Impairment of Fertility:* Studies have not been performed to ascertain whether Anthrax Vaccine Adsorbed has carcinogenic action, or any effect on fertility.
3. *Pregnancy:* PREGNANCY CATEGORY C. ANTHRAX VACCINE ADSORBED Animal reproduction studies have not been conducted with Anthrax Vaccine Adsorbed. It is also not known whether Anthrax Vaccine Adsorbed can cause fetal harm when administered to a pregnant woman or

can affect reproduction capacity. Anthrax Vaccine Adsorbed should be given to pregnant women only if clearly needed.

4. *Pediatric Use:* This antigen should be administered only to healthy men and women from 18 to 65 years of age because investigations to date have been conducted exclusively in that population.

ADVERSE REACTIONS

Local Reactions: Mild local reactions occur in approximately thirty per cent of recipients and consist of a small ring of erythema, 1-2 cm in diameter, plus slight local tenderness(1). This reaction usually occurs within 24 hours and begins to subside by 48 hours. Occasionally, the erythema increases to 3 to 5 cm in diameter. Local reactions tend to increase in severity by the 5th injection and then may decrease in severity with subsequent doses.

Moderate local reactions which occur in 4 per cent of recipients of a second injection are defined by an inflammatory reaction greater than 5 cm diameter.

These may be pruritic. Subcutaneous nodules may occur at the injection site and persist for several weeks in a few persons. A moderate local reaction can occur if the vaccine is given to anyone with a past history of anthrax infection.

More severe local reactions are less frequent and consist of extensive edema of the forearm in addition to the local inflammatory reaction. All local reactions have been reversible.

Systemic Reactions: Systemic reactions which occur in fewer than 0.2 per cent of recipients have been characterized by malaise and lassitude. Chills and fever have been reported in only a few cases. In such instances, immunization should be discontinued.

All adverse reactions thought by a physician possibly to have been related to this product should be directed to the BioPort Corporation (517) 327-1500 during regular working hours and (517) 327-7200 during off hours.

DOSAGE AND ADMINISTRATION

Dosage

Primary immunization consists of three subcutaneous injections, 0.5 mL each, given 2 weeks apart followed by three additional subcutaneous injections, 0.5 mL each, given at 6, 12 and 18 months(1).

If immunity is to be maintained, subsequent booster injections of 0.5 mL of anthrax vaccine at one year intervals are recommended.

Administration

1. Use a separate sterile needle and syringe for each patient to avoid transmission of viral hepatitis and other infectious agents.
2. Shake the bottle thoroughly to ensure that the suspension is homogeneous during withdrawal. The rubber stopper should be treated with an appropriate disinfectant and allowed to dry before inserting the needle.
3. This preparation must be give subcutaneously after cleansing the overlying skin with an antiseptic.
4. Follow the usual precautions to avoid intravenous injection.
5. After withdrawing the needle, the injection site may be massaged briefly and gently to promote dispersal of the vaccine.
6. The same site should not be used for more than one injection of this vaccine.
7. Do not syringe-mix with any other product.
8. Parenteral drug products should be inspected visually for particulate matter and discoloration prior to administration, whenever solution and container permit.

HOW SUPPLIED

Anthrax Vaccine Adsorbed is supplied in 5 mL vials containing 10 doses each.

STORAGE

THIS PRODUCT SHOULD BE STORED AT AT 2 TO 8 degrees C (35.6 to 46.4 degrees F). Do not freeze. Do not use after the expiration date given on the package.

REFERENCES

1. Brachman, P. S., et. al. Field Evaluation of a Human Anthrax Vaccine. Amer. J. Pub. Health, 52:632-645 (1962).
2. Editorial: Vaccine Against Antrax. Brit. Med, J., 2:717-718(1965).
3. Advisory Committee for Immunization Practices. Adult Immunization, Morbidity and Mortality Report, 33(15):33-34, 1984.
4. Committee on Immunization, *Guide for Adult Immunization, 1985,* Amer. Col. Physicians, Philadelphia, PA (1985).
5. Report of Committee on Infectious Diseases, 19th Edition, Amer. Acad. Pediatrics, Evanston, IL (1982).

These recommendations are prepared by the BioPort Corporation only for the guidance of the physician. They do not replace the experience and judgement of the physician, who should be familiar with the recent pertinent medical literature before administering any biologic product.

Manufactured by
BIOPORT CORPORATION Lansing, Michigan 48909
U.S. License No. 1260

All rights reserved © 1999 BioPort Corporation

31 JAN 2002

ANTHRAX VACCINE ADSORBED (BIOTHRAX™)

DESCRIPTION
Anthrax Vaccine Adsorbed, (BioThrax™) is a sterile, milky-white suspension (when mixed) made from cell-free filtrates of microaerophilic cultures of an avirulent, nonencapsulated strain of *Bacillus anthracis*. The production cultures are grown in a chemically defined protein-free medium consisting of a mixture of amino acids, vitamins, inorganic salts and sugars. The final product, prepared from the sterile filtrate culture fluid contains proteins, including the 83kDa protective antigen protein, released during the growth period. The final product contains no dead or live bacteria. The final product is formulated to contain 1.2 mg/mL aluminum, added as aluminum hydroxide in 0.85% sodium chloride. The product is formulated to contain 25 μg/mL benzethonium chloride and 100 μg/mL formaldehyde, added as preservatives.

CLINICAL PHARMACOLOGY
Epidemiology
Anthrax occurs globally and is most common in agricultural regions with inadequate control programs for anthrax in livestock. Anthrax is a zoonotic disease caused by the Gram-positive, spore-forming bacterium *Bacillus anthracis*. The spore form of *Bacillus anthracis* is the predominant phase of the bacterium in the environment and it is largely through the uptake of spores that anthrax disease is contracted. Spore forms are markedly resistant to heat, cold, pH, desiccation, chemicals and irradiation. Following germination at the site of infection, the bacilli can also enter the blood and lead to septicemia. Antibiotics are effective against the germinated form of *Bacillus anthracis*, but are not effective against the spore form of the organism.

The disease occurs most commonly in wild and domestic animals, primarily cattle, sheep, goats and other herbivores. In humans, anthrax disease can result from contact with animal hides, leather or hair products from contaminated animals, or from other exposures to *Bacillus anthracis* spores. It occurs in three forms depending upon the route of infection: cutaneous anthrax, gastrointestinal anthrax and inhalation anthrax.

Cutaneous anthrax is the most commonly reported form in humans (> 95% of all anthrax cases). It can occur when the bacterium enters a cut or abrasion on the skin, such as when handling contaminated meat, wool, hides, leather or hair products from infected animals or other contaminated materials. The symptoms of cutaneous anthrax begin with an itchy reddish-brown papule on exposed skin surfaces and may appear approximately 1-12 days after contact. The lesion soon develops a small vesicle. Secondary vesicles are sometimes seen. Later the vesicle ruptures and leaves a painless ulcer that typically develops a blackened eschar with surrounding swollen tissue. There are often associated systemic symptoms such as swollen glands, fever, myalgia, malaise, vomiting and headache. The case fatality rate for cutaneous anthrax is estimated to be 20% without antibiotic treatment.

Gastrointestinal anthrax usually begins 1-7 days after ingestion of meat contaminated with anthrax spores. There is acute inflammation of the intestinal tract with nausea, loss of appetite, vomiting and fever followed by abdominal pain, vomiting of blood and bloody diarrhea. There can also be involvement of the pharynx with sore throat, dysphagia, fever, lesions at the base of the tongue or tonsils and regional lymphadenopathy. The case fatality rate is unknown but estimated to be 25% to 60%.

Inhalation (pulmonary) anthrax has been reported to occur from 1-43 days after exposure to aerosolized spores.[1] Studies in rhesus monkeys indicate that a small number of inhaled spores may remain viable for at least 100 days following exposure.[2] However, information on how long spores remain viable in the lungs of humans is unavailable and the incubation period for inhalation anthrax is unknown. Initial symptoms are non-specific and may include sore throat, mild fever, myalgia, coughing and chest discomfort lasting up to a few days. The second stage develops abruptly with

31 JAN 2002

findings such as sudden onset of fever, acute respiratory distress with pulmonary edema and pleural effusion followed by cyanosis, shock and coma. Meningitis is common. The fatality rate for inhalation anthrax in the U.S. is estimated to be approximately 45% to 90%. From 1900 to October 2001, there were 18 identified cases of inhalation anthrax in the U.S., the latest of which was reported in 1976, with an 89% (16/18) mortality rate. Most of these exposures occurred in industrial settings, i.e., textile mills.[3] From October 4, 2001, to December 5, 2001, a total of 11 cases of inhalation anthrax linked to intentional dissemination of *Bacillus anthracis* spores were identified in the U.S. Five of these cases were fatal.[4]

Mechanism of Action
Virulence components of *Bacillus anthracis* include an antiphagocytic polypeptide capsule and three proteins known as protective antigen (PA), lethal factor (LF) and edema factor (EF). Individually these proteins are not cytotoxic but the combination of PA with LF or EF results in the formation of the cytotoxic lethal toxin and edema toxin, respectively. Although an immune correlate of protection is unknown, antibodies raised against PA may contribute to protection by neutralizing the activities of these toxins.[5] The contribution of *Bacillus anthracis* proteins other than PA, that may be present in BioThrax, to the protection against anthrax has not been determined.

CLINICAL STUDIES
A controlled field study using an earlier version of a protective antigen–based anthrax vaccine, developed in the 1950's, that consisted of an aluminum potassium sulfate-precipitated cell free filtrate from an aerobic culture, was conducted from 1955-1959. This study included 1,249 workers [379 received anthrax vaccine, 414 received placebo, 116 received incomplete inoculations (with either vaccine or placebo) and 340 were in the observational group (no treatment)] in four mills in the northeastern United States that processed imported animal hides.[6] During the trial, 26 cases of anthrax were reported across the four mills - five inhalation and 21 cutaneous. Prior to vaccination, the yearly average number of human anthrax cases was 1.2 cases per 100 employees in these mills. Of the five inhalation cases (four of which were fatal), two received placebo and three were in the observational group. Of the 21 cutaneous cases, 15 received placebo, three were in the observational group, and three received anthrax vaccine. Of those three cases in the vaccine group, one case occurred just prior to administration of the scheduled third dose, one case occurred 13 months after an individual received the third of the scheduled 6 doses (but no subsequent doses), and one case occurred prior to receiving the scheduled fourth dose of vaccine. In a comparison of anthrax cases between the placebo and vaccine groups, including only those who were completely vaccinated, the calculated vaccine efficacy level against all reported cases of anthrax combined was 92.5% (lower 95% CI = 65%).

From 1962 to 1974, based on information reported to Centers for Disease Control and Prevention (CDC), 27 cases of anthrax occurred in mill workers or those living near mills in the United States. Of those, 24 cases occurred in unvaccinated individuals, one case occurred after the person had been given one dose of anthrax vaccine and two cases occurred after individuals had been given two doses of anthrax vaccine. No documented cases of anthrax were reported for individuals who had received the recommended six doses of anthrax vaccine. These individuals received either an earlier version of a protective antigen-based anthrax vaccine or BioThrax.

In an open-label safety study conducted by the CDC, BioThrax was administered in 0.5 mL doses according to a 0, 2, 4 week initial dose schedule followed by additional doses at 6, 12 and 18 months to complete the 6 dose vaccination series. Annual boosters were administered thereafter. In this study, 15,907 doses of BioThrax were administered to approximately 7,000 textile employees, laboratory workers and other at risk individuals and the incidence rates of local and systemic adverse reactions were recorded. (See ADVERSE REACTIONS*)*

A randomized clinical study was conducted by the U.S. Army Medical Research Institute of Infectious Diseases (USAMRIID) from 1996-1999 in 173 volunteers to evaluate changes to the vaccination schedule and route of vaccine administration. Of those, 28 were enrolled into the study arm to receive the licensed schedule (initial injections at 0, 2 and 4 weeks followed by additional doses at 6, 12 and 18 months) and were subsequently monitored for the occurrence of local and systemic adverse events. (See ADVERSE REACTIONS)

INDICATIONS AND USAGE
BioThrax is indicated for the active immunization against *Bacillus anthracis* of individuals between 18 and 65 years of age who come in contact with animal products such as hides, hair or bones that come from anthrax endemic areas, and that may be contaminated with *Bacillus anthracis* spores. BioThrax is also indicated for individuals at high risk of exposure to *Bacillus anthracis* spores such as veterinarians, laboratory workers and others whose occupation may involve handling potentially infected animals or other contaminated materials.

Since the risk of anthrax infection in the general population is low, routine immunization is not recommended.

The safety and efficacy of BioThrax in a post-exposure setting has not been established.

CONTRAINDICATIONS
The use of BioThrax is contraindicated in subjects with a history of anaphylactic or anaphylactic-like reaction following a previous dose of BioThrax, or any of the vaccine components.

WARNINGS
Preliminary results of a recent unpublished retrospective study of infants born to women in the U.S. military service worldwide in 1998 and 1999 suggest that the vaccine may be linked with an increase in the number of birth defects when given during pregnancy (unpublished data, Department of Defense). Although these data are unconfirmed, pregnant women should not be vaccinated against anthrax unless the potential benefits of vaccination have been determined to outweigh the potential risk to the fetus.

Animal reproduction studies have not been conducted with BioThrax.

PRECAUTIONS
Before administration, the patient's medical immunization history should be reviewed for possible vaccine sensitivities and/or previous vaccination-related adverse events, in order to determine the existence of any contraindications to immunization.

Pregnant women should not be vaccinated against anthrax unless the potential benefits of vaccination clearly outweigh the potential risks to the fetus.

BioThrax should not be administered to individuals with a history of Guillain-Barré Syndrome (GBS) unless there is a clear benefit that outweighs the potential risk of a recurrence.

History of anthrax disease may increase the potential for severe local adverse reactions.

Patients with impaired immune responsiveness due to congenital or acquired immunodeficiency, or immunosuppressive therapy may not be adequately immunized following administration of BioThrax. Vaccination during chemotherapy, high dose corticosteroid therapy of greater than 2-week duration, or radiation therapy may result in a suboptimal response. Deferral of vaccination for 3 months after completion of such therapy may be considered.[7]

The administration of BioThrax to persons with concurrent moderate or severe illness should be postponed until recovery. Vaccination is not contraindicated in subjects with mild illnesses with or without low-grade fever.[7]

31 JAN 2002

This product should be administered with caution to patients with a possible history of latex sensitivity since the vial stopper contains dry natural rubber.

Epinephrine solution, 1:1000, should always be available for immediate use in case an anaphylactic reaction should occur.

Pregnancy
PREGNANCY CATEGORY D.
See Warnings.

Nursing Mothers
It is not known whether exposure of the mother to BioThrax poses a risk of harm to the breast-feeding child. However, administration of non-live vaccines (e.g., anthrax vaccine) during breast-feeding is not medically contraindicated.[7]

Pediatric Use
Safety and effectiveness in pediatric patients have not been established.

Geriatric Use
No data regarding the safety of BioThrax are available for persons aged > 65 years.

ADVERSE REACTIONS

Pre Licensure
Local Reactions- In an open-label safety study, 15,907 doses of BioThrax were administered to approximately 7,000 textile employees, laboratory workers and other at risk individuals *(See Clinical Studies)*. Over the course of the 5-year study, there were 24 reports (0.15% of doses administered) of severe local reactions (defined as edema or induration measuring greater than 120 mm in diameter or accompanied by marked limitation of arm motion or marked axillary node tenderness). There were 150 reports (0.94% of doses administered) of moderate local reactions (edema or induration greater than 30 mm but less than 120 mm in diameter) and 1373 reports (8.63% of doses administered) of mild local reactions (erythema only or induration measuring less than 30 mm in diameter).

Systemic Reactions- In the same open label study, four cases of systemic reactions were reported during a five-year reporting period (<0.06% of doses administered). These reactions, which were reported to have been transient, included fever, chills, nausea and general body aches.

31 JAN 2002

Post Licensure
Recently (1996-1999), an assessment of safety was conducted as part of a randomized clinical study conducted by the U.S. Army Medical Research Institute of Infectious Diseases (USAMRIID) *(See Clinical Studies)*. A total of 28 volunteers were enrolled to receive subcutaneous doses of BioThrax according to the licensed schedule. Each volunteer was observed for approximately 30 minutes after administration of AVA and scheduled for follow-up evaluations at 1-3 days, 1 week and 1 month after vaccination. Four volunteers reported seven acute adverse events within 30 minutes after the subcutaneous administration of BioThrax. These included erythema (3), headache (2), fever (1) and elevated temperature (1). Of these events, a single patient reported the simultaneous occurrence of headache, fever and elevated temperature (100.7°F).

Local Reactions- The most common local reactions reported after the first dose (n=28) in this study were tenderness (71%), erythema (43%), subcutaneous nodule (36%), induration (21%), warmth (11%) and local pruritus (7%). The most frequently reported local reactions after the second dose (n=28) were tenderness (61%), subcutaneous nodule (39%), erythema (32%), induration (18%), local pruritus (14%), warmth (11%) and arm motion limitation (7%). After the third dose (n=26), the most frequently reported local reactions were tenderness (58%), warmth (19%), local pruritus (19%), erythema (12%), arm motion limitation (12%), induration (8%), edema (8%) and subcutaneous nodule (4%). Local reactions were found to occur more often in women. No abscess or necrosis was observed at the injection site.

Systemic Reactions- All systemic adverse events reported in this study were transient in nature. The systemic reactions most frequently reported after the first dose (n=28) were headache (7%), respiratory difficulty (4%) and fever (4%). After the second dose (n=28), the most frequently reported systemic reactions were malaise (11%), myalgia (7%), fever (7%), headache (4%), anorexia (4%) and nausea or vomiting (4%). After the third dose (n=26), the most frequently reported systemic reactions were headache (4%), malaise (4%), myalgia (4%) and fever (4%). There was one report of delayed hypersensitivity reaction beginning with lesions 3 days after the first dose. The subject was reported to have diffuse hives by day 17, 3 days after the second dose, and had swollen hands, face and feet by day 18 and discomfort swallowing. The subject did not receive any subsequent scheduled doses.

Post Licensure Adverse Event Surveillance
Data regarding potential adverse events following anthrax vaccination are available from the Vaccine Adverse Event Reporting System (VAERS).[8] The report of an adverse event to VAERS is not proof that a vaccine caused the event. Because of the limitations of spontaneous reporting systems, determining causality for specific types of adverse events, with the exception of injection-site reactions, is often not possible using VAERS data alone. The following four paragraphs describe spontaneous reports of adverse events, without regard to causality.

From 1990 to October 2001, over 2 million doses of BioThrax have been administered in the United States. Through October 2001, VAERS received approximately 1850 spontaneous reports of adverse events. The most frequently reported adverse events were erythema, headache, arthralgia, fatigue, fever, peripheral swelling, pruritus, nausea, injection site edema, pain/tenderness and dizziness.

Approximately 6% of the reported events were listed as serious. Serious adverse events include those that result in death, hospitalization, permanent disability or are life-threatening. The serious adverse events most frequently reported were in the following body system categories: general disorders and administration site conditions, nervous system disorders, skin and subcutaneous tissue disorders, and musculoskeletal, connective tissue and bone disorders. Anaphylaxis and/or other generalized hypersensitivity reactions, as well as serious local reactions, were reported to occur occasionally following administration of BioThrax. None of these hypersensitivity reactions have been fatal.

Other infrequently reported serious adverse events that have occurred in persons who have received BioThrax have included: cellulitis, cysts, pemphigus vulgaris, endocarditis, sepsis, angioedema and

APPENDIX D

31 JAN 2002

other hypersensitivity reactions, asthma, aplastic anemia, neutropenia, idiopathic thrombocytopenia purpura, lymphoma, leukemia, collagen vascular disease, systemic lupus erythematosus, multiple sclerosis, polyarteritis nodosa, inflammatory arthritis, transverse myelitis, Guillain-Barré Syndrome, immune deficiency, seizure, mental status changes, psychiatric disorders, tremors, cerebrovascular accident (CVA), facial palsy, hearing and visual disorders, aseptic meningitis, encephalitis, myocarditis, cardiomyopathy, atrial fibrillation, syncope, glomerulonephritis, renal failure, spontaneous abortion and liver abscess. Infrequent reports were also received of multisystem disorders defined as chronic symptoms involving at least two of the following three categories: fatigue, mood-cognition, musculoskeletal system.

Reports of fatalities included sudden cardiac arrest (2), myocardial infarction with polyarteritis nodosa (1), aplastic anemia (1), suicide (1) and central nervous system (CNS) lymphoma (1).

Post Licensure Survey Studies
In addition to the VAERS data, adverse events following anthrax vaccination have been assessed in survey studies conducted by the Department of Defense in the context of their anthrax vaccination program. These survey studies are subject to several methodological limitations, e.g., sample size, the limited ability to detect adverse events, observational bias, loss to follow-up, exemption of vaccine recipients with previous adverse events and the absence of unvaccinated control groups. Overall, the most reported events were localized, minor and self-limited and included muscle or joint aches, headache and fatigue. Across these studies, systemic reactions were reported in 5-35% of vaccine recipients and included reports of malaise, chills, rashes, headaches and low-grade fever. Women reported these symptoms more often than men.

Reporting Adverse Events
Adverse events following immunization with BioThrax should be reported to the Medical Affairs Division of BioPort Corporation (517) 327-1675 during regular working hours and (517) 327-7200 during off hours. Adverse events may also be reported to the U. S. Department of Health and Human Services (DHHS) Vaccine Adverse Event Reporting System. Report forms and reporting requirement information can be obtained from VAERS through a toll free number 1-800-822-7967.

DOSAGE AND ADMINISTRATION
Dosage
Immunization consists of three subcutaneous injections, 0.5 mL each, given 2 weeks apart followed by three additional subcutaneous injections, 0.5 mL each, given at 6, 12, and 18 months. Subsequent booster injections of 0.5 mL of BioThrax at one-year intervals are recommended.

Administration
Use a separate 5/8-inch, 25- to 27-gauge sterile needle and syringe for each patient to avoid transmission of viral hepatitis and other infectious agents. Use a different site for each sequential injection of this vaccine and do not mix with any other product in the syringe.
 1. Shake the bottle thoroughly to ensure that the suspension is homogeneous during withdrawal and visually inspect the product for particulate matter and discoloration. If the product appears discolored or has visible particulate matter, DISCARD THE VIAL.
 2. Wipe the rubber stopper with an alcohol swab and allow to dry before inserting the needle.
 3. Clean the area to be injected with an alcohol swab or other suitable antiseptic.
 4. Holding the needle at a 45° angle to the skin, inject the vaccine subcutaneously.
 5. DO NOT inject the product intravenously. Follow the usual precautions to ensure that you have not entered a vein before injecting the vaccine.
 6. After injecting, withdraw the needle and briefly and gently massage the injection site to promote dispersal of the vaccine.

HOW SUPPLIED/STORAGE
Anthrax Vaccine Adsorbed (BioThrax™) is supplied in 5 mL multidose vials.

THIS PRODUCT IS TO BE STORED AT 2°C TO 8°C (36 TO 46°F). Do not freeze. Do not use after the expiration date given on the package.

Nonclinical Toxicology
Carcinogenesis, Mutagenesis, Impairment of Fertility
Animal studies have not been performed to ascertain whether BioThrax has carcinogenic action, or any effect on fertility.

REFERENCES
1. Meselson, M., et al., 1994. The Sverdlosk anthrax outbreak of 1979. *Science* 266:1201-8.
2. Henderson, D.W., Peacock, S., Belton, F.C., 1956. Observations on the prophylaxis of experimental pulmonary anthrax in the monkey. *J. Hygiene*, 54:28-36.
3. Brachman, P.S., 1980. Inhalation Anthrax. *Ann. NY Acad. Science*, 353:83-93.
4. Update: Investigation of bioterrorism-related anthrax—Connecticut, 2001. *MMWR.* 2001; 50:1077-9.
5. Brachman, P.S., & A. M. Friedlander. 1999. Anthrax. In Vaccines, Third Edition, Plotkin & Orenstein (eds.), pp. 629-637.
6. Brachman, P.S., et al., 1962. Field Evaluation of a Human Anthrax Vaccine. *Amer. J. Public Health*, 52:632-645.
7. Centers for Disease Control and Prevention. General recommendations on immunization recommendations of the Advisory Committee on Immunization Practices (ACIP). *MMWR.* 1994; Vol. 43 (No. RR-1).
8. Chen, R.T., et al., 1994. The Vaccine Adverse Event Reporting System (VAERS). *Vaccine* 12(6): 542-550.

Revision: January 31, 2002

Rx Only---Federal (U.S.A.) law prohibits dispensing without a prescription.

Manufactured by
BIOPORT CORPORATION
Lansing, Michigan 48906
U.S. License No. 1260

50483-04

Appendix E

Vaccine Adverse Event Reporting System (VAERS) Form

APPENDIX E

VACCINE ADVERSE EVENT REPORTING SYSTEM

VAERS
24 Hour Toll Free Information 1-800-822-7967
P.O. Box 1100, Rockville, MD 20849-1100
PATIENT IDENTITY KEPT CONFIDENTIAL

For CDC/FDA Use Only
VAERS Number _____
Date Received _____

Patient Name: _____
Last   First   M.I.
Address _____
_____
_____
City   State   Zip
Telephone no. (___) _____

Vaccine administered by (Name): _____
Responsible Physician _____
Facility Name/Address _____
_____
_____
City   State   Zip
Telephone no. (___) _____

Form completed by (Name): _____
Relation to Patient   ☐ Vaccine Provider ☐ Patient/Parent
                      ☐ Manufacturer   ☐ Other
Address *(if different from patient or provider)*
_____
_____
City   State   Zip
Telephone no. (___) _____

| 1. State | 2. County where administered | 3. Date of birth mm/dd/yy | 4. Patient age | 5. Sex ☐M ☐F | 6. Date form completed mm/dd/yy |

7. Describe adverse events(s) (symptoms, signs, time course) and treatment, if any

8. Check all appropriate:
☐ Patient died   (date ___/___/___ mm/dd/yy)
☐ Life threatening illness
☐ Required emergency room/doctor visit
☐ Required hospitalization (_____days)
☐ Resulted in prolongation of hospitalization
☐ Resulted in permanent disability
☐ None of the above

9. Patient recovered ☐ YES ☐ NO ☐ UNKNOWN

12. Relevant diagnostic tests/laboratory data

| 10. Date of vaccination mm/dd/yy Time ___ AM/PM | 11. Adverse event onset mm/dd/yy Time ___ AM/PM |

13. Enter all vaccines given on date listed in no. 10

Vaccine (type)	Manufacturer	Lot number	Route/Site	No. Previous Doses
a.				
b.				
c.				
d.				

14. Any other vaccinations within 4 weeks prior to the date listed in no. 10

Vaccine (type)	Manufacturer	Lot number	Route/Site	No. Previous doses	Date given
a.					
b.					

15. Vaccinated at:
☐ Private doctor's office/hospital ☐ Military clinic/hospital
☐ Public health clinic/hospital   ☐ Other/unknown

16. Vaccine purchased with:
☐ Private funds ☐ Military funds
☐ Public funds   ☐ Other/unknown

17. Other medications

18. Illness at time of vaccination (specify)

19. Pre-existing physician-diagnosed allergies, birth defects, medial conditions(specify)

20. Have you reported this adverse event previously?
☐ No
☐ To doctor
☐ To health department
☐ To manufacturer

Only for children 5 and under
22. Birth weight ___ lb. ___ oz.
23. No. of brother and sisters

21. Adverse event following prior vaccination (check all applicable, specify)

	Adverse Event	Onset Age	Type Vaccine	Dose no. in series
☐ In patient				
☐ In brother or sister				

Only for reports submitted by manufacturer/Immunization project
24. Mfr./imm. proj. report no.
25. Date received by mfr./imm.proj.
26. 15 day report? ☐ Yes ☐ No
27. Report type ☐ Initial ☐ Follow-Up

Health care providers and manufacturers are required by law (42 USC 300aa-25) to report reactions to vaccines listed in the Table of Reportable Events Following Immunization Reports for reactions to other vaccines are voluntary except when required as a condition of immunization grant awards.

Form VAERS-1(FDA)

"Fold in thirds, tape & mail - DO NOT STAPLE FORM"

NO POSTAGE
NECESSARY
IF MAILED
IN THE
UNITED STATES
OR APO/FPO

BUSINESS REPLY MAIL
FIRST-CLASS MAIL   PERMIT NO. 1895   ROCKVILLE, MD
POSTAGE WILL BE PAID BY ADDRESSEE

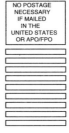

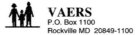 **VAERS**
P.O. Box 1100
Rockville MD 20849-1100

DIRECTIONS FOR COMPLETING FORM
(Additional pages may be attached if more space is needed)

GENERAL

Use a separate form for each patient. Complete the form to the best of your abilities. Items 3, 4, 7, 8, 10, 11, and 13 are considered essential and should be completed whenever possible. Parents/Guardians may need to consult the facility where the vaccine was administered for some of the information (such as manufacturer, lot number or laboratory data.)
Refer to the Reportable Events Table (RET) for events mandated for reporting by law. Reporting for other serious events felt to be related but not on the RET is encouraged.
Health care providers other than the vaccine administrator (VA) treating a patient for a suspected adverse event should notify the VA and provide the information about the adverse event to allow the VA to complete the form to meet the VA's legal responsibility. These data will be used to increase understanding of adverse events following vaccination and will become part of CDC Privacy Act System 09-20-0136, "Epidemiologic Studies and Surveillance of Disease Problems". Information identifying the person who received the vaccine or that person's legal representative will not be made available to the public, but may be available to the vaccinee or legal representative.
Postage will be paid by addressee. Forms may be photocopied (must be front & back on same sheet).

SPECIFIC INSTRUCTIONS

Form Completed By: To be used by parents/guardians, vaccine manufacturers/distributors, vaccine administrators, and/or the person completing the form on behalf of the patient or the health professional who administered the vaccine.

Item 7: Describe the suspected adverse event. Such things as temperature, local and general signs and symptoms, time course, duration of symptoms diagnosis, treatment and recovery should be noted.
Item 9: Check "YES" if the patient's health condition is the same as it was prior to the vaccine, "NO" if the patient has not returned to the pre-vaccination state of health, or "UNKNOWN" if the patient's condition is not known.
Item 10: Give dates and times as specifically as you can remember. If you do not know the exact time, please
Item 11: indicate "AM" or "PM" when possible if this information is known. If more than one adverse event, give the onset date and time for the most serious event.
Item 12: Include "negative" or "normal" results of any relevant tests performed as well as abnormal findings.
Item 13: List ONLY those vaccines given on the day listed in Item 10.
Item 14: List any other vaccines that the patient received within 4 weeks prior to the date listed in Item 10.
Item 16: This section refers to how the person who gave the vaccine purchased it, not to the patient's insurance.
Item 17: List any prescription or non-prescription medications the patient was taking when the vaccine(s) was given.
Item 18: List any short term illnesses the patient had on the date the vaccine(s) was given (i.e., cold, flu, ear infection).
Item 19: List any pre-existing physician-diagnosed allergies, birth defects, medical conditions (including developmental and/or neurologic disorders) for the patient.
Item 21: List any suspected adverse events the patient, or the patient's brothers or sisters, may have had to previous vaccinations. If more than one brother or sister, or if the patient has reacted to more than one prior vaccine, use additional pages to explain completely. For the onset age of a patient, provide the age in months if less than two years old.
Item 26: This space is for manufacturers' use only.

Appendix F

Anthrax Vaccine Expert Committee (AVEC) Case Assessment Form

AVEC Case Assessment Form

VAERS Number | **Date AVEC Initial Review** | **Date of Most Recent AVEC Review** | **Insufficient Data**

Other Vaccinations Administered | **Concomitant or Preceding Medical Condition** | **Concomitant or Preceding Drug Therapy** | **Contributing Factors** | **Type of Event(s)** | **Seen by HCP**

Event(s) for Reporting

Event for reporting

Dose | **Lot** | **Category Code** | **Possible New Entity** | **SAE OMIAE** | **Onset** | **Duration** | **Recovery Status** | **Patient Had Similar Symptom(s) to Previous Anthrax Vaccination**

Positive Rechallenge | **Patient Had Similar Symptom(s) to Prior Vaccination(s)** (excluding anthrax) | **Patient Had Similar Symptom(s) in Past NOT Following Vaccination** | **Vaccine-Event Onset Interval Compatibility With Event** | **Causal Relation or Association** | **Due To Physical Act of Vaccination**

Additional Info Needed

Comments

Re-review Comments

Form Printed Friday, January 18, 2002

Appendix G
DMSS Analyses Requested by the IOM Committee to Assess the Safety and Efficacy of the Anthrax Vaccine

TABLE G-1 Among Service Members Receiving at Least One Dose of AVA Hospitalization Diagnoses with Rate Ratios Above 1.0, U.S. Armed Forces, Active Duty, 1998 to 2000

ICD-9-CM Code(s)	Description	Anthrax Immunization Status				Adjusted Rate Ratio	95% Confidence Intervals	
		Post		Pre				
		Number	Rate per 100,000	Number	Rate per 100,000			
193	Malignant neoplasm of thyroid gland	41	5.6	9	1.9	2.40	1.05	5.49
233	Carcinoma in situ of breast and genitourinary system	19	2.6	5	1.0	5.14	1.81	14.57
250	Diabetes mellitus	67	9.1	8	1.7	3.46	1.51	7.90
296	Affective psychoses	600	81.3	120	25.1	2.15	1.71	2.71
298	Other nonorganic psychoses	69	9.3	14	2.9	2.50	1.29	4.83
309	Adjustment reaction	1,219	165.1	403	84.3	1.38	1.20	1.59
311	Depressive disorder, not elsewhere classified	167	22.6	46	9.6	1.79	1.21	2.66
374	Other disorders of eyelids	16	2.2	7	1.5	2.71	1.05	7.00
550	Inguinal hernia	293	39.7	172	36.0	1.31	1.04	1.65
569	Other disorders of intestine	34	4.6	6	1.3	2.94	1.23	7.07
724	Other and unspecified disorders of back	108	14.6	38	7.9	1.51	1.04	2.20
726	Peripheral enthesopathies and allied syndromes	213	28.8	97	20.3	1.29	1.01	1.64
732	Osteochondropathies	38	5.1	11	2.3	2.03	1.03	3.98
808	Fracture of pelvis	53	7.2	16	3.3	1.81	1.03	3.20
823	Fracture of tibia and fibula	169	22.9	60	12.5	1.63	1.14	2.32

TABLE G-2 Among Service Members Receiving at Least One Dose of AVA, Hospitalization Diagnoses with Rate Ratios Above 1.0, by Number of Days after Immunization, U.S. Armed Forces, Active Duty, 1998 to 2000

ICD-9-CM Code(s)	Description	Anthrax Immunization Status							Comparison*					
		Pre		0–45 days		>45 days		0–45 / Pre			>45 / Pre		
		Number	Rate per 100,000	Number	Rate per 100,000	Number	Rate per 100,000	Adjusted Rate Ratio	95% CI		Adjusted Rate Ratio	95% CI	
193	Malignant neoplasm of thyroid gland	9	1.88	10	6.04	31	5.41	2.88	1.12	7.37	2.16	0.90	5.17
220	Benign neoplasm of ovary	9	1.88	8	4.83	12	2.10	2.61	1.01	6.77	1.13	0.48	2.68
233	Carcinoma in situ of breast and genitourinary system	5	1.05	5	3.02	14	2.44	4.12	1.17	14.49	5.85	1.95	17.58
250	Diabetes mellitus	8	1.67	13	7.85	54	9.43	3.49	1.39	8.79	3.44	1.47	8.06
296	Affective psychoses	120	25.10	102	61.56	498	86.96	1.84	1.39	2.43	2.31	1.82	2.94
298	Other nonorganic psychoses	14	2.93	9	5.43	60	10.48	1.52	0.64	3.62	3.08	1.55	6.13
304	Drug dependence	6	1.25	2	1.21	33	5.76	.	.	.	3.06	1.08	8.66
309	Adjustment reaction	403	84.29	258	155.72	961	167.80	1.37	1.16	1.62	1.38	1.19	1.61
311	Depressive disorder, not elsewhere classified	46	9.62	35	21.12	132	23.05	1.78	1.11	2.84	1.80	1.19	2.72
312	Disturbance of conduct, not elsewhere classified	6	1.25	0	0.00	12	2.10	.	.	.	1.41	1.41	1.41
414	Other forms of chronic ischemic heart disease	18	3.76	20	12.07	81	14.14	2.15	1.09	4.23	1.65	0.89	3.07
429	Ill-defined descriptions and complications of heart disease	6	1.25	0	0.00	12	2.10	.	.	.	1.32	1.32	1.32
451	Phlebitis and thrombophlebitis	5	1.05	0	0.00	12	2.10	.	.	.	1.58	1.58	1.58
470	Deviated nasal septum	45	9.41	23	13.88	90	15.72	1.19	0.72	1.97	1.47	1.02	2.11
493	Asthma	41	8.58	30	18.11	64	11.18	1.83	1.14	2.93	1.10	0.74	1.64
541	Appendicitis, unqualified	47	9.83	19	11.47	77	13.45	1.15	0.68	1.97	1.46	1.01	2.11
550	Inguinal hernia	172	35.98	76	45.87	217	37.89	1.24	0.93	1.65	1.36	1.05	1.76
569	Other disorders of intestine	6	1.25	10	6.04	24	4.19	4.16	1.51	11.49	2.61	1.06	6.44
598	Urethral stricture	22	5.18	8	5.38	51	9.89	0.96	0.43	2.16	1.66	1.00	2.75
622	Noninflammatory disorders of cervix	15	28.20	22	129.54	48	84.26	2.64	1.30	5.35	1.55	0.78	3.09
724	Other and unspecified disorders of back	38	7.95	19	11.47	89	15.54	1.25	0.72	2.18	1.59	1.08	2.33
733	Other disorders of bone and cartilage	95	19.87	45	27.16	194	33.87	1.12	0.77	1.62	1.45	1.06	1.98
735	Acquired deformities of toe	34	7.11	20	12.07	83	14.49	1.15	0.66	2.01	1.58	1.06	2.37
808	Fracture of pelvis	16	3.35	11	6.64	42	7.33	1.66	0.77	3.60	1.86	1.04	3.34
823	Fracture of tibia and fibula	60	12.55	36	21.73	133	23.22	1.53	0.99	2.37	1.68	1.15	2.46
865	Injury to spleen	9	1.88	10	6.04	19	3.32	2.83	1.15	6.99	1.61	0.72	3.58
999	Complications of medical care, not elsewhere classified	7	1.46	5	3.02	5	0.87	3.70	1.05	13.04	1.25	0.30	5.11

TABLE G-3 Among Service Members Receiving at Least One Dose of AVA, Hospitalization Diagnoses with Rate Ratios Above 1.0, by Number of Doses After Immunization, U.S. Armed Forces, Active Duty, 1998 to 2000

ICD-9-CM	Description	Anthrax Immunization Status							Comparison			
		Pre		1 to 3 doses		4 or more doses		1 to 3 doses/Pre		4 or more/Pre	
		Number	Rate/100,000	Number	Rate/100,000	Number	Rate/100,000	Adjusted Rate ratio	95%CI	Adjusted Rate ratio	95%CI
193	Malignant neoplasm of thyroid gland	9	1.88	12	6.51	29	5.23	2.55	0.94-6.94	2.35	1.01-5.48
225	Benign neoplasm of brain and other parts of nervous system	6	1.25	8	4.34	6	1.08	2.99	1.02-8.77	0.70	0.22-2.19
250	Diabetes mellitus	8	1.67	24	13.02	43	7.76	4.98	2.02-12.25	3.05	1.31-7.09
296	Affective psychoses	120	25.10	229	124.27	371	66.95	3.65	2.81-4.74	1.79	1.42-2.27
298	Other nonorganic psychoses	14	2.93	26	14.11	43	7.76	4.08	1.92-8.68	2.11	1.07-4.18
300	Neurotic disorders	69	14.43	70	37.99	101	18.23	2.20	1.46-3.30	0.92	0.64-1.32
301	Personality disorders	64	13.39	115	62.41	81	14.62	1.95	1.32-2.87	0.69	0.46-1.02
304	Drug dependence	6	1.25	13	7.05	22	3.97	4.20	1.37-12.91	1.81	0.64-5.07
309	Adjustment reaction	403	84.29	460	249.63	759	136.98	2.28	1.94-2.69	1.16	1.00-1.34
311	Depressive disorder, not elsewhere classified	46	9.62	49	26.59	118	21.30	2.60	1.62-4.20	1.63	1.09-2.44
346	Migraine	36	7.53	30	16.28	46	8.30	1.82	1.12-2.98	0.90	0.58-1.40

348	Other conditions of brain	7	1.46	9	4.88	8	1.44	2.80	1.03-7.63	0.78	0.28-2.19
410	Acute myocardial infarction	22	4.60	24	13.02	44	7.94	2.60	1.42-4.75	1.15	0.69-1.94
470	Deviated nasal septum	45	9.41	18	9.77	95	17.14	1.15	0.65-2.00	1.47	1.02-2.10
493	Asthma	41	8.58	36	19.54	58	10.47	2.18	1.37-3.47	1.00	0.67-1.51
550	Inguinal hernia	172	35.98	55	29.85	238	42.95	1.24	0.88-1.75	1.32	1.04-1.68
555	Regional enteritis	5	1.05	19	10.31	20	3.61	4.90	1.55-15.44	1.96	0.65-5.95
569	Other disorders of intestine	6	1.25	6	3.26	28	5.05	2.05	0.66-6.41	3.24	1.33-7.89
724	Other and unspecified disorders of back	38	7.95	26	14.11	82	14.80	1.78	1.06-2.98	1.45	0.98-2.13
726	Peripheral enthesopathies and allied syndromes	97	20.29	57	30.93	156	28.15	1.49	1.07-2.09	1.04	0.80-1.34
732	Osteochondropathies	11	2.30	6	3.26	32	5.78	1.50	0.55-4.12	2.17	1.09-4.32
733	Other disorders of bone and cartilage	95	19.87	68	36.90	171	30.86	1.77	1.22-2.56	1.23	0.91-1.66
735	Acquired deformities of toe	34	7.11	12	6.51	91	16.42	0.93	0.48-1.82	1.60	1.07-2.39
808	Fracture of pelvis	16	3.35	15	8.14	38	6.86	2.47	1.20-5.09	1.64	0.91-2.98
813	Fracture of radius and ulna	102	21.33	54	29.30	114	20.57	1.62	1.10-2.37	1.13	0.83-1.54
823	Fracture of tibia and fibula	60	12.55	50	27.13	119	21.48	1.93	1.24-3.01	1.55	1.07-2.23
844	Sprains and strains of knee and leg	113	23.64	64	34.73	167	30.14	1.67	1.22-2.29	1.10	0.86-1.39
851	Cerebral laceration and contusion	8	1.67	2	1.09	22	3.97	-	-	2.43	1.08-5.47
891	Open wound of knee, leg [except thigh], and ankle	18	3.76	18	9.77	28	5.05	2.10	1.08-4.11	1.26	0.70-2.29
998	Other complications of procedures, not elsewhere classified	157	32.84	112	60.78	250	45.12	1.51	1.13-2.02	1.11	0.87-1.41

TABLE G-4 Among all Service Members, Hospitalization Diagnoses with Rate Ratios Above 1.0, U.S. Armed Forces, Active Duty, 1998 to 2000

ICD-9-CM Code(s)	Description	Anthrax Immunization Status				Adjusted Rate Ratio	95% Confidence Intervals	
		Pre		Never				
		Number	Rate per 100,000	Number	Rate per 100,000			
084	Malaria	18	3.8	62	2.1	1.76	1.04	2.99
695	Erythematous conditions	9	1.9	22	0.8	2.74	1.25	6.00
913	Superficial injury of elbow, forearm, and wrist	10	2.1	17	0.6	3.37	1.53	7.45
986	Toxic effect of carbon monoxide	8	1.7	8	0.3	7.49	2.74	20.46
993	Effects of air pressure	11	2.3	46	1.6	2.05	1.01	4.17

Appendix H
An Assessment of the Safety of the Anthrax Vaccine: A Letter Report

An Assessment of the Safety of the Anthrax Vaccine

A Letter Report

Committee on Health Effects Associated with
Exposures During the Gulf War

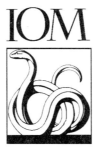

INSTITUTE OF MEDICINE
Washington, D.C.

An Assessment of the Safety of the Anthrax Vaccine

A Letter Report

March 30, 2000

Major General Randall L. West, USMC
Special Advisor for Biological Defense Affairs
Under Secretary of Defense for Personnel and Readiness
Department of Defense
4000 Defense Pentagon
Washington, DC 20301-4000

Dear General West:

In February of this year, the Department of Defense (DoD) requested that the Institute of Medicine (IOM) provide a report on the safety and efficacy of the anthrax vaccine that could be used to answer questions raised by Congress. The IOM has agreed to undertake this comprehensive study, which will require approximately 24 months to complete. The questions include the types and severity of adverse reactions, including gender differences; long-term health implications; efficacy of the vaccine against inhalational anthrax; correlation of animal models to safety and effectiveness in humans; validation of the manufacturing process; definition of vaccine components in terms of the protective antigen and other bacterial products and constituents; and identification of gaps in existing research.

Because of immediate concern over anthrax vaccine safety issues, the IOM offered to draw relevant information from an ongoing study of Gulf War exposures funded by the Department of Veterans Affairs. The opportunity to provide limited information relating to the safety of anthrax vaccine is possible due to the ongoing work of the IOM Committee on Health Effects Associated with Exposures During the Gulf War, which was tasked with conducting literature reviews on six Gulf War exposures (including the anthrax vaccine). This committee began its work in January 1999, and it is scheduled to provide its report in August of this year. With the agreement of the Department of Veterans Affairs, the IOM was able to produce this letter report that summarizes the committee's literature review on the safety of the anthrax vaccine. This information, while very narrowly focused, may be helpful now to Congress, the DoD, and others before the IOM begins its comprehensive assessment of the anthrax vaccine. Although DoD requested the IOM's consideration of safety and efficacy, the current IOM committee was not tasked with issues of vaccine efficacy. The report that follows therefore addresses only the limited peer-reviewed literature on the safety of the anthrax vaccine.

The committee evaluated the primary peer-reviewed literature and did not draw conclusions from the secondary literature (e.g., reviews). Publications that were not peer reviewed had no evidentiary value for the committee, and they were not used as a basis for conclusions about the degree of association between an exposure and a health effect. The ability of the IOM to conduct the more comprehensive study of the anthrax vaccine requested by the DoD assumes that the significant body of work that has been conducted by the DoD on this subject will be released for publication in peer-reviewed scientific journals.

INTRODUCTION

Currently there are two types of anthrax vaccine available for human use: a live attenuated spore vaccine that has been tested and used widely in the countries of the former Soviet Union (Shlyakhov and Rubinstein, 1994) and protective-antigen vaccines that were developed in the United States and the United Kingdom in the 1950s using filtrates of attenuated strains of the anthrax bacillus. Protective antigen, one of the three toxin proteins produced by the anthrax bacillus, is the protective component of the British and U.S. vaccines, which differ in their method of production and in the strains of the bacillus used (Ibrahim et al., 1999). The committee decided to base its conclusions solely on studies of the protective-antigen vaccines because the live attenuated spore vaccine differs substantially in terms of composition, reactogenicity, and potential residual virulence.

The U.S. anthrax vaccine, which was used in the Gulf War and is currently still in use, was granted product licensure on November 10, 1970. In 1985, a Food and Drug Administration (FDA) advisory panel reviewing the status of bacterial vaccines and toxoids categorized the anthrax vaccine in Category 1 (safe, effective, and not misbranded) (FDA, 1985). The current dosing schedule is 0.5 ml administered subcutaneously at 0, 2, and 4 weeks and 6, 12, and 18 months, followed by yearly boosters. It is estimated that 68,000 doses of the U.S. anthrax vaccine were distributed from 1974 to 1989; 268,000 doses in 1990; and 1.2 million doses from 1991 to July 1999 (Ellenberg, 1999). The exact number of people who received the vaccine is not known. The following sections provide a synthesis of the available peer-reviewed studies.

ANIMAL STUDIES

Few studies have explicitly looked for adverse health effects of the protective-antigen anthrax vaccine in animals. In a study by Wright and colleagues (1954), 25 rabbits were administered five 0.5-ml intracutaneous injections of anthrax vaccine on alternate days. The rabbits were sacrificed 23 days later. Complete autopsies including gross and microscopic examination of all organs revealed no adverse effects. In studies conducted in nonhuman primates, no remarkable local or systemic reactions were seen (Darlow et al., 1956; Ivins et al., 1998). Few meaningful conclusions regarding adverse effects in humans can be drawn from the animal studies of the vaccine; the primary goal of the majority of those studies has been to determine the vaccine's efficacy.

HUMAN STUDIES

There are only a few published peer-reviewed studies examining the safety of the anthrax vaccine in humans. The studies discussed below, with the exception of the Ft. Detrick studies, administered only the anthrax vaccine and were not intended to examine the effects of multiple vaccinations. The committee notes a recent literature review (Demicheli et al., 1998) on anthrax vaccine studies conducted according to the Cochrane Collaboration guidelines for systematic reviews of health care interventions. Only the Brachman study (described below) met the Cochrane criteria for prospective randomized or quasi-randomized studies of a protective antigen anthrax vaccine.

Short-Term Studies

During the development of the anthrax vaccine, several studies examined adverse reactions in humans. These studies used early versions of the culture filtrate (protective-antigen) vaccine. Wright and colleagues (1954) described the reactions of 660 persons who received a total of 1,936 injections. They found that 0.7% of the vaccinated subjects reported systemic reactions—typically consisting of mild muscle aches, headaches, and mild-to-moderate malaise lasting 1 to 2 days. Significant local reactions—typically swelling (5–10 cm in diameter) and local pruritus (itching)—were reported for 2.4% of the injections. The incidence of local reactions increased with the number of previous injections. Two additional early studies also showed low rates of mild, brief local reactions (Darlow et al., 1956; Puziss and Wright, 1963). There is no long-term follow-up reported on the subjects in these studies.

Brachman Study

Brachman and colleagues (1962) conducted the only randomized clinical trial of vaccination with a protective-antigen anthrax vaccine. Although the vaccine used in this study was similar to the vaccine currently available in the United States in that it was a protective-antigen vaccine, the manufacturing process has since changed and a different strain of anthrax bacillus is now used (GAO, 1999a).

The clinical trial was conducted among 1,249 eligible workers[1] at four goat hair processing mills in which some raw materials were contaminated by the anthrax bacillus. After the initial series of three injections, the study had to be terminated at the largest mill, which employed nearly half of the subjects, because of an outbreak of inhalation anthrax that required the immunization of all employees. At the remaining mills, 480 participants completed the series of injections (230 of whom were randomized to active vaccination and 250 of whom were randomized to receive placebo injections) and 81 participants did not complete the series of injections.[2] The study subjects did not know

---

[1]Employees who had a previous case of anthrax were not eligible for the study. Of the 1,249 eligible participants, 340 refused to participate in the study.

whether they had received the active vaccine or placebo; the article does not state whether the investigators were also blinded.

The report of the study does not always clearly distinguish the results in the three mills for the 480 subjects who completed the vaccination series from the 81 subjects who did not complete the series. Neither does it clearly distinguish the results for the 480 subjects in the three mills who completed the series from results for the subjects from the largest mill who had been randomized, received the initial injections, and were partially evaluated prior to the mill's withdrawal from the study.

The participants were examined 24 and 48 hours following each vaccination to assess both local and systemic reactions to the vaccine. There was no report of subsequent active or passive surveillance for possible adverse effects beyond 48 hours after each vaccination (there was further monitoring for the vaccine's efficacy, however). The typical reaction is described as a ring of erythema (1–2 cm in diameter) at the injection site, with local tenderness that lasted 24–48 hours. Some subjects (a number was not given) reported more extensive edema, erythema (>5 cm in diameter), pruritus, induration, or small painless nodules at the injection site (lasting up to several weeks). Twenty-one persons had moderate local edema that lasted up to 48 hours. Three individuals had edema extending from the deltoid to the mid-forearm (in one case, to the wrist) that dissipated within 5 days. The only systemic reactions were reported in two individuals (0.9% of the actively vaccinated subjects), who experienced "malaise" lasting 24 hours following vaccination. The study notes that three individuals who received the placebo (0.1% alum) had mild reactions.

Long-Term Studies

The committee located only one published series of studies that discussed long-term follow-up of individuals who received multiple vaccinations, including the anthrax vaccine, due to the nature of their employment. A group of employees at Fort Detrick, Maryland, were followed for an average of 25 years to investigate the potential subclinical effects of intensive vaccination.[3] The participants underwent physical examinations and/or laboratory testing in 1956 ($n = 93$), 1962 ($n = 76$), and 1971 ($n = 77$) (Peeler et al., 1958, 1965; White et al., 1974).

No clinical sequelae attributable to intense long-term immunization could be identified in this cohort. None of the subjects suffered unexplained clinical symptoms requiring them to take sick leave that could be attributed to the vaccination program. There was some evidence of a chronic inflammatory response, as characterized by certain laboratory test abnormalities: elevated levels of hexosamine, an acute-phase reactant, and polyclonal

---

[2]The authors state that there was a gradual decline in participation in the study, partly because of changes in the nature of the textile business and partly because some of the employees withdrew from the program.

[3]Prior to 1956, all 99 persons had been vaccinated against botulism, tularemia, Rocky Mountain spotted fever, Q fever, plague, typhus, psittacosis, and Eastern, Western, and Venezuelan equine encephalitis; in addition, 95 of the subjects were also immunized against smallpox, 37 against brucellosis, 28 against anthrax, and 25 against diphtheria. By 1962, 72 of the 76 study subjects had been vaccinated against anthrax (in addition to other vaccinations) (Peeler et al., 1958, 1965).

elevations in levels of gamma globulins. These changes cannot necessarily be attributed to the vaccinations, as the workers studied were occupationally exposed to a number of virulent microbes. However, the studies did not report any clear adverse clinical consequences, such as neoplasms, amyloidosis, or autoimmune diseases.

This series of longitudinal clinical studies had several shortcomings. There was no comparison cohort and no random sampling of the employees. Therefore, the results may not be applicable to a broader population. Further, the outcomes may be due in part to the healthy worker effect, since the subjects were selected for the intensity and length of their immunization history, and individuals who left employment were not considered. Thus, the studies may have inadvertently focused on the most resilient individuals. Moreover, it would be difficult, if not impossible, to attribute adverse effects to any one vaccine, since the study subjects received multiple vaccines.

Non-Peer-Reviewed, Unpublished Information

The committee reviewed summaries of data from the Vaccine Adverse Event Reporting System (VAERS).[4] We did not, however, review the individual VAERS forms submitted by health care providers, people receiving the vaccination, family members, or others. VAERS data are useful as a sentinel for adverse events but are limited in their usefulness for assessing the rate or causality of adverse events since the information may be underreported, incomplete, or duplicative and may not always have been confirmed by medical personnel (IOM, 1994). From its inception in 1990 through July 1, 1999, there have been 215 VAERS reports regarding anthrax vaccination (Ellenberg, 1999). The majority of the reports describe local or systemic symptoms including injection site edema, injection site hypersensitivity, rash, headache, and fever. Twenty-two of the VAERS reports are considered serious events and were described as occurring (or being diagnosed) from 45 minutes to 4½ months after the vaccination. The reports of serious events include severe injection site reactions, a widespread allergic reaction, a case of aseptic meningitis, an onset of lupus, an onset of inflammatory demyelinating disease, a diagnosis of bipolar disease, and two cases of Guillain-Barré syndrome (Ellenberg, 1999). FDA and CDC are responsible for monitoring the VAERS data to detect unusual trends and occurrences of adverse health effects. That monitoring assists the FDA and CDC in responding appropriately to adverse events. In recent congressional testimony, FDA stated that "the reports on the anthrax vaccine received thus far do not raise any specific concerns about the safety of the vaccine" (Ellenberg, 1999).

Additionally, there are a number of unpublished studies with data on the safety of the anthrax vaccine (Table 1). However, these studies are either ongoing or have not been published in the peer-reviewed literature, and they were therefore not considered in the committee's conclusions regarding the strength of the evidence for associations with adverse health outcomes. In its full report, the committee uses these studies in determining its recommendations for future research directions. The studies are currently described

---

[4]VAERS is a passive surveillance system that is overseen jointly by the Centers for Disease Control and Prevention (CDC) and the FDA. Reports may be sent in to VAERS at any time following vaccination.

only in secondary sources (e.g., reviews, congressional testimony, and reports from the General Accounting Office). The publication of these studies would substantially increase the available body of information on which conclusions regarding health effects can be made.

TABLE 1. Unpublished and Ongoing Studies of the Anthrax Vaccine

Study	Brief Description
Licensure Safety Study	Data submitted in support of the application for licensure describes approximately 7,000 persons who received approximately 16,000 doses
Special Immunization Program Safety Study	Follow-up study on 1,590 workers at the U.S. Army Medical Research Institute of Infectious Diseases (USAMRIID) who received 10,451 doses since 1973
Ft. Bragg Booster Study	An assessment of the safety of booster shots given to 486 male military personnel who had received initial anthrax vaccinations during the Gulf War
Canadian Forces Safety Survey	Active monitoring of 576 persons in the Canadian military who received the anthrax vaccine in 1998
USAMRIID Reduced Dose and Route Change Study	Pilot study involving 173 persons who received a reduced dose schedule or vaccination via a different route (intramuscular)
Tripler Army Medical Center Survey	Survey of 603 health care personnel who were vaccinated at Tripler Army Medical Center in 1998–1999
U.S. Air Force Vision Study	A comparison of visual acuity in 354 vaccinated aircrew members with 363 unvaccinated aircrew personnel
Korea Survey	Survey of military personnel at the time they received subsequent doses of the vaccine

SOURCES: Claypool, 1999; GAO, 1999b.

Conclusions on Human Studies

There is a paucity of published peer-reviewed literature on the safety of the anthrax vaccine. The committee located only one randomized peer-reviewed study of the type of anthrax vaccine used in the United States (Brachman et al., 1962). However, the formulation of the vaccine used in that study differs from the vaccine currently in use. The series of Ft. Detrick studies shows no clinical sequelae from multiple vaccinations, including the anthrax vaccination, over 25 years of intermittent observation in a highly selected cohort. However, there was no active surveillance for chronic symptoms in these studies, which raises the possibility of underreporting of symptoms.

The published studies have found transient local and systemic effects (primarily erythema, edema, or induration) of the anthrax vaccine. There have been no studies of the anthrax vaccine in which the long-term health outcomes have been systematically evaluated with active surveillance. That is not unusual, however, as few vaccines for any disease have been actively monitored for adverse effects over long periods of time. The committee strongly encourages the development of active monitoring studies that evaluate long-term safety in recipients of the anthrax vaccine.

The committee concludes that in the peer-reviewed literature there is inadequate/ insufficient evidence to determine whether an association does or does not exist between anthrax vaccination and long-term adverse health outcomes. This finding means that the evidence reviewed by the committee is of insufficient quality, consistency, or statistical power to permit a conclusion regarding the presence or absence of an association between the vaccine and a health outcome in humans. Reviewing the large body of results that have not yet been published would enable more definitive conclusions about the vaccine's safety. The committee strongly urges the investigators conducting studies on the safety of the anthrax vaccine to submit their results to peer-reviewed scientific journals for publication. The proposed IOM study to evaluate the safety and efficacy of the anthrax vaccine will be able to examine a more extensive literature, as the DoD has agreed to make its studies of the vaccine available.

To date, published studies have reported no significant adverse effects of the vaccine, but the literature is limited to a few short-term studies. The committee's findings are best regarded as an early step in the complex process of understanding the vaccine's safety, which began with the vaccine's licensure in 1970 and the 1985 FDA advisory panel finding that categorized the anthrax vaccine as safe and effective. Active long-term monitoring of large populations will provide further information for documenting the relative safety of the anthrax vaccine.

Sincerely,

Institute of Medicine Committee on Health Effects
Associated with Exposures During the Gulf War

REFERENCES

Brachman PS, Gold H, Plotkin S, Fekety FR, Werrin M, Ingraham NR. Field evaluation of a human anthrax vaccine. *American Journal of Public Health.* 1962;52:632–645.

Claypool GR, Deputy Assistant Secretary for Health Operations Policy, U.S. Army Medical Corps. *The Anthrax Vaccine Immunization Program.* Statement at the July 21, 1999 Hearing of the Subcommittee on National Security, Veterans Affairs, and International Relations, Committee on Government Reform, U.S. House of Representatives, 1999.

Darlow HM, Belton FC, Henderson DW. The use of anthrax antigen to immunise man and monkey. *Lancet.* 1956;2:476–479.

Demicheli V, Rivetti D, Deeks JJ, Jefferson T, Pratt M. The effectiveness and safety of vaccines against human anthrax: A systematic review. *Vaccine.* 1998;16:880–884.

Ellenberg SS, Center for Biologics Evaluation and Research, Food and Drug Administration. Statement at the July 21, 1999, Hearing of the Subcommittee on National Security, Veterans Affairs, and International Relations, Committee on Government Reform, U.S. House of Representatives, 1999.

FDA (Food and Drug Administration). Biological products: Bacterial vaccines and toxoids; implementation of efficacy review. *Federal Register.* 1985;50(240):51002–51117.

8 AN ASSESSMENT OF THE SAFETY OF THE ANTHRAX VACCINE

GAO (General Accounting Office). *Medical Readiness: Safety and Efficacy of the Anthrax Vaccine. Testimony.* GAO/T-NSAID-99-148. Washington, DC: GAO. 1999a.

GAO. *Medical Readiness: Issues Concerning the Anthrax Vaccine. Testimony.* GAO/T-NSAID-99-226. Washington, DC: GAO. 1999b.

Ibrahim KH, Brown G, Wright DH, Rotschafer JC. *Bacillus anthracis*: Medical issues of biologic warfare. *Pharmacotherapy.* 1999;19(6):690–701.

IOM (Institute of Medicine). *Adverse Effects of Pertussis and Rubella Vaccines.* Washington, DC: National Academy Press, 1994.

Ivins BE, Pitt ML, Fellows PF, Farchaus JW, Benner GE, Waag DM, Little SF, Anderson GW Jr, Gibbs PH, Friedlander AM. Comparative efficacy of experimental anthrax vaccine candidates against inhalation anthrax in rhesus macaques. *Vaccine.* 1998;16:1141–1148.

Peeler RN, Cluff LE, Trever RW. Hyper-immunization of man. *Bulletin of the Johns Hopkins Hospital.* 1958;103:183–198.

Peeler RN, Kadull PJ, Cluff LE. Intensive immunization of man: Evaluation of possible adverse consequences. *Annals of Internal Medicine.* 1965;63(1):44–57.

Puziss M, Wright GC. Studies on immunity in anthrax. X. Gel-adsorbed protective antigen for immunization of man. *Journal of Bacteriology.* 1963;85:230–236.

Shlyakhov EN, Rubinstein E. Human live anthrax vaccine in the former USSR. *Vaccine.* 1994;12:727–730.

White CS, Adler WH, McGann VG. Repeated immunization: Possible adverse effects. *Annals of Internal Medicine.* 1974;81(5):594–600.

Wright GG, Green TW, Kanode RG Jr. Studies on immunity in anthrax. V. Immunizing activity of alum-precipitated protective antigen. *Journal of Immunology.* 1954;73:387–391.

COMMITTEE ON HEALTH EFFECTS ASSOCIATED WITH EXPOSURES DURING THE GULF WAR

HAROLD C. SOX, Jr. (*Chair*), Professor and Chair, Department of Medicine, Dartmouth-Hitchcock Medical Center
MICHAEL ASCHNER, Professor, Department of Physiology and Pharmacology, Wake Forest University School of Medicine
PATRICIA A. BUFFLER, Professor of Epidemiology, University of California at Berkeley School of Public Health
LUCIO GUIDO COSTA, Professor, Department of Environmental Health, University of Washington
FIRDAUS DHABHAR, Assistant Professor, College of Dentistry, The Ohio State University
ANTHONY L. KOMAROFF, Professor of Medicine, Harvard Medical School, and Editor-in-Chief, Harvard Medical Publications
JANICE L. KRUPNICK, Professor, Department of Psychiatry, Georgetown University
HERBERT LOWNDES, Professor, College of Pharmacy, Rutgers University
ERNEST L. MAZZAFERRI, Emeritus Professor and Chairman, Department of Internal Medicine, The Ohio State University
DEMETRIOS J. MOSCHANDREAS, Professor, Department of Environmental Engineering, Illinois Institute of Technology
CHARLES E. PHELPS, Provost, University of Rochester
SAMUEL J. POTOLICCHIO, Professor, Department of Neurology, George Washington University Medical Center
JEAN REGAL, Professor, Department of Pharmacology, School of Medicine, University of Minnesota at Duluth
MARC SCHENKER, Professor, Epidemiology and Preventive Medicine, University of California at Davis School of Medicine
PETER H. SCHUR, Professor of Medicine, Harvard University, Brigham and Women's Hospital
FRANCOISE SEILLIER-MOISEIWITSCH, Associate Professor, Department of Biostatistics, University of North Carolina School of Public Health
WALTER C. WILLETT, Professor and Chairman, Department of Nutrition, Harvard University School of Public Health
SCOTT L. ZEGER, Professor and Chair, Department of Biostatistics, Johns Hopkins University School of Public Health

Staff

CAROLYN E. FULCO, Study Director
CATHARYN T. LIVERMAN, Study Director
SANDRA AU, Research Assistant
KYSA CHRISTIE, Senior Project Assistant
ROSE MARIE MARTINEZ, Director, Division of Health Promotion and Disease Prevention

THE NATIONAL ACADEMIES

National Academy of Sciences
National Academy of Engineering
Institute of Medicine
National Research Council

The **National Academy of Sciences** is a private, nonprofit, self-perpetuating society of distinguished scholars engaged in scientific and engineering research, dedicated to the furtherance of science and technology and to their use for the general welfare. Upon the authority of the charter granted to it by the Congress in 1863, the Academy has a mandate that requires it to advise the federal government on scientific and technical matters. Dr. Bruce M. Alberts is president of the National Academy of Sciences.

The **National Academy of Engineering** was established in 1964, under the charter of the National Academy of Sciences, as a parallel organization of outstanding engineers. It is autonomous in its administration and in the selection of its members, sharing with the National Academy of Sciences the responsibility for advising the federal government. The National Academy of Engineering also sponsors engineering programs aimed at meeting national needs, encourages education and research, and recognizes the superior achievements of engineers. Dr. William A. Wulf is president of the National Academy of Engineering.

The **Institute of Medicine** was established in 1970 by the National Academy of Sciences to secure the services of eminent members of appropriate professions in the examination of policy matters pertaining to the health of the public. The Institute acts under the responsibility given to the National Academy of Sciences by its congressional charter to be an adviser to the federal government and, upon its own initiative, to identify issues of medical care, research, and education. Dr. Kenneth I. Shine is president of the Institute of Medicine.

The **National Research Council** was organized by the National Academy of Sciences in 1916 to associate the broad community of science and technology with the Academy's purposes of furthering knowledge and advising the federal government. Functioning in accordance with general policies determined by the Academy, the Council has become the principal operating agency of both the National Academy of Sciences and the National Academy of Engineering in providing services to the government, the public, and the scientific and engineering communities. The Council is administered jointly by both Academies and the Institute of Medicine. Dr. Bruce M. Alberts and Dr. William A. Wulf are chairman and vice chairman, respectively, of the National Research Council.

INSTITUTE OF MEDICINE • 2101 Constitution Avenue, N.W. • Washington, DC 20418

NOTICE: Preparation of this report was approved by William Colglazier, Executive Officer of the National Research Council, on behalf of its Governing Board, whose members are drawn from the councils of the National Academy of Sciences, the National Academy of Engineering, and the Institute of Medicine. The members of the Committee on Health Effects Associated with Exposures During the Gulf War, which are responsible for the report, were chosen for their special competences and with regard for appropriate balance.

This work is supported by the U.S. Army Medical Research and Material Command under Contract No. DAMD17-00-C-003. The views, opinions, and/or findings contained in this report are those of the Institute of Medicine Committee on Health Effects Associated with Exposures During the Gulf War and should not be construed as an official Department of the Army position, policy, or decision unless so designated by other documentation.

Additional copies of this letter report are available in limited quantities from the Division of Health Promotion and Disease Prevention, Institute of Medicine, 2101 Constitution Avenue, N.W., Washington, DC 20418. The full text of this letter report is available on line at **www.nap.edu/readingroom.**

For more information about the Institute of Medicine, visit the IOM home page at **www.iom.edu.**

Copyright 2000 by the National Academy of Sciences. All rights reserved.

Printed in the United States of America

The serpent has been a symbol of long life, healing, and knowledge among almost all cultures and religions since the beginning of recorded history. The image adopted as a logotype by the Institute of Medicine is based on a relief carving from ancient Greece, now held by the Staatliche Museen in Berlin.

APPENDIX H

INDEPENDENT REPORT REVIEWERS

This report has been reviewed in draft form by individuals chosen for their diverse perspectives and technical expertise, in accordance with procedures approved by the National Research Council's Report Review Committee. The purpose of this independent review is to provide candid and critical comments that will assist the Institute of Medicine in making the published report as sound as possible and to ensure that the report meets institutional standards for objectivity, evidence, and responsiveness to the study charge. The review comments and draft manuscript remain confidential to protect the integrity of the deliberative process. The committee wishes to thank the following individuals for their participation in the review of this report:

Donald A. Henderson, Johns Hopkins University
Richard Johnston, University of Colorado
Joyce Lashof, University of California, Berkeley
Robert Miller, (retired) National Cancer Institute
Gregory Poland, Mayo Clinic and Foundation
Hugh Tilson, University of North Carolina at Chapel Hill
Mary Wilson, Mount Auburn Hospital, Cambridge, MA

While the individuals listed above have provided constructive comments and suggestions, responsibility for the final content of this report rests solely with the authoring committee and the Institute of Medicine.